Health Informatics

(formerly Computers in Health Care)

Kathryn J. Hannah   Marion J. Ball
Series Editors

Health Informatics Series

(formerly Computers in Health Care)

Series Editors
Kathryn J. Hannah Marion J. Ball

Dental Informatics
Integrating Technology into the Dental Environment
L.M. Abbey and J. Zimmerman

Ethics and Information Technology
A Case-Based Approach to a Health Care System in Transition
J.G. Anderson and K.W. Goodman

Aspects of the Computer-Based Patient Record
M.J. Ball and M.F. Collen

Performance Improvement Through Information Management
Health Care's Bridge to Success
M.J. Ball and J.V. Douglas

Strategies and Technologies for Healthcare Information
Theory into Practice
M.J. Ball, J.V. Douglas, and D.E. Garets

Nursing Informatics
Where Caring and Technology Meet, Third Edition
M.J. Ball, K.J. Hannah, S.K. Newbold, and J.V. Douglas

Healthcare Information Management Systems
A Practical Guide, Second Edition
M.J. Ball, D.W. Simborg, J.W. Albright, and J.V. Douglas

Clinical Decision Support Systems
Theory and Practice
E.S. Berner

Strategy and Architecture of Health Care Information Systems
M.K. Bourke

Information Networks for Community Health
P.F. Brennan, S.J. Schneider, and E. Tornquist

Informatics for the Clinical Laboratory
A Practical Guide
D.F. Cowan

Introduction to Clinical Informatics
P. Degoulet and M. Fieschi

Behavioral Healthcare Informatics
N.A. Dewan, N.M. Lorenzi, R.T. Riley, and S.R. Bhattacharya

(continued after Index)

Kathryn J. Hannah Marion J. Ball
Margaret J.A. Edwards

Introduction to Nursing Informatics

Third Edition

With 45 Figures

Springer

Kathryn J. Hannah, PhD, RN
President, Hannah Educational & Consulting Services, Inc.
Calgary, Alberta, T3B 4ZB
Canada
and
Professor, Department of Community Health Sciences
Faculty of Medicine
University of Calgary
Calgary, Alberta T2N 4N1
Canada

Marion J. Ball, EdD
Vice President, Clinical Informatics Strategies
Healthlink, an IBM company
Baltimore, Maryland 21210
USA
and
Professor, Johns Hopkins University School of Nursing
Baltimore, Maryland, 21205
USA

Margaret J.A. Edwards, PhD, RN
Professor and Coordinator, Graduate Programs
Centre for Nursing and Health Studies
Athabasca University
Athabasca, Alberta T9S 3A3
Canada
and
President, Margaret J.A. Edwards & Associates, Inc.
Calgary, Alberta T2W 2A6
Canada

Library of Congress Control Number: 2005929460

ISBN -10: 0-387-26096-X
ISBN -13: 978-0387-26096-9

Printed on acid-free paper.

Printed in the United States of America. (TB/SBA)

9 8 7 6 5 4 3 2 1

springeronline.com

The three authors of this book share many experiences, interests, and values. The strongest of these shared values is a firm belief in marriage and family. We dedicate this book to our husbands, Richard Hannah, John Ball, and Craig Edwards, who are our respective life partners, our friends, and our greatest individual sources of support. We also dedicate this book to our families, especially the youngest generation, which represents the future: Richard Steven Hannah, Cameron Robert Hannah, Kyle James Hannah, Alexis Marion Concordia, Michael John Concordia, Erica Adelaide Concordia, Alexander John Ball, Ryan Jokl Ball, Maryn Joy Edwards, and John Kurt Edwards.

Series Preface

This series is directed to healthcare professionals who are leading the transformation of healthcare by using information and knowledge. Launched in 1998 as Computers in Health Care, the series offers a broad range of titles: some addressed to specific professions such as nursing, medicine, and health administration; others to special areas of practice such as trauma and radiology. Still other books in the series focus on interdisciplinary issues, such as the computer-based patient record, electronic health records, and networked healthcare systems.

Renamed Health Informatics in 1998 to reflect the rapid evolution in the discipline now known as health informatics, the series will continue to add titles that contribute to the evolution of the field. In the series, eminent experts, as editors or authors, offer their accounts of innovations in health informatics. Increasingly, these accounts go beyond hardware and software to address the role of information in influencing the transformation of healthcare delivery systems around the world. The series also will increasingly focus on "peopleware" and the organizational, behavioral, and societal changes that accompany the diffusion of information technology in health services environments.

These changes will shape health services in the new millennium. By making full and creative use of the technology to tame data and to transform information, health informatics will foster the development of the knowledge age in health care. As coeditors, we pledge to support our professional colleagues and the series readers as they share advances in the emerging and exciting field of Health Informatics.

Kathryn J. Hannah
Marion J. Ball

Preface

The first book in the Computers in Health Care series, *Introduction to Nursing Informatics*, was published more than a decade ago. The third edition of this book is intended to be a primer for those just beginning to study nursing informatics, providing a thorough introduction to basic terms and concepts. We have listened to feedback about the two earlier editions from readers. The book has been reorganized and restructured. New material has been added and new information incorporated. The book introduces terms and concepts foundational to nursing informatics and provides an introduction to the Internet. An overview of nursing use of information systems is provided. The book includes an exploration of the most common applications of nursing informatics in clinical nursing practice (both community and facility settings), nursing education, nursing administration, and nursing research. It also provides insight into practical aspects of the infrastructure elements of the informatics environment. An overview of professional nursing informatics education and the future for nurses in health informatics concludes the book.

Although readers will no doubt find diverse uses for this book, we have written it with three principal uses in mind:

University and College Baccalaureate Nursing Programs and Health Information Science Programs: to acquaint undergraduate students in nursing and health information science with the field of nursing informatics. This book provides students with a fundamental understanding of the field of nursing informatics necessary for them to be able to use computers and information management strategies in their practices, to make informed choices related to software/hardware selection and implementation strategies, and to use the more advanced volumes in the Springer series.

Nursing Administrators: to familiarize themselves with the field of nursing informatics in preparation for implementing computerized solutions for information management in their institutions. Practical guidelines will assist the manager in making informed decisions regarding system selection/development, implementation, and use.

Reference: to involve nursing unit managers and staff in the implementation of computer applications and automated information management strategies in their workplaces. This book would be used to familiarize staff with the field of nursing informatics. In addition, the practical information facilitates implementation and use of computer applications.

We believe that this book, *Introduction to Nursing Informatics*, Third Edition, and the companion volume, *Nursing Informatics: Where Caring and Technology Meet*, provide comprehensive coverage of nursing informatics.

We hope that through this book we can introduce newcomers to the excitement of nursing informatics and share our enthusiasm for this rapidly evolving field.

Calgary, Alberta, Canada — *Kathryn J. Hannah*
Baltimore, Maryland, USA — *Marion J. Ball*
Calgary, Alberta, Canada — *Margaret J.A. Edwards*

Contents

PART IV INFRASTRUCTURE ELEMENTS OF THE INFORMATICS ENVIRONMENT

PART V PROFESSIONAL NURSING INFORMATICS

APPENDICES

Contributors

James Cato
Chief Nursing Officer, Eclipsys Corporation, Boca Raton, FL 33487, USA

Ann Casebeer, BA, MPA, PhD
Associate Professor, Department of Community Health Sciences; Associate Director, Centre for Health and Policy Studies; Faculty Director, AHFMR SEARCH Program, University of Calgary, Calgary, Alberta T2N 1N4, Canada

Hélène Clément, RN, BScN, MHA
Vice President, Canadian Operations, GRASP Systems International Companies, Richmond Hill, Ontario L4C 9Y5, Canada

Jane Curry
Information Architect, Health Information Strategies, Inc., St. Albert, Alberta T8N 6M5, Canada

Linda Dietrich, MSN, RN
Director, Practice Transformation, Clinical Practice Model Resource Center, a Subsidiary of Eclipsys Corporation, Grand Rapids, MI 49509, USA

Diana Domonkos
Healthlink, an IBM company, Houston, TX 77098, USA

Judith V. Douglas, MA, MHS
Adjunct Faculty, Johns Hopkins University School of Nursing, Baltimore, MD 21205, USA

Craig Edwards, CIO
Margaret J.A. Edwards & Associates, Calgary, Alberta T2W 2A6, Canada

Richard S. Hannah, PhD
Professor Emeritus, Faculty of Medicine, University of Calgary, Calgary, Alberta T2N 1N4, Canada

Eleanor Callahan Hunt, RN, MSN, BC
Clinical Informatics, EMR Solutions R&D, Misys Healthcare Systems, Raleigh, NC 27615, USA

Rebecca Rutherford Kitzmiller, RN, MSN, MHR, BC
Director of Nursing Informatics, Duke University Health System, Durham, NC 27710, USA

Jo Ann Klein, MS, RN-C
Forum Manager, The Nursing Network Forum; Member, Curriculum Committee, Johns Hopkins University School of Nursing, Baltimore, MD 21205, USA

Susan K. Newbold, MS, RNBC, FAAN, FHIMSS
Lecturer in Nursing, Vanderbilt University School of Nursing, Nashville, TN 37203, USA

Paul E. Pancoast, MD
Senior Manager, Clinical Specialist, Deloitte Consulting LLC, Austin, TX 78701, USA

Helen Lee Robertson, MLIS
Document Delivery/Liaison Librarian, University of Calgary, Calgary, Alberta T2N 1N4, Canada

Joyce Sensmeier
Vice President of Informatics, HIMSS, Chicago, IL 60611, USA

Sara Breckenridge Sproat, RN, MSN, BC
Lieutenant Colonel, US Army Nurse Corps, Deputy Director, Division of Regulated Activities, Walter Reed Army Institute of Research, Silver Spring, MD 20910, USA

Carole Stephens
Coustal Physician Services, Durham, NC 27705, USA

Lorraine Toews, MLIS
Head, Public Services, Health Sciences Library, University of Calgary, Calgary, Alberta T2N 1N4, Canada

Part I
Foundations of Nursing Informatics

1 Nurses and Informatics

We have entered the information age. Home computers, laptops, handheld computers, and iPODs are pervasive. Banks and stock markets move and track billions of dollars around the world every day through information systems. Factories and stores buy, build, sell, and account for the products in our lives through information systems. In schools, computers are being used as teaching tools and as instructional resources for students in such varied disciplines as astronomy, Chinese, and chemistry. The airline industry uses information systems to book seats, calculate loads, order meals, determine flight plans, determine fuel requirements, and even fly the planes and control air traffic.

The information age has not left the health industry untouched. Moving beyond standard data processing for administrative functions common to all organizations such as human resources, payroll, and financial information systems now play an important role in patient care by interpreting electrocardiograms, scheduling, entering orders, reporting results, and preventing drug interactions (by cross-referencing drug compatibility and warning appropriate staff). We are beginning to see the advent of lifetime electronic health records in many countries. In addition, information systems are now being more widely used in support of population health and public health activities related to health protection (e.g., immunization), health promotion (e.g., well baby clinics), disease prevention (e.g., smoking cessation or needle exchange programs), and health monitoring or surveillance (e.g., restaurant inspection or air quality monitoring).

Nurses have always had a major communication role at the interface between the patient/client and the health system. This role is now labeled information management, and nurses are increasingly using information systems to assist them to fulfill this role in clinical practice, administration, research, and education. Before attempting to talk about the role of nursing in informatics, let us first establish definitions of nursing and "nursing informatics."

What Is Nursing?

Nursing is emerging as a professional practice discipline. Based on the work of theorists, nursing practitioners see its goals as the promotion of adaptation in health and illness and the facilitation of achievement of the highest possible individual state of health (Rogers, 1970; Roy, 1976). These early theoretical models have provided the impetus for the development of current approaches to the classification of phenomena of concern to nursing care (see Chapter 12 for a detailed discussion of nursing classification and nomenclature systems).

The practitioner of nursing has many roles and responsibilities. Among these roles are those of an interface between the client and the healthcare system and that of client advocate in the healthcare system. Nursing functions can be considered under three major categories.

- Managerial, which includes establishing nursing care plans, keeping charts, transcribing orders and requisitions, and scheduling patient appointments for diagnostic procedures or therapy
- Delegated tasks, which include physical treatments and administration of medications under the direction of a physician
- Autonomous nursing functions, which include interpersonal communication skills, application of the psychological principles of client care, and providing physical care to patients.

It is the third category of nursing activities that is the core of nursing practice. In this category of autonomous activity nurses use their knowledge, skills, judgment, and experience to exercise independent decision making related to the phenomena for which nurses provide care and the nursing interventions that effect those phenomena and influence patient care outcomes.

What Is "Medical/Healthcare Informatics?"

Before we explore the nature of hospital and nursing information systems, we need to review the definitions of health, medical, and nursing informatics. Francois Gremy of France is widely credited with coining the term *informatique medical*, which was translated into English as *medical informatics*. Early on, the term medical informatics was used to describe "those collected informational technologies which concern themselves with the patient care, medical decision making process" (Greenburg, 1975). Another early definition, in the first issue of the *Journal of Medical Informatics*, proposed that medical informatics was "the complex processing of data by a computer to produce new kinds of information" (Anderson, 1976). As our understanding of this discipline developed, Greenes and Shortliffe (1990) redefined medical informatics as "the field that concerns itself with the cognitive, information processing and communication tasks of medical practice, education, and research, including the information science and the technology to support these tasks. An intrinsically interdisciplinary field... [with] an applied focus, ... [addressing] a number of fundamental research problems as well as planning and policy issues." More recently, Shortliffe et al. (2001) defined medical informatics as "the scientific field that deals with biomedical information, data, and knowledge—their storage, retrieval and optimal use for problem-solving and decision-making."

One question consistently arose: "Does the word *medical* refer only to physicians, or does it refer to all healthcare professions?" In the first edition of this book, the premise was that *medical* referred to all healthcare professions and that a parallel definition of medical informatics might be "those collected informational technologies that concern themselves with the patient care decision-making process performed by healthcare practitioners." Thus, because nurses are healthcare practitioners who are involved in the patient care and the decision-making process that uses information captured by and extracted from the information technologies, there clearly was a place for nursing in medical informatics. Increasingly, as research was conducted and medical informatics evolved, nurses realized there was a discrete body of knowledge related to nursing and the use of informatics. During the early 1990s, other health professions began to explore the use of informatics in their disciplines. Mandil (1989) coined the phrase "health informatics," which he defined as the use of information technology (including both hardware and software) in combination with information management concepts and methods to support the delivery of healthcare. Thus, health informatics has become the umbrella term encompassing medical, nursing, dental, and pharmacy informatics among others. Health informatics focuses attention on the recipient of care rather than on the discipline of the caregiver.

Nursing's Early Role in Medical Informatics

The nurse's early role in medical informatics was that of a consumer. The literature clearly shows the contributions of medical informatics to the practice of nursing and patient care. Early developments in medical informatics and their advantages to nursing have been thoroughly documented (Hannah, 1976; see also Chapter 3, this volume). These initial developments were fragmentary and generally restricted to automating existing functions or activities such as automated charting of nurses' notes, automated nursing care plans, automated patient monitoring, automated personnel time assignment, and the gathering of epidemiological and administrative statistics. Subsequently, an integrated approach to medical informatics resulted in the development and marketing of sophisticated hospital information systems that included nursing applications or modules. As models of health services delivery have shifted toward integrated care delivery across the entire spectrum of health services, integrated information systems have developed. These enterprise systems provided an integrated clinical record within a complex integrated healthcare organization. Such systems support evidence-based nursing practice, facilitate nurses' participation in the healthcare team, and document nurses' contribution to patient care outcomes. They have failed, however, to meet the challenge of providing a nationwide comprehensive, lifelong, electronic health record that integrates the information generated by all of a person's contacts with the healthcare system.

Development of Nursing Informatics

Nursing informatics, as originally defined (Hannah, 1985, p. 181) referred to the use of information technologies in relation to those functions within the purview of nursing that are carried out by nurses when performing their duties. Therefore, any use of information technologies by nurses in relation to the care of patients, the administration of healthcare facilities, or the educational preparation of individuals to practice the discipline is considered nursing informatics. For example, nursing informatics would include, but not be limited to the following.

- Use of artificial intelligence or decision-making systems to support the use of the nursing process
- Use of a computer-based scheduling package to allocate staff in a hospital or healthcare organization
- Use of computers for patient education
- Use of computer-assisted learning in nursing education
- Nursing use of a hospital information system
- Research related to what information nurses use when making patient care decisions and how those decisions are made

As the field of nursing informatics has evolved, the definition of nursing informatics has been elaborated and refined. Graves and Corcoran (1989) suggested that nursing informatics is "a combination of computer science, information science, and nursing science designed to assist in the management and processing of nursing data, information and knowledge to support the practice of nursing and the delivery of nursing care." An Expert Panel of the American Nurses Association (2001) promoted nursing informatics as

> a specialty that integrates nursing science, computer science, and information science to manage and communicate data, information, and knowledge in nursing practice. Nursing informatics facilitates the integration of data, information and knowledge to support patients, nurses and other providers in their decision-making in all roles and settings. This support is accomplished through the use of information structures and information technology.

In an extensive review and analysis of the evolution of definitions of nursing informatics, Staggers and Thompson (2002, p. 259) concluded that after three decades as a specialty there was still a proliferation of definitions for nursing informatics. Staggers and Thompson (2002) modified the ANA definition and proposed a revised definition of nursing informatics as

> a specialty that integrates nursing science, computer science, and information science to manage and communicate data, information and knowledge to support patients, nurses and other providers in their decision making in all roles and settings. This support is accomplished through the use of information structures, information processes and information technology.

Furthermore, Staggers and Thompson (2002, p. 259–260) built on the ANA work to propose that the goal of nursing informatics is

> to improve the health of populations, communities, families and individuals by optimizing information management and communication. This includes the use of information and technology in the direct provision of care, in establishing effective administrative systems, in managing and delivering educational experiences, in supporting lifelong learning, and in supporting nursing research.

Impact of Informatics on Nursing

As we mentioned earlier, nursing informatics has moved beyond merely the use of computers and is increasingly referring to the impact of information and information management on the discipline of nursing. Staggers and Thompson (2002) affirmed our long-held position that nurses are "information integrators at the patient level." Nurses form the largest group of healthcare professionals in any setting to have a health information system. Therefore, when providing patient care, nurses make use of information management more often than any other group of healthcare professionals. (The advantages to the practice of nursing that come from information systems and information management are described in detail in Chapters 7 and 8.)

The nursing profession is recognizing the potential of informatics to improve nursing practice and the quality of patient care. New roles are evolving for nurses. The American Nurses Association (2001) recognized nursing informatics as a nursing specialty in 2001. Hospitals and other healthcare organizations are now hiring informatics nurse specialists and informatics nurse consultants to help in the design and implementation of information systems. Nurse educators are using information systems to manage the educational environment. Computer-based information systems are used to instruct, evaluate, and identify problem areas of specific students; gather data on *how* each student learns; process data for research purposes; and carry out continued education. Nurse researchers, who have been using computerized software for data manipulation for years, are turning their attention to the problems of identifying variables for data sets essential to the diagnosing of nursing problems, choosing nursing actions, and evaluating patient care. As Figures 1.1 and 1.2 illustrate, there is no doubt that *we have reached the information age in nursing*. We must now prepare for the full impact of informatics on nursing.

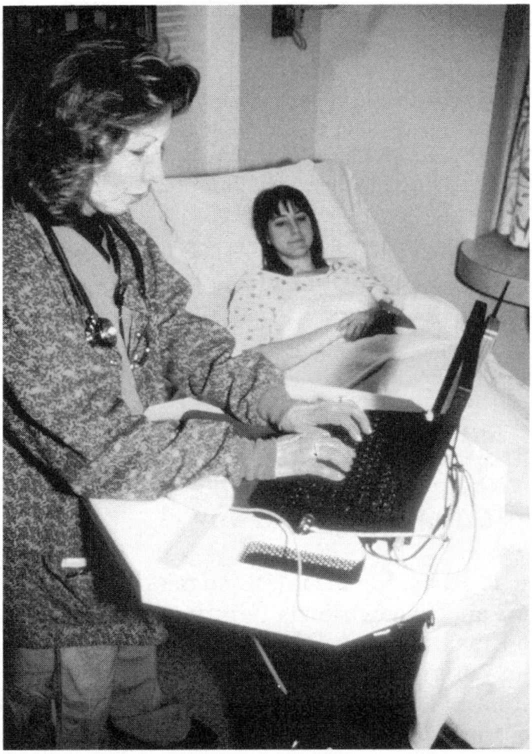

Figure 1.1. Nursing informatics at the bedside. (Photograph courtesy of Aironet Wireless Communications, Inc.)

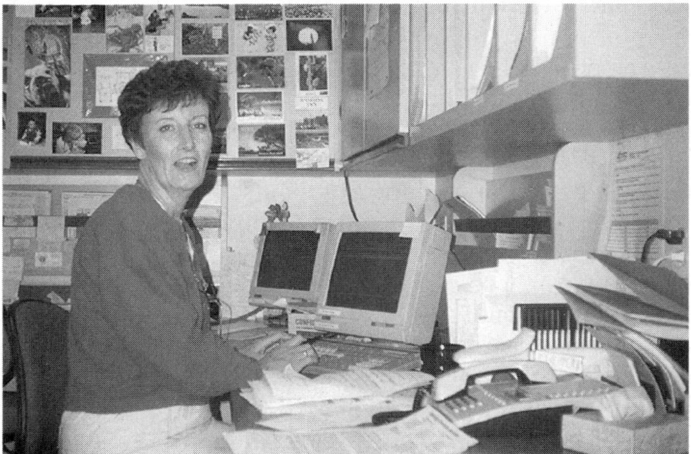

Figure 1.2. Nursing informatics at the nursing station. (Photograph courtesy of Clinicare Corporation.)

Future Implications

Technology has historically relieved people of backbreaking drudgery and dreary monotony, providing them with more free time to pursue personal relations and creative activities. Nurses, too, when relieved of routine and time-consuming clerical or managerial paper handling chores, can devote more time to the unique problems and needs of individual patients or clients. Increasingly, across the world, the managerial and clerical paper-handling tasks of nursing are being performed by information systems. In addition, robotics (e.g., lifting and turning patients, delivering medications or meals, and recording temperature, pulse, and other physiological measurements) might assist with the physical care category of nursing tasks. Similarly, decision support systems may actively assist with nursing judgments.

Relieved of routine and less complex chores, the professional nurse having enhanced information management skills and working in an environment enhanced by information systems will be expected to carry out higher level, more complex activities that cannot be programmed. Nurses are being held responsible and accountable for the systematic planning of holistic and humanistic nursing care for patients and their families. Nurses are also increasingly responsible for the continual review and examination of nursing practice (using innovative, continuous quality improvement approaches), as well as applying basic research to finding creative solutions for patient care problems and the development of new models for the delivery of nursing care. Increasingly, nurses will provide more primary care through community-based programs providing health promotion and early recognition and prevention of illness. Nurses' role as patient educator is being extended by means of multimedia programs and the Internet. At the same time nurses must assume greater responsibility for assisting the public to become discriminating users of information as they select, sort, interpret, evaluate, and use the vast volumes of facts available across the Internet.

Nurses still must assess, plan, carry out, and evaluate patient care, but advances in the use of information management, information processes, and technology will continue to create a more scientific, complex approach to the nursing care process. They will have to be better equipped by their education and preparation to have a more inquiring and investigative approach to patient care. Evidence-based nursing practice is becoming the standard. As information systems assume more routine clerical functions, nurses will have more time for direct patient care. Accordingly, nursing must be part of future developments in nursing informatics with strong input regarding such decisions as the following.

1. Which patient care-related nursing functions could be accomplished by nursing informatics?
2. What information do nurses require to make patient care decisions?

3. What information do caregivers from other health professions require from nursing?
4. To what extent can nursing informatics support improvements in the quality of nursing care received by patients?
5. How can the financial and emotional costs of care to patients be reduced using nursing informatics?
6. What is the impact of nursing on client outcomes?
7. What do nursing interventions contribute to patient outcomes?

The implication is that nursing must continually reassess its status and reward systems. Presently, a nurse gains status and financial reward by moving away from the bedside into supervisory and managerial roles. If more of these coordinating functions are taken over by the computer, nursing must reappraise its value system and reward quality of care at the bedside with prestige and money. Some movement in this direction is already beginning: for example, the movement toward employment of clinical nurse specialists prepared at the master's degree level to work at the bedside. However, currently this movement seems to be too little and too slow.

Summary

The role of the nurse will intensify and diversify with the widespread integration of computer technology and information science into healthcare agencies and institutions. Redefinition, refinement, and modification of the practice of nursing will intensify the nurse's role in the delivery of patient care. At the same time, nurses will have greater diversity by virtue of employment opportunities in the nursing informatics field.

Nursing's contributions can and will influence the evolution of healthcare informatics. Nursing will also be influenced by informatics, resulting in a better understanding of our knowledge and a closer link of that knowledge to nursing practice (Turley, 1997). As a profession, nursing must anticipate the expansion and development of nursing informatics. Leadership and direction must be provided to ensure that nursing informatics expands and improves the quality of healthcare received by patients within the collaborative interdisciplinary venue of health informatics.

References

American Nurses Association. (2001). Scope and Standards of Nursing Informatics Practice. Washington, D.C., ANA.

Anderson, J. (1976). Editorial. *Journal of Medical Informatics 1*:1.

Graves, J.R., & Corcoran, S. (1989). The study of nursing informatics. *Image*; *21*:227–231.

Greenburg, A.B. (1975). *Medical informatics: Science or science fiction.* unpublished.

Greenes, R.A., & Shortliffe, E.H. (1990). Medical informatics: an emerging academic discipline and institutional priority. *Journal of American Medical Association 263*(8):1114–1120.

Hannah, K.J. (1976). The computer and nursing practice. *Nursing Outlook 24*(9): 555–558.

Hannah, Kathryn J., Guillemin, Evelyn J., & Conklin, Dorothy, N. (eds.) (1985). *Nursing Use of Computers and Information Science*. Amsterdam: North Holland.

Mandil, S. (1989). Health informatics: New solutions to old challenges. *World Health* 2 (Aug/Sept):5.

Rogers, M.E. (1970). *An Introduction to the Theoretical Base of Nursing Practice.* Philadelphia: Davis.

Roy, C. (1976). *Introduction to Nursing: An Adaptation Model.* Englewood Cliffs, N.J.: Prentice-Hall.

Shortliffe, E.H., Perreault, L.E., Wiederhold, G., & Fagan, L.M. (eds.) (2001). *Medical Informatics: Computer Applications in healthcare and Biomedicine, 2nd Edition.* New York: Springer-Verlag, p. 21.

Staggers, N., & Thompson, C.B. (2002). The evolution of definitions for nursing informatics: a critical analysis and revised definition. *Journal of the American Medical Informatics Association* 9(May/June):255–261.

Turley, J.P. (1997). Developing informatics as a discipline. In: Gerdin, U., Tallberg, M., Wainwright, P. (eds.) *Nursing Informatics: The Impact of Nursing Knowledge on healthcare Informatics.* Amsterdam: IOS Press, pp. 69–74.

2
Anatomy and Physiology of Computers

CRAIG EDWARDS

Basic Computer Ideas

For most people the inner workings of a television are a mystery, but that does not stop them from using and enjoying television. In the same way, it is not necessary to understand all the details of computer technology before it can be used to great advantage. This chapter is intended to give an adequate but not exhaustive understanding of computers, thus enabling the reader to take confident advantage of whatever computer technology is available.

There are generally two main parts to any computer system.

1. *Hardware* is the term that describes the physical pieces of the computer, commonly grouped in five categories.
   - Input: Data must be placed into the computer before the computer can be useful.
   - Memory: All data processing takes place in memory.
   - Central processing unit (CPU): This is the "brain" of the computer, which coordinates all the activities and does the actual data processing.
   - Storage: The data and programs can be saved for future use.
   - Output: Processed data are of little value to people unless they can see the data in some form.

   Hardware can be considered the anatomy of a computer, its physical, mechanical portion.
2. *Software* is the term that describes the nonphysical pieces. It can be grouped into two categories.
   - Operating system: This is the collection of standard computer activities that need to be done consistently and reliably. These processes are the building blocks for computer functions and programs.
   - Application programs: These are packages of instructions that combine logic and mathematical processing using the building blocks of the computer. Programs are what make computers valuable to people by transforming raw data into information.

Software can be considered the physiology of a computer, the instructions that make its anatomy function properly. These pieces of a computer are described later in more detail, but it is important to have a mental picture of a "computer" before we proceed. It is also helpful to understand some computer terminology (or jargon) that often overwhelms or confuses.

Common Computer Terms

- *Chip* refers to a small piece of silicon that has electronic logic circuits built into it. A chip can hold thousands of circuits in something that is about one-quarter of an inch on each side (Fig. 2.1). The chip is the fundamental physical piece used for computer memory and central processing units (see later in the chapter).
- *RAM* and *ROM* are the two types of memory that a computer uses. ROM stands for *R*ead-*O*nly *M*emory. This memory has information already stored in it by the computer manufacturer, and nothing is allowed to change that information. RAM stands for *R*andom-*A*ccess *M*emory. This memory has no information in it but is available for any program to store information.
- *Bit* is the smallest part of computer memory. It can hold exactly one piece of information that has only two possible values, either a one (1) or a zero (0). This "two-value" system is called a binary system.
- *Byte* is the fundamental grouping of bits used to make up computer memory. By grouping bits together and setting these bits to either 0 or 1 in different combinations, a coding scheme can be built to represent information. The byte is the basic measuring unit for memory capacity or storage capacity.
- *Kilo*, *mega*, and *giga* are prefixes that represent certain multipliers. Although "kilo" in scientific notation means "1000" (10^3), its value is changed to "1024" (2^{10}) when talking about computer memory or storage. Numbers that are powers of 2 (e.g., 4 is a power of 2, being 2^2) are chosen because the

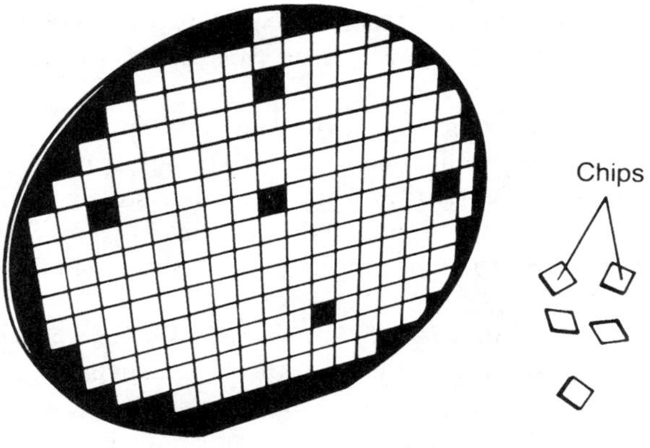

FIGURE 2.1. Silicon wafer.

computer uses a binary system. Thus, one kilobyte of computer memory represents 1024 (1×1024) bytes, two kilobytes represent 2048 (2×1024) bytes, and so on. One megabyte represents 1,048,576 (1024×1024) bytes, and one gigabyte represents 1,073,741,824 bytes ($1024 \times 1024 \times 1024$). Although it is not accurate, most people tend to still give kilo, mega, and giga their normal values of 10^3,10^6, and 10^9 when referring to computers.
- *Megahertz* (MHz) and *gigahertz* (GHz) describe the frequency that the central processing unit's internal clock uses for its timing control (see later in the chapter).

Computer technology has had an explosive growth during the past several decades. The large computers that used to fill their own special-purpose rooms have in many cases been replaced by computers small enough to fit on a desk ("desktop" model), on one's lap ("laptop" model), or in the palm of one's hand ("palmtop" computers). This trend is expected to continue. It is probable that what is described next will be considered obsolete within just a few years.

Hardware

Input

- *Keyboard* is the most common way a person gives information and commands to a computer. It looks like a typewriter; its surface is filled with keys that are either numbers, letters, or control functions (such as "Home" and "Delete").
- *Touchscreen* is a technique that lets people do what comes naturally—point with a finger. When a special sensing device is fitted around the perimeter of a monitor, the computer can calculate where someone's finger has touched the screen.
- *Light pen* is another pointing technique. Using special types of monitors, an attached pen (Fig. 2.2.) can be used (instead of a finger) to point to places on the screen.
- *Mouse* is yet another pointing device and perhaps the most common one. By moving a mouse around on a flat surface, a person also causes a marker (called the "cursor") on the computer screen to move. When that marker is resting on the desired place on the screen, a button on the mouse is pressed to signal the computer that something has been "pointed to."
- *Voice* is a technology that is evolving rapidly. Using a microphone and some special application programs, a person can speak in a natural way and have that speech recognized by the computer. The words could be numbers (i.e., "One"), commands (i.e., "Print"), or just text (e.g., "The" "dog," "was"...).

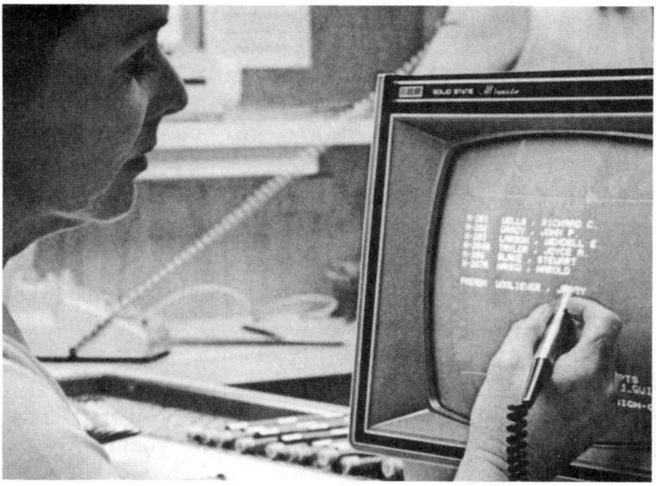

Figure 2.2. Light pen.

- *Pen-based* technology translates the normal model of pen and paper for use with a computer system. With special computer screens and pens, a person can print or write on the screen with the pen and have the computer recognize what is written. Nothing is physically marked on the screen by the pen, but the computer senses and traces out the pen's movements. It then tries to recognize letters or numbers from those traces or it can just store what has been traced out as an image file, a picture of the pen's movements.

Memory

The two basic types of memory, ROM and RAM, were defined earlier. Generally, a computer has a sufficient amount of ROM built in by the manufacturer. ROM is preloaded with the low-level logic and processes needed to start the computer when its power is turned on (a process called "booting up"). Most computers also have a starting amount of RAM preinstalled. RAM can be purchased separately, though, and installed as needed. Application programs are loaded, when called for, into RAM. The program executes there and stores information in other parts of RAM as is needed. Today, application programs have growing RAM requirements as more logic and functions are packed in them.

Central Processing Unit

There are several types of CPU chips. In the personal computer world, the Intel Corporation is probably the most recognized manufacturer with, first, its 80 × 86 series of CPU chips (i.e., 80386, 80486, . . .) and then its Pentium™ chip (i.e., Pentium 4 or P4) series. In the large computer world, IBM (International Business Machines) is probably the most recognized name.

One measure of CPU processing capacity is called MIPS ("*m*illions of *i*nstructions *p*er *s*econd.") Although not a totally accurate measure, it is useful to see the growth of processing capacity over time. Intel's 80386 chip, produced in 1985, was rated at 5 MIPS. Intel's Pentium chip, introduced 8 years later in 1993, was rated at 100 MIPS—about 20 times faster. Intel's Pentium 4 chip, made 7 years later in 2000, was rated at 1700 MIPS.

All CPUs have three basic elements: a control unit, an arithmetic logic unit (ALU), and an internal memory unit. The ALU performs all the mathematical operations, the control unit determines where and when to send information being used by the ALU, and the internal memory is used to hold and store information for those operations. The CPU has an internal system clock that it uses to keep everything in synchronized order. The clock's speed is described in terms of frequency, using megahertz (MHz) or gigahertz (GHz), so a CPU might be described as having a clock speed of 450 MHz or 2.4 GHz. Generally, the faster the clock, the faster the CPU can process information.

Storage

The memory of a computer is not the place to store information and programs for a long time. ROM is read-only (unwriteable) and therefore not of any use. RAM holds programs and information but only so long as the computer is turned on; once turned off, all information in RAM is gone. Therefore other means are used for long-term storage, the most common technologies being magnetic, optical, and special nonvolatile memory.

- *Floppy Disk* (or "floppy") is the term that describes a material that can be magnetically encoded to store information and programs. This material is housed in a protective case. Floppy disks most commonly are 3.5 inches ("three and a half") in size. The computer has a specially sized slot or opening where these floppy disks can be inserted as needed. The amount of information these disks can hold varies. The 3.5 inch floppy disk holds 1.44 megabytes of data. Some manufacturers have experimented with floppy drives and disks that can store 120 megabytes of information. Floppies are reusable; old information on the floppy can be erased and new information stored in its place. Floppies are removable from the computer.
- *Hard Disk Drive* (or simply "Hard Drive") is the term that describes a device that magnetically encodes much more information than a floppy can but is not removable from the computer. A typical hard drive size on personal computers, for example, is 40 to 80 gigabytes of capacity. Most often, a person does not see a hard drive; the drives are usually inside a computer and not removable. Hard disks are reusable.

- *Removable Disk Drive* is the same kind of device as a hard disk drive with similar storage capabilities. The difference is that the magnetic storage media can be removed and replaced, just as with a floppy disk.
- *Tape* describes a medium that can magnetically encode a lot of information. In many ways, tape in a computer system is used like audio tape. Computer tape is typically used to store a copy of important information, to be recovered in case of a major problem with the computer. Tape is packaged in various ways, from large reels to small cartridges. Tape is reusable.
- *Optical Storage* is a term that covers several devices that store information optically, not magnetically. Common examples are CD-R (Compact Disc-Recordable) and CD-RW (Compact Disc-Rewritable). Capacities of 500 megabytes or more are available. Reusable optical storage is becoming more common as manufacturers agree on storage standards.
- *Flash Drive* is a removable device that uses special nonvolatile memory to hold information. Unlike RAM, this memory retains its information when the device is removed from the computer. When the device is connected, the computer sees and uses it as a removable hard drive. Flash drives can store gigabytes of information.

Output

- *Monitor* is the most common way a person sees the information and instructions on a computer. Historically, on desktop computers the monitor looks like a television screen and uses the same display technology as a television. On laptop computers ("small enough to fit in your lap"), the monitor is a flat screen that uses liquid crystal display (LCD) technology. This LCD technology is increasingly being used in desktop monitors as well. Some other names for the monitor are VDT (video display terminal), CRT (cathode ray tube), screen, and display. Illustrations of what a monitor and keyboard may look like are shown in Figure 2.3.
- *Printers* and *plotters* are two ways by which the computer can put the processed information, such as a report or a chart, onto paper for people. The most common output device in offices is the laser printer, capable of putting either text (e.g., a report) or graphics (e.g., a chart) onto standard-size paper.

Software

Operating Systems

Operating systems are the basic control programs for a computer. All the basic logic required for using a computer's hardware, such as the monitor, the

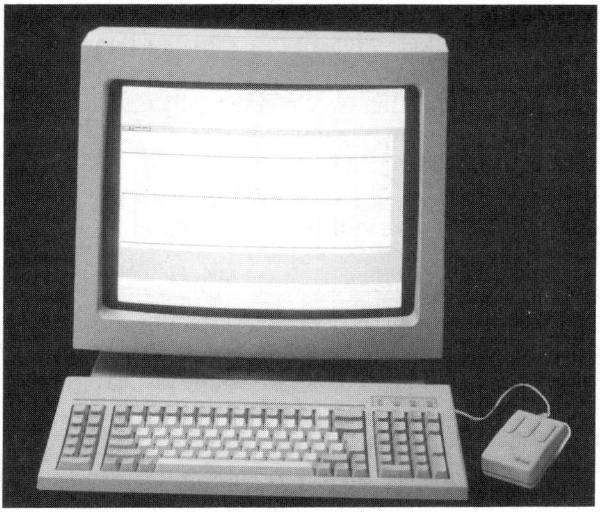

FIGURE 2.3. A. Monitor, keyboard, and mouse.

printer, and the hard drive, is contained in the operating system. Because the operating system handles those computer parts, it is unnecessary for application programs to do so. An example in the personal computer world is Microsoft Corporation's Windows™ operating system.

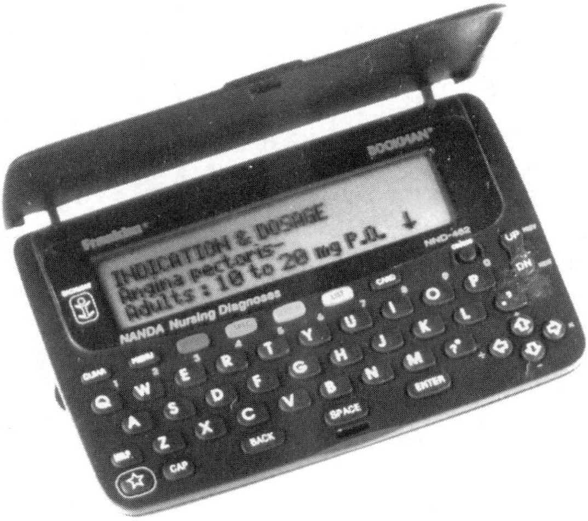

FIGURE 2.3. B. Another type of monitor and keyboard. (Photograph courtesy of Franklin Electronic Publishing.)

Application Programs

Application programs are packages of instructions and operations that take raw data and process them into information. Applications focus on working with people to produce information that is important to them. Some examples of applications are word processing, spreadsheets, and desktop publishing.

Graphical User Interface (GUI) Software

The graphical user interface (GUI) is a special type of software in common use today. It can be part of the operating system software, or it can be a complete application program on its own; at times, a GUI (pronounced "gooey") seems to straddle the line between operating and application software. The basic design of any GUI is that it stands between the operator of the computer and the computer itself and acts as the go-between. Any GUI has two primary goals: (1) to shield the operator from needing a great amount of technical knowledge to use the computer effectively and correctly; and (2) to give a consistent "look-and-feel" to application programs (if they are designed for it).

Accomplishing the first goal means that an operator can perform all necessary technical tasks (e.g., copying data files between disks, backing up information) by pointing at icons (small pictures) on the screen. These icons represent the tasks that can be done. For example, by pointing to an icon that represents a desired data file and then dragging that icon over onto another icon that represents a printer, a person can print the file. Note that because of the GUI's capabilities, the person did not have to know the correct operating system commands to print the file.

Accomplishing the second goal means that any application program can be designed so it is less difficult for a person to learn how to use it. Basically, the GUI defines a standard set of functions that it can provide (e.g., open a data file, save a data file, print a data file) and gives standard ways for application programs to use these functions. If application programs are designed and built to use these functions, a person has to learn only *once* how to open a data file. Any other program that uses the GUI functions has the same "look-and-feel"; that is, a person can open a data file in the same manner. Doing things in a consistent, predictable way not only reduces a person's learning time but increases a person's comfort level and productivity. Figure 2.4 is an example of a main menu for a nursing software package.

Databases and Relational Database Management Systems

A database is a data file whose information is stored and organized so it can be easily searched and retrieved. A simple analogy is a filing cabinet drawer.

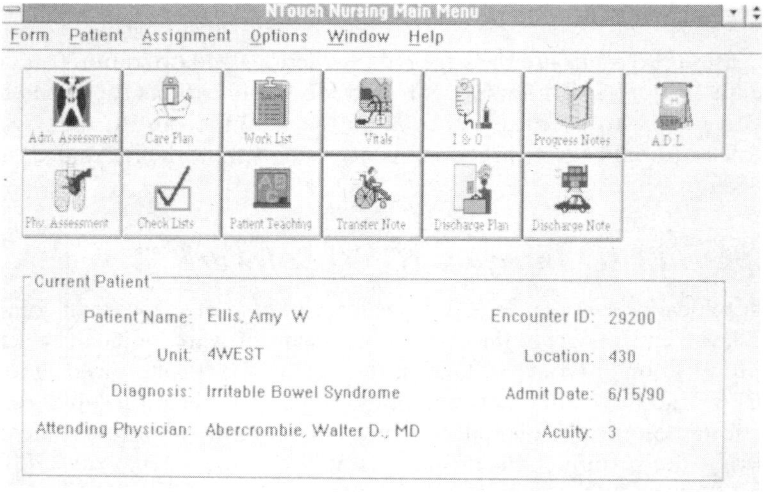

FIGURE 2.4. Graphical user interface (GUI)-type menu.

The difference between a file and a database is the same difference between a file drawer that has reports dumped into it in any old way and a drawer that has neatly labeled file folders, arranged in meaningful order, with an index that shows where to store a report. In both cases, we know the information we need is in the file drawer—only in the second case (i.e., the database) we are confident that we can find that information quickly and easily.

A database management system (DBMS) is a set of functions that application programs use to store and retrieve information in an organized way. Over the years, various ways to organize information have been used (e.g., hierarchical, network, indexed). The way it is used most frequently now is called *relational.* A relational DBMS stores information in tables (i.e., rows and columns of information). This approach allows powerful searches to be done quite easily.

Terminals, Workstations, Stand-alone, Networks

Terminals

In the early days of computer technology, an organization usually required only a single large-capacity computer to handle its information needs. These computers were called "mainframes." They required a trained staff to maintain and run them and were quite expensive to purchase and upgrade (e.g., add more memory, more disk storage). People gave information and commands to the mainframe through a "terminal," essentially just a keyboard and monitor; the terminal had no processing capability of its own. The number of terminals a mainframe could handle was limited, which created lineups of people waiting their turn to submit computer requests.

Workstations

Advances in computer technology, such as IBM's personal computer introduced in 1981, dramatically changed this situation. Now it was possible to have a powerful computer right in the office and for far less money. What is more, all its resources and power were under the control of, and totally available to, its user. As people began to move toward personal computing, computer manufacturers built more powerful workstations. Soon, these powerful workstations became small enough to be easily moved, promoting the idea of "mobile computing." Today, laptop computers easily allow computer technology to be available at the point of care (Fig. 2.5) (see Chapter 7 for more discussion).

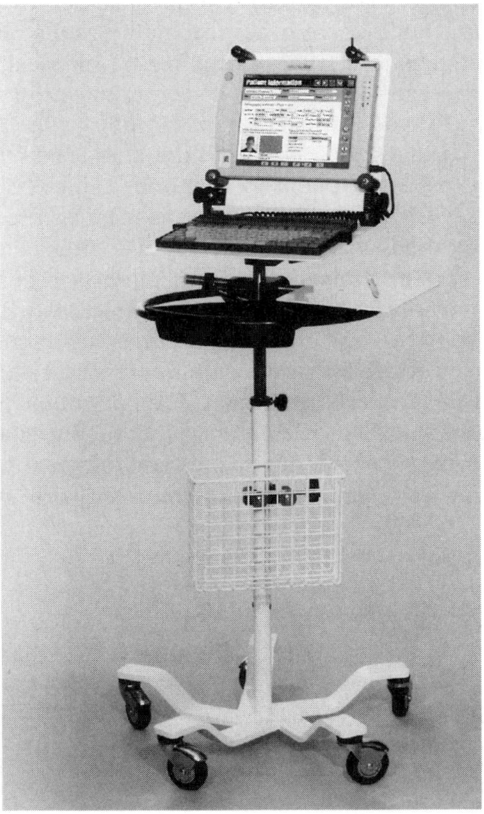

Figure 2.5. Portable terminal. (Photograph courtesy of Prologix.)

Stand-alone

By "stand-alone" we mean that all the pieces of a computer that are needed to gather, process, display, possibly store, and provide an output of the information are physically connected; moreover, if needed, they can be moved as a complete unit to another location. This is the usual setup for most home and small business computer systems. Such a setup is inexpensive and quite simple to manage. Although it makes sense to use a "stand-alone" computer, it is often better for a computer to be part of a network.

Local Area Networks

Definition

A network is a way to connect computers so several benefits can be realized. Local Area Networks (LANs) connect computers that are physically close together (i.e., in the same local area). This means not only in the same room but also in the same building, or in several buildings that are close together. LANs use three things to connect computers: a physical connection (e.g., wire), a network operating system, and a communication scheme.

There are several ways to connect computers physically. The most common method is to use coaxial cable, similar to the kind used by cable television. Another way is to use wire similar to telephone cable ("twisted pair"), and the latest way uses fiberoptic cable (light is used in place of electricity). The very latest methods are wireless; they use either radio transmission or infrared light for the connection. Each method is suited for different situations and is part of the consideration when a network is built.

There are several network operating systems available today that provide the necessary processes to allow computers to talk with each other and to share information and programs. The communication schemes are properly called *protocols*. This is a standard method by which the computers in a network to talk with each other and pass information around. There are three main ways to connect computers in a network: star, ring, and bus

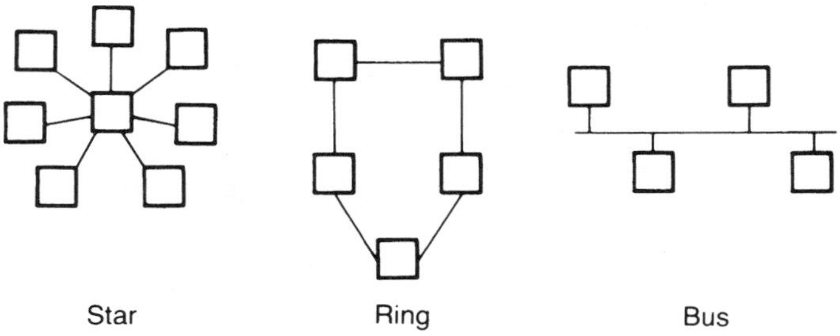

Figure 2.6. Network typologies.

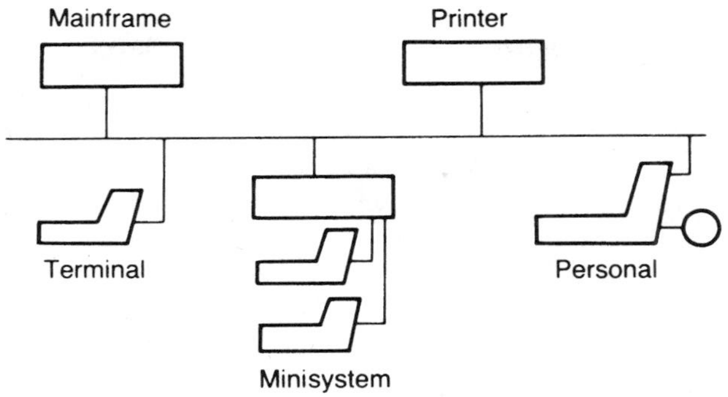

Figure 2.7. Example of resource sharing on a network.

configurations. These are called network topologies and represent different physical arrangements of the computers (Fig. 2.6). As with the physical connecting medium (i.e., coaxial cable vs. twisted pair), each topology has its strengths and weaknesses, which must be considered when a network is built.

Benefits of a Network

The important benefits of a network are shared information, shared programs, shared equipment, and easier administration. It is technically possible for any computer on a network to read and write information that another computer has in its storage (i.e., its hard disk). Whether that computer is *allowed* to do so is an administrative matter. This means, though, that information can be shared among the computers on the network. Programs can also be used by computers on the network, regardless of where those programs are physically stored. It is also possible (and usually desirable) for computers on a network to share equipment such as printers. A diagram of how a system might be connected is shown in Figure 2.7. Technically, any computer on the network can print its information on a printer that is physically connected to another computer somewhere else. By sharing expensive office equipment, an organization reduces its expenses. Finally, administration of computers on a network is simplified because all the other computers can be examined, helped, and maintained from one computer.

Wide Area Networks

Wide Area Networks (WANs) are extensions of Local Area Networks. There are two kinds of WAN. The first one attaches or connects a single computer to a preexisting LAN; this kind is called "remote LAN attachment." The second one connects, or "bridges," two or more preexisting LANs. Both WANs allow a computer to use information or equipment no matter where they are located in the organization. An interesting point about WANs is the options that can be used to connect the LANs. Instead of being limited by the length of cable that can be placed between computers, WANs can communicate via satellite and earth stations. This literally means that a person could be using a computer in Africa and working with information that is on a computer in Iceland—without knowing or caring about its origin. To that person, the information appears to be on his or her computer.

Open Systems

"Open systems" is the idea that it should be possible to do two things: run a particular program on any brand of computer and connect any collection of computers together in a network. However, because of the development of computer technology, this is difficult to accomplish.

Most computers were initially developed as "closed" systems; that is, a manufacturer built the computer, wrote the operating system, and wrote the application programs to run on the computer. Each computer manufacturer saw tremendous sales advantage from this strategy. The result was several computers that were similar in function but very different in how those functions were executed. It was not easy to buy an application program from a vendor and run it on two different brands of computers. It was a torturous exercise to get any two computer brands to "talk" with each other.

For people who simply want to buy and use computer technology, "plug and play" is the ideal mode. This means that a computer could be purchased from vendor X, a second computer from vendor Y, a program from vendor Z, and a printer from vendor A, and all these parts could be connected and used with the same ease that people expect with stereo system components. The way to achieve this ideal is through standards. Just as stereo components are built to use a standard voltage, produce or use a standard type of signal, and connect with standard plugs and cables, computers and application programs need to use certain standards for communication protocols and file access. This "plug and play" mode is getting closer today because of vendors' and manufacturers' support and adoption of standards.

Client/Server Computing

As we have seen, computers come in a variety of sizes and with various processing capacities. Some computers are better suited than others for different tasks. For example, personal computers, because of the physical size of their hard drives, have a limit to their storage capacity. On the other hand, the large, mainframe-type computer was designed to handle tremendous amounts of information and therefore has large storage capacity. Where does it make more sense to store a large data set?

This brings us to client/server computing. The essence of "client/server computing" is to assign to each computer the tasks for which it is best qualified or, in other words, to use the right tool for the job. Capitalize on the strengths of one computer for task A and use a different computer more suited for task B. A personal computer works well with people; it is fast and has color and good graphics display capability. It could be the primary interface device for people and computer systems. Mainframe computers have huge storage capacity, great speed, and large processing power. This could be the place to store, process, and retrieve information from the vast amount of data accumulated by a large organization. In a network, client/server computing makes sense.

Remote Access Computing

Computers can be connected together in a network; but, increasingly, mobile computing requires that computers be able to access and connect to other computers from almost anywhere. This is possible through the use of telephone or cable systems and special computer communication devices called "modems" (Fig. 2.8.) "Modem" is short for "modulate-demodulate." The computer that, at the moment, is sending information uses its modem to "modulate" its electronic signal into a form that can be carried over the telephone or cable system; the computer receiving that information uses its modem to "demodulate" the signal. Information can be exchanged at speeds that allow effective long-distance computing.

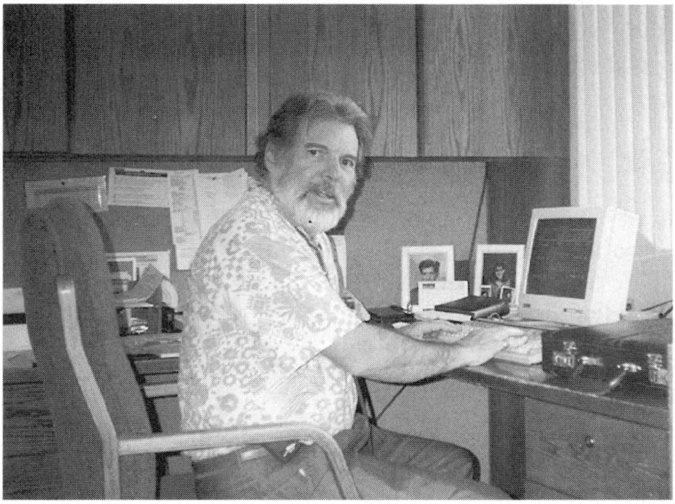

FIGURE 2.8. Remote access from clinic office. (Photograph courtesy of Clinicare Corporation and Health Plus Medical Clinic, Calgary, Alberta, Canada.)

Computing Hygiene for E-mail

The advent of the Internet and of "E-mail" (electronic mail; see Chapter 4) has allowed us to exchange ideas and information remotely, easily, and to great advantage. Unfortunately, there are those who try to introduce problems into this situation.

"Spam" refers to e-mail containing information on products and services that are sent out to many people at the same time. The problem is that the people rarely asked for this information. These recipients then spend significant time reviewing their incoming electronic mail, discarding the unrequested e-mails and keeping the valuable ones. Most e-mail programs have some kind of filtering tool that can be used to reduce the number of "junk" e-mails a person sees.

In addition, e-mails can have files attached to them. This is one way information can be exchanged electronically. The problem is that when an attached file is opened, it can run a program called a "virus" or a "worm" without notifying the operator of the computer. If the creator of the attached file intends harm, opening that file can cause problems for the computer operator. There are several antivirus programs available that can scan e-mails as they are received and try to remove any attached files that carry viruses or worms.

There are some general rules of computing hygiene for handling e-mail.

- Purchase an antivirus program and use it. Make sure it is scanning the incoming mail. Keep its "virus recognition" files up-to-date.
- Do not open an e-mail message if you do not recognize the sender—just delete the e-mail.
- Even if the sender is known, do not open or run any attached files until you know the purpose or content of the file.

Summary

As promised, we have not gone into great detail about computer technology. We have also not included a bibliography because technology is changing every day. We recommend that the interested reader visit any library or local bookstore to find up-to-date information on computer technology. For the very latest information, the Internet is the place to search.

3
History of Healthcare Computing

Since the beginning of time, people have invented tools to help them. Tracing the evolution of computers gives us a clearer historical vantage point from which to view our rapidly changing world. This approach also identifies informatics as a tool that can advance the goal of high quality nursing care. From a historical perspective, however, it is difficult to identify the true origin of computers. For instance, we could go back in time to the devices introduced by Moslem scientists and to the mathematicians of the fifteenth century. An example is Al-Kashi, who designed his plate of conjunctions to calculate the exact hour at which two planets would have the same longitude (De and Price, 1959; Goldstine, 1972). A more familiar example is the first rudimentary calculating tool, the Chinese abacus. This is still a rapid and efficient method of handling addition and subtraction.

Historical Development of Computers

Before 1950

The early nineteenth century had its share of men and women whose ideas were far ahead of the engineering, technological, and tooling abilities necessary to build calculating or computing machines. The groundwork for computerization was laid by Boole (1815–1864), who expanded the Leibnitz mathematic logic (binary numbers), and by Babbage (1791–1871), who invented the analytical machine in 1842.

It was not until the twentieth century that manufacturing made it possible to carry out those ideas. Differential analyzers were developed in Germany and Russia during the 1930s. By 1940 there were about seven of these primitive analog computers in operation throughout the world. In 1939, Howard H. Aiken of Harvard University and Claire D. Lake of IBM developed an automatic sequence-controlled calculator. In 1944 they developed the Harvard Mark I. The Mark I was an electromechanical digital machine that would do arithmetic computations (using punched cards) and store results. One hundred times faster than any manual operation, it could run 24 hours per day and accomplish 6 months' work during those 24 hours.

George R. Stibitz, at the Bell Telephone Laboratories, set up yet another type of electromechanical computer using relay machines. It was possible, using this device, to calculate and produce firing and bombing tables and related gun control data. This prompted the Ordnance Department of the U.S. War Department to underwrite a development program at the Moore School of Electrical Engineering, University of Pennsylvania, which resulted in the production of the ENIAC in 1946. The ENIAC, using vacuum tubes and electronic circuits, received much publicity as the first electrical computer with no moving parts. However, it has subsequently been revealed that Konrad Zuse, an aircraft engineer, had built the world's programmable binary based electric computer in Germany in 1941 (Lee, 1994). Similarly, the English code breakers at Bletchley Park developed and built the COLOSSUS Mark I computer that began breaking code in January 1944 (Sale, 2004).

Augusta, Lady Lovelace, daughter of Lord Byron, is known as the "mother of programming" because of her pioneering work on the mathematic logic for Babbage's difference engine, his analytic machine (Fig. 3.1). John von Neumann is widely credited with the concept of the stored computer program that revolutionized programming techniques based on his theoretical paper in 1945 (Lee, 2002). However, Tom Kilburn at the University of Manchester in England wrote the first computer program that first worked on June 21, 1948 on the first electronic stored-program computer (affectionately called "Baby") (University of Manchester, 2001).

The invention of the general purpose, high speed electronic computer and the work by von Neumann and Kilburn mark the close of the early development of the computer. These first-generation computers, although

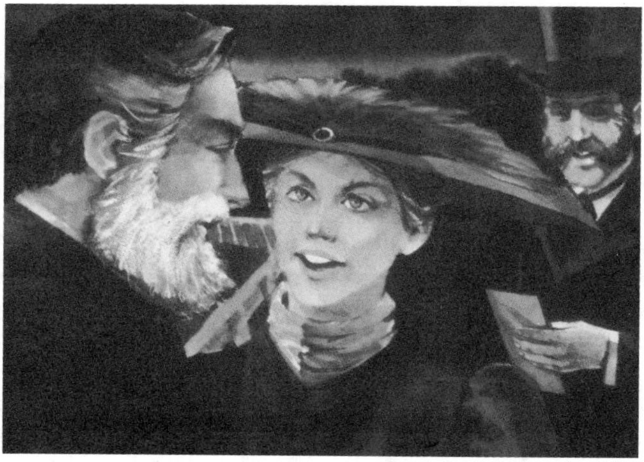

FIGURE 3.1. Augusta, Lady Lovelace, the mother of programming.

bulky, expensive, and less than totally reliable, provided useful results and excellent experience for both users and developers of the computer.

The 1950s

The transistor, invented by Shockley in 1947 (WGBH, 2004), was used to develop a second generation of computers and ultimately the transistor lead to the silicon chip. Second-generation computers were smaller, produced less heat, were more reliable, and were much easier to operate and maintain. Second-generation computers moved into the business and industrial world where they were used for data-processing functions such as payroll and accounting. The rapidly expanding healthcare industry began using computers to track patient charges, calculate payrolls, control inventory, and analyze medical statistics.

During the 1950s, Blumberg (1958) foresaw the possibilities of automating selected nursing activities and records. Little action was taken then because the existing computer programs were inflexible, computer manufacturers had a general lack of interest in the healthcare market, and hospital administrators and nursing management had a general lack of interest and knowledge about such equipment.

The 1960s

During the 1960s, universities were bursting at the seams as members of the post-World War II baby boom entered college. The philosophy of "education for all" left educators searching for a way to provide more individualized and self-paced instruction. The computer seemed to hold great promise. At the University of Illinois, Dr. Donald Bitzer was working on a display screen that would increase the graphics resolution available on the PLATO (programmed logic for automated teaching operations) computer system he developed.

During 1965 and 1966, the "third generation" of computers was introduced. These third-generation computers were identifiable by their modular components, increased speed, ability to service multiple users simultaneously, inexpensive bulk storage devices that allowed more data to be immediately accessible, and rapid development of systems.

The 1970s

The development of the silicon chip paved the way for the development of minicomputers and personal computers. The silicon chip allowed large amounts of data to be stored in an extremely small space. This development allowed the total size of computers to be significantly reduced. The first mass-market personal computer, the MITS Altair 8800, was sold in 1975 as a hobbyist kit; the Apple I, another personal computer kit marketed to hobbyists by Stephen Wozniak and Steve Jobs, followed in 1976.

Soon the vision of connecting computers to share information began to spread, and many computer networks were being developed all over the world, but they could not communicate with one another because they used different protocols, or standards, for transmitting data. In 1974, Vint Cerf (sometimes known as the "father of the Internet"), along with Bob Kahn, wrote a new protocol, TCP (transmission control protocol), which became the accepted international standard. The implementation of TCP allowed the various networks to connect and become the Internet as we know it.

The 1980s

Personal computer technology augmented and replaced the large, cumbersome hardware of the 1970s. In 1981 IBM debuted the PC with an Intel 8088 microprocessor, 16K of RAM, and a 5.25 disk drive with two choices of operating system. The Apple Mac was launched in 1984, and in 1986 Intel introduced the 486 Processor. Research and development in computer technology was aimed at "open systems." This additional technological advance served the nursing profession because it systematized and simplified the process of data entry, storage, and retrieval.

The 1990s

During the 1990s, information technologies, including personal computers and workstations, combined with telecommunications technologies such as local and wide area networks to create client/server architectures. Client/server architecture integrated and capitalized on the strengths of the hardware, software, and telecommunications capacities, allowing users to navigate through data across many systems. These linkages were vital to breaking the barriers between different systems. The open flow of information among systems (see Chapter 2 for details) contributed to many developments in nursing informatics.

In 1990 Tim Berners-Lee created a new way to interact with the Internet—the World Wide Web. His system made it much easier to share and find data on the Internet. Others augmented the World Wide Web by creating new software and technologies to make it more functional. For example, Marc Andreesen led the team that created Netscape Navigator (Griffin, 2000).

The New Millennium (2000)

The dawning of the twenty-first century saw pervasive digital proliferation. Digital cameras, music players, and videos became widely available. Handheld devices of all sorts and for highly diverse purposes multiplied and became widely available and affordable. Handheld wireless communication devices such as Blackberry are bringing convergence of digital telecommunications.

Introduction of Computers into Healthcare

Healthcare trailed government and industry in the initial exploration of the feasibility of computer usage and in installation of computers. One reason for the delay was that first- and second-generation computers were not well suited for the data processing needs of hospitals. A second reason was that only about 250 of the largest hospitals had in-hospital punch card installations. These hospitals were usually the first targets of computer salesmen. The computer manufacturers simply did not understand the potential of the hospital market or ultimately the healthcare market.

When focusing on the use of computers in healthcare, computers traditionally gained entry through the accounting area, where most hospital computer systems still have their roots. Patient care requires continuous and instantaneous response in contrast to the fiscal methodology where timing is less critical. To achieve successful utilization of computers in healthcare, both needs must be addressed.

The 1950s

During the late 1950s a few pioneering hospitals installed computers and began to develop their application software. Some hospitals had help from computer manufacturers, especially IBM. Then, in 1958–1959, John Diebold and Associates undertook an in-depth feasibility study of hospital computing at Baylor University Medical Center. The final report identified two major hospital wide needs for computerization: (1) a set of business and financial applications, and (2) a set of hospital–medical applications that would require on-line terminals at nursing stations and departments throughout the hospital. Such a system could be used for the following purposes.

- As a communications and message-switching device to route physicians' orders and test results to their proper destinations
- As a data-gathering device to capture charges and patient medical information
- As a scheduler to prepare such items as nursing station medication schedules
- As a database manager with report preparation and inquiry capabilities

These functions are often collectively called hospital information systems (HISs), medical information systems (MISs), and sometimes hospital–medical information systems (HMISs). The first term (or its acronym, HIS) is used in this book.

The 1960s

Although a few hardware manufacturers offered some business and financial application packages for in-hospital processing during the early 1960s, it was not until the mid-1960s that other vendors began to see the potential of the hospital data-processing market. The hardware vendors during the 1960s (e.g., IBM, Burroughs, Honeywell, UNIVAC, NCR, CDC) were committed primarily to selling large general-purpose computers to support clinical, administrative, communication, and financial systems of the hospitals.

The 200 to 400 bed hospitals that installed computers during the late 1960s for accounting applications found their environments growing more complex, which resulted in a constant battle just to maintain and update existing systems to keep pace with regulating agencies. Many hospitals of this size turned to shared computer services.

In 1966, Honeywell announced the availability of a business and financial package for a shared hospital data-processing center. IBM followed quickly the next year with SHAS (shared hospital accounting system). The availability of this software was an important factor in establishing not-for-profit and for-profit shared centers during the next 5 years. There are still many shared-service companies (e.g., SMS, McAuto) specializing in hospital data processing. These companies continue to provide useful services, particularly to smaller hospitals. The companies prospered not only because of their computer and systems products and services but because smaller, single hospitals were unable to justify, employ, and retain the varied technical and management skills required for this complex and constantly changing environment.

The first hospital computer systems for other than accounting services were developed during the late 1960s. The technology that attempted to address clinical applications was unsuccessful. Terminal devices such as keyboard overlays, early cathode-ray tubes, and a variety of keyboard and card systems were expensive, unreliable, and unwieldy. Also, hardware and software were scarce, expensive, and inflexible. Database management systems, which are at the heart of good information software today, had not yet appeared. During this period, some hospitals installed computers in offices to do specific jobs (Ball and Jacobs, 1980). The most successful of these early clinical systems were installed in the clinical pathology laboratory (Ball, 1973). Most of the hospitals that embarked on these dedicated clinical programs were large teaching institutions with access to federal funding or foundation research money. Limited attempts were made to integrate the accounting computer with these stand-alone systems.

During the mid-1960s, Lockheed Missile and Space Company and National Data Communications (then known as Reach) began the development of HISs that would require little or no modification by individual hospitals. This was the forerunner to the product that is now marketed by Eclipsys.

About 1965, the American Hospital Association (AHA) began to conduct four or five conferences per year to acquaint hospital executives with the potential the computer holds for improving hospital administration. The AHA also devoted two issues of its journal solely to data processing. These AHA activities served to crystallize a market (i.e., hospitals ready for data processing) and to encourage existing and new firms to enter the marketplace.

The 1970s

During the early 1970s, with inflation problems and with cost reimbursement becoming stricter, some large hospitals that had installed their own computers with marginal success changed to the shared service. By this time the shared companies had improved earlier accounting software and could carry out tighter audit controls. Most importantly, however, the companies developed personnel who understood hospital operations and could communicate and translate the use of computer systems into results in their client hospitals. This added a dimension of service that is seldom offered or understood by the major hardware vendors. As a result, the business opportunities for the service companies increased. Over time, these companies have expanded their scope of services from fiscal applications and administrative services to clinical and communication applications.

Major hardware changes took place as the minicomputer entered the scene. This was quickly followed by the introduction of the personal computer during the late 1970s. Technologic developments have resulted in a steady trend toward microminiaturization of computers. Personal computers are now more powerful than the original ENIAC. These personalcomputers have invaded homes, schools, offices, nursing stations, and administrative offices to a degree never dreamed possible. The linking of these personal computers, using local area networking technology, provided a better alternative to many of the processes formerly carried out by one large general-purpose computer.

Many major mainframe hardware companies moved rapidly into the personal computer field as well. Simultaneously, the service companies began to develop on-site networking systems to handle data communications and specialized nonfinancial applications. They began to expand their scope of data retention to support clinical applications that required a historical patient database.

The 1980s

During the 1980s, specific personal computer-based systems were developed. These systems did not replace but, instead, complemented a variety of alternatives in various healthcare environments. Thus, awareness of computer concepts by healthcare professionals became even more essential.

The 1990s

During the 1990s, the advent of powerful, affordable, portable personal computers made information management tools accessible to support highly mobile, remote activities, especially in community health. At the same time, the power of networks and database technology has made possible linkages of health data in widely separated locations. There also was a growing emphasis on information management across health enterprises. Accompanying this was recognition of the importance of patient/client-centered, integrated data in contrast to departmental focused data. Such linkages and shift in focus created the possibility of a longitudinal, lifelong health record encompassing healthcare encounters by individuals with all sectors of the healthcare system.

History of Nursing Use of Computers

Nursing Education

The seminal work in the use of computers in nursing education was conducted by Maryann Drost Bitzer. During the early 1960s, Bitzer wrote a program that was used to teach obstetric nursing. Her program was a simulation exercise. It was the first simulation in nursing and one of the first in the healthcare field. (Bitzer's 1963) master's thesis showed that students learned and retained the same amount of material using the computer simulation in one-third the time it would take using the classic lecture method. This thesis (Bitzer, 1963) has become a classic model for subsequent work by her and many others, including two of the authors (K.J.H. and M.J.E.) of this volume. Bitzer's early findings have been consistently confirmed. She was later project director on two Department of Health Education and Welfare (HEW)-funded research projects. These projects undertook evaluative studies that documented the efficacy of teaching nursing content using a computer. Until 1976 Bitzer was associated with the Computer-Based Education Research Laboratory at the University of Illinois in Urbana, where she continued to develop computer-assisted instruction lessons to teach nursing.

During the 1970s many individual nursing faculties, schools, and units developed and evaluated computer-assisted instruction (CAI) lessons to meet specific institutional student needs. Most of the software created was used solely by the developing institution.

The use of computers to teach nursing content has been a focal point of informatics activity in nursing education. However, the need to prepare nurses to use informatics in nursing practice is just as important. This aspect was pioneered in 1975 by Judith Ronald of the School of Nursing, State University of New York at Buffalo. Ronald developed the course that served as a model and inspiration for courses developed later. Ronald's enthusiasm and her willingness to share her course materials and experiences have greatly facilitated the implementation of other such courses throughout North America. In Scotland, Christine Henney of the University of Dundee undertook similar activities aimed at promoting computer literacy among nurses.

Nursing Administration

The use of computers to provide management information to nurse managers in hospitals has been promoted on both sides of the Atlantic. Marilyn Plomann of the Hospital Research and Educational Trust (an affiliate of the American Hospital Association) in Chicago was actively involved for many years in the design, development, and demonstration of a planning, budgeting, and control system (PB CS) for use by hospital managers. In Glasgow (Scotland) Catherine Cunningham was actively involved in the development of nurse-manpower planning projects on microcomputers. Similarly, Elly Pluyter-Wenting (from 1976 to 1983 in Leiden, Holland), Christine Henney (from 1974 to 1983 in Dundee, Scotland), Phyllis Giovanetti (from 1978 to the time of writing in Edmonton, Canada), and Elizabeth Butler (from 1973 to 1983 in London, England) have been instrumental in developing and implementing nurse scheduling and staffing systems for hospitals in their areas.

In the public health area of nursing practice, Virginia Saba (a nurse consultant to the Division of Nursing, Bureau of Health Manpower, Health Resources Administration, Public Health Service, Department of Health and Human Services) was instrumental in promoting the use of management information systems for public health nursing services. The objective of all these projects has been to use computers to provide management information to help in decision-making by nurse administrators.

Nursing Care

Much research on the development of computer applications for use in patient care was conducted during the 1960s. Projects were designed to provide justification for the initial costs of automation and to show improved patient care. Hospital administrators became aware of the possibilities of automating healthcare activities other than business office procedures. Equipment became more refined and sophisticated. Healthcare professionals began to develop patient care applications, and the manufacturers recognized the sales potential in the healthcare market.

Nurse pioneers who have contributed to the use of computers in patient care activities have been active on both sides of the Atlantic. In the United Kingdom, Maureen Scholes, chief nursing officer at The London Hospital (Whitechapel), began her involvement with computers and nursing in 1967 as the nurse member of the steering team that directed and monitored The London Hospital Real-Time Computer Project. This project resulted in a hospital communication system that provided patient administration services, laboratory services, and radiography services using 105 visual display units in all hospital wards and departments.

Elizabeth Butler was associated with the Kings College Hospital from 1970 to 1973. As the nursing officer on a medical unit, Butler was involved in developing and implementing the computerized nursing care plan system for the Professional Medical Unit and for the nursing care plan system for all wards and specialties in the 500-bed general area of the hospital. In Dundee, Scotland, Christine Henney worked with James Crooks (from 1974) on the design and implementation of a real-time nursing system at Ninewells Hospital.

In the United States, Carol Ostrowski and Donna Gane McNeill were both associated with the development of the Problem Oriented Medical Information System (PROMIS) at Medical Center Hospital of Vermont under the direction of Lawrence Weed. From 1969 to 1979, Donna Gane McNeill was a nurse clinician on the PROMIS project. As such, McNeill managed the first computerized nursing unit, developed content for PROMIS, and developed functions and tasks for the computer. She also conducted a comparison between computerized and noncomputerized units. From June 1976 to December 1977, Carol Ostrowski served as director of audit for the PROMIS system. She was responsible for implementing the components that supported concurrent audit of medical and nursing care and the environment that guided and evaluated patient care.

In the United States, Margo Cook also began her association with computers in nursing in 1970 when she was employed at El Camino Hospital, Mountain View, California. Cook participated as the nursing representative on the team that developed and implemented the Medical Information System (still marketed by Elipsys). As nursing implementation coordinator, Cook was responsible for identifying and addressing the needs of all nursing units at El Camino. Often she functioned as interpreter between the computer analysts and nurses. Eventually she assumed senior level responsibility for the MIS maintenance and development. In 1983 Cook left El Camino to become senior consultant of Hospital Productivity Management Services.

In 1976 Dickey Johnson became computer coordinator at Latter Day Saints Hospital in Salt Lake City, Utah. Johnson's responsibilities involved coordination between the computer department and other hospital users in planning, development, implementation, and maintenance of all programs either used by, or affecting, nursing personnel. In 1983, Johnson was the nursing representative on the hospital's Computer Committee, which was actively involved in planning, designing, and implementing a hospital-wide computer system. Johnson was responsible for projects that included order entries, nursing care plans, nurse acuity, and nurse staffing.

In Canada, from 1978 to 1983, Joy Brown and Marjorie Wright, systems coordinators at York Central Hospital in Richmond Hill, Ontario, were actively involved in designing, coding, and implementing the computerized patient care system at their hospital. They were also responsible for training many nurse users on the system. Beginning in 1982 at Calgary General Hospital in Calgary, Alberta, Wendy Harper, assistant director, Nursing Systems, was responsible for all aspects of the nursing applications on the hospital information system being installed in that hospital.

Nurses have recognized the potential for improving nursing practice and the quality of patient care through nursing informatics. These applications facilitate charting, care planning, patient monitoring, interdepartmental scheduling, and communication with the hospital's other computers. New roles for nurses have emerged. Nurses have formed computer and nursing informatics interest groups (see Appendix B) to provide a forum through which information about computers and information systems is communicated worldwide.

Nursing Research

During the 1960s, nursing researchers began using computers to store data and maintain complex data sets without error.

Communicating Nursing Developments

Kathryn Hannah, of the University of Calgary, was the first nurse elected to the Board of Directors of the Canadian Organization for the Advancement of Computers in Health (COACH). In that capacity, with the assistance of David Shires of Dalhousie University (and at that time program chairman for the International Medical Informatics Association), Hannah was instrumental in establishing the first separate nursing section at an International Medical Informatics Association (IMIA) meeting (Medinfo '80, Tokyo). Previously, nursing presentations at this international conference had been integrated within other sections. In 1982, based on the success of this Tokyo workshop, which Hannah also chaired, a contingent of British nurses led by Maureen Scholes mounted an International Open Forum and Working Conference on "The Impact of Computers on Nursing." The international symposium on the impact of computers on nursing was convened in London, England, in the fall of 1982, followed immediately by an IMIA-sponsored working conference. One outcome of the working conference was a book that documented the developments related to nursing uses of computers from their beginning until 1982. The second outcome was a consensus that nurses needed a structure within an international organization to promote future regular international exchanges of ideas related to the use of computers in nursing and healthcare. Consequently, in the spring of 1983, a proposal to establish a permanent nursing working group (Group 8) was approved by the General Assembly of IMIA. In August 1983, the inaugural meeting of the IMIA Working Group on Nursing Informatics (Group 8) was held in Amsterdam.

In 1992, the working group recommended a change of bylaws and began its transformation to a nursing informatics society within the IMIA. This society continues the organization of symposia every 3 years for exchange of ideas about nursing informatics, dissemination of new ideas about nursing informatics through its publications, provision of leadership in the development of nursing informatics internationally, and promotion of awareness and education of nurses about nursing informatics.

In the United States in 1981, Virginia Saba was instrumental in establishing a nursing presence at the Symposium on Computer Applications in Medical Care (SCAMC). This annual symposium, although not a professional organization, provided opportunities for nurses in the United States to share their experiences. In 1982 the American Association for Medical Systems and Informatics (AAMSI) established a Nursing Professional Specialty Group. This group, which was chaired by Carol Ostrowski, provided the benefits of a national professional organization as a focal point for discussion, exchange of ideas, and leadership for nurses involved in the use of computers. Subsequently, AAMSI merged with SCAMC to become the American Medical Informatics Association (AMIA). This organization continues to have a highly active nursing professional specialty group.

Summary

Despite their wide usage, computers are historically young and did not come into prominence until 1944 when the IBM-Harvard project called Mark I was completed. This was followed closely by the development, in 1946 at the University of Pennsylvania, of the ENIAC I, the first electronic computer with no moving parts. Subsequent refinement of computer technology, development of the silicon chip in 1976, development of the Internet, and the World Wide Web have made personal computers as common in our homes as television sets. Handheld wireless digital telecommunications devices are now pervasive.

During the 1950s computers entered the healthcare professions. They were primarily used for the purposes of tabulating patient charges, calculating payrolls, controlling inventory, and analyzing medical statistics. A few farsighted individuals saw the possibilities of automating selected nursing activities and records. However, little action was taken because of the inflexibility and slowness of the equipment, the general disinterest of the manufacturers in the healthcare market, and the lack of knowledge concerning such equipment among hospital management, hospital administrators, and nursing management.

By the 1960s, hospital administrators had been exposed to the possibility of automating healthcare activities; in addition to existing business office automation, equipment had become more refined and sophisticated, and the manufacturers had recognized the sales potential in the healthcare market. The major focus during the 1960s was on the research aspect of computer applications for patient care; the business applications for auditing functions in the healthcare industry were becoming well established. Projects were designed to provide justification for the initial costs of automation and to display the variety of areas in which computers could be used to facilitate and improve patient care. Nurses began to recognize the potential of computers for improving nursing practice and the quality of patient care, especially in the areas of charting, care plans, patient monitoring, interdepartmental scheduling, and communication and personnel time assignment. These individual computer applications or modules, which were developed to support selected nursing activities, were later integrated in modular fashion into various hospital information systems. Today these hospital information systems are widely promoted and marketed by computer vendors.

Simultaneously, advances in the uses of computers in educational environments were initiated during the 1960s. The major focus during this decade was on showing the efficacy of computers as teaching methods. During the 1970s, many projects were designed to compare student learning via computer with learning via traditional teaching methods. The mid-1970s also saw the development of the personal microcomputer and during the latter years of that decade their widespread dissemination throughout society. During the 1980s nursing educators were scrambling to develop software for use with this technology. In fact, the hardware technology has advanced beyond nursing educators' capacity to use it all.

Major contributions by nurses to developments leading to the use of computers in nursing were also discussed. Our apologies to those nurses whose activities were unknown to us. If readers know of other nurses whose contributions merit inclusion in future editions, the authors would be pleased to receive such information.

The future demands that computer technology be integrated into the clinical practice environment, education, and research domains of the nursing profession. The ultimate goal is always the best possible care for the patient.

References

Ball, M.J. (1973). *How to Select a Computerized Hospital Information System.* New York: Karger.

Ball, M.J., & Jacobs, S.E. (1980). Information systems: the status of level 1. *Information Systems,* 179–186.

Bitzer, M.D. (1963). *Self-Directed Inquiry in Clinical Nursing Instruction by Means of PLATO Simulated Laboratory.* Report R-184, Co-ordinated Science Laboratory. Urbana: University of Illinois.

Blumberg, M.S. (1958). Automation offers savings opportunities. *Modern Hospital* 91:59.

de S. Price, D.J. (1959). An ancient Greek computer. *Scientific American 200*(6):60–67.

Goldstine, H.H. (1972). *The Computer from Pascal to von Neumann.* Princeton: Princeton University Press, pp. 5, 69.

Griffin, S. *Internet Pioneers*. (2000). http://www.ibiblio.org/pioneers/index.html (accessed December 14, 2004).

Lee, J.A.N. (1994). *Konrad Zuse*. http://ei.cs.vt.edu/~history/Zuse.html (accessed December 14, 2004).

Lee, J.A.N. (2002). *John von Neuman*. http://ei.cs.vt.edu/~history/VonNeumann.html (accessed December 14, 2004).

Sale, T. *The COLOSSUS; Its Purpose and Operation.* http://www. codesandciphers.org.uk/lorenz/colossus.htm (accessed December 14, 2004).

University of Manchester. (2001). *Tom Kilburn*. http://www.computer50.org/mark1/kilburn.html (accessed December 14, 2004).

WGBH. People and Discoveries: *William Schockley* 1910–1989. http://www.pbs.org/wgbh/aso/databank/entries/btshoc.html (accessed December 14, 2004).

4
Telecommunications and Informatics

The convergence of telecommunications and informatics has opened up a new world of communication service delivery and health information for consumers and health professionals. This chapter is designed to provide a basic understanding of the Internet, intranets, and extranets.

What Is the Internet?

At the most basic level, the Internet is the name for a group of worldwide computer-based information resources that are connected. It is often defined as a network of networks of computers. According to the Internet Systems Consortium, there are more than 171 million hosts (computers) connected throughout the world (http://www.isc.org/index.pl?/ops/ds/host-count-history.php). These sites support more than 2 billion indexable Web pages. It is estimated that more than 1 million sites join the Internet every day.

One of the major challenges when using the Internet is that there is no clear map of how all those networks are connected. There is also no master list of what information or resource is available where. Because there is no overall structured grand plan, the shape and face of the Internet is constantly changing to meet the needs of the people who use it. The Internet can be likened to a cloud in this way; it is amorphous, without boundaries and constantly changing shape and space.

Although the thought of all those computers joined together is mind boggling, the real power of the Internet is in the people and information that all those computers connect. The Internet is a people-oriented community that allows millions of individuals around the world to communicate with one another. The computers move the information around and execute the programs that allow us to access the information. However, it is the information itself and the people connected to the information that make the Internet useful.

Connecting to the Internet

There are three basic ways to connect to the Internet: make a direct connection over dedicated communications lines; use your computer to connect to a university or hospital computer system that has Internet access; or buy time and connections from a commercial Internet service provider.

Direct Connection to the Internet

A direct or dedicated connection wires a personal computer directly to the Internet through a dedicated machine called a *router* or *gateway*. The connection is made over a special kind of telephone line. The gateway identifies the personal computer as an "official" Internet computer that must remain on-line all the time. This type of direct connection is extremely expensive to install and maintain. For this reason, it is usually used only by large companies or institutions rather than by individuals or small businesses.

Connecting Through Another's Gateway

Another way to connect to the Internet is to use a gateway that another company or institution has established. In this case, a company or university or hospital that has an Internet gateway allows individuals to connect to the Internet using their system. The connection is usually made through a modem or remote terminal. This type of access is often available to students through the computing services department of their university. Many hospitals and health services organizations also allow staff access to the Internet through the institution's facilities. To use an institution's access, each user needs a login identification and password. For the individual, this is the best type of access to have if full Internet access is available. An organization maintains the computer system and the Internet connection and, most importantly, pays for the connection.

Connecting Through a Commercial Service Provider

Connecting to the Internet through a service provider is much the same process as using another's gateway. The service provider builds and maintains the gateway and sells Internet connection access to individuals and organizations. The service provider supplies a user name and password to connect to its gateway. Service providers usually charge a flat fee to provide a certain amount of Internet access per month or year and a personal e-mail address. Some providers, such as America Online (AOL), also offer access to other interesting software or participation in unique discussion groups through their own system.

Ways to Connect to a Commercial Service Provider

Today there are four main ways to connect your computer to an Internet Service Provider: dial-up, DSL, cable, or wireless. Each method has its pros and cons. For example, the DSL, cable, and wireless connection methods are not available to everyone. When choosing a connection type, you can be guided by your own needs, the available choices, and your budget. For example, if you only need e-mail service, a dial-up connection is probably sufficient.

Dial-up Connection

Dial-up was the first and probably is still the most common method of connecting to the Internet. Using software that is a normal part of your computer and an inexpensive modem in your computer, you can establish an Internet connection over your telephone line through your Internet Service Provider (ISP). Your ISP gives you a local telephone number for your computer to call. The dial-up software on your computer makes a telephone call to that number, and your modem establishes an Internet connection through the ISP's computer. Most ISPs charge a flat monthly or yearly fee for unlimited access to the Internet using this method. An advantage to this approach is that you probably have a telephone already and your computer likely has a modem already installed. A drawback is that you lose the normal use of your telephone while you are connected to the Internet. Another major drawback is that regular telephone lines cannot pass digital information faster than about 22.8 kilobits per second. Although that seems like a large number, it strongly limits the speed at which graphics information from the Internet is displayed. This may limit your ability to view large graphics files.

DSL Connection

To increase the speed of regular telephone lines for Internet use, telecommunication companies developed the digital subscriber line (DSL) technology. This technology allows information to move at speeds of up to 6 megabits per second. Your DSL provider installs a network interface card in your computer, connects it to a DSL modem, and then connects it to your telephone line. So long as your computer is turned on and plugged in, you have an "always on" Internet connection through your telephone line. An advantage, in addition to the transmission speed, is that you can use your telephone normally even while accessing the Internet. Another advantage is that, unlike a cable connection (see below), you do not share your telephone line with others to access the Internet. The immediate problem with this technology today is that there are distance limitations with DSL. You must be located within a certain distance from your telephone company's internal systems for DSL to work. The only way to find out if DSL is possible for you is to ask a DSL provider (likely a local ISP or your local telephone company).

Cable Connection

The other approach to having fast Internet service uses the cable that delivers cable television into your home. A cable company installs a network interface card in your computer, connects it to a cable modem, and then connects the modem to the cable television line in your house. As with the DSL technology, so long as your computer is turned on and plugged in, you have an "always on" Internet connection. An advantage, beyond the speed of Internet access, is that this approach does not affect your telephone in any way. There are several possible problems with this approach, however. For example, you may not have cable television installed in your house or your cable company may not offer Internet access. Also, it is possible that, as more people in an area share the service, performance in that area may degrade.

Wireless Connection

A fourth approach is Internet access using cellular phones and other portable wireless information devices. Many locations such as hospitals, airports, hotels and cyber cafes have put in place a "wireless access point" that uses radio transmitter-receiver technology. Computers, personal digital assistants (PDAs), and cell phones that are equipped with a wireless communication card, can take advantage of these access points, or "hotspots." The organization supporting the wireless access point control what is accessible. For example, some hospitals allow access to internal intranets but do not allow access to the Internet. Wireless access is limited by the speed of information flow. Wired networks are 2 to 10 times faster than wireless access. In addition, because radio transmission is used, interference can be an issue. There may be places in a building where reception is better than in other places.

What to Look for When Choosing an Internet Provider

There are several basic elements to consider when obtaining access to the Internet through a provider. First, what kind of personal computer (PC) is to be used for the connection? Generally, providers are most comfortable supporting PC-compatible computers. The processing power and storage capacity of the computer are also important.

Second, what is the individual's level of technical knowledge and comfort when working with the computer? There may be levels of technical details not understood by computing nonprofessionals. Some Internet providers, for a fee, help you install the connection software on your computer and get it working.

Third, look for a provider with a local telephone number that is used to connect. Some providers advertise 1–800 numbers. The point here is to avoid additional telephone charges. Without a local number, additional charges to a telephone company result.

Fourth, what set of Internet services or tools does the provider offer? Be sure to check the details of what is offered and what, if any, additional charges there might be for things such as the number of e-mail messages sent.

Fifth, what is the cost of this connection? Be sure that all the restrictions and assumptions are fully identified. Last, what kind of technical support does the provider offer? Make sure of the support policy of the provider (i.e., 24 hours a day, business hours only).

Security Issues

Connecting to the Internet gives others the opportunity to cause trouble for you. There are two ways your computer can be attacked: directly and indirectly.

Hacking or Cracking—Direct Attack

The news continually has reports about people who break into computer systems. The news reports often call these people "hackers", but to be strictly correct these people are "crackers." *Hacker* is a term that applies to anyone who writes computer program code. *Cracker* is a term that applies to people who use their skills to attempt to access other computers without permission. There are even programs, shared across the Internet, that allow people with little skill to mount an attack.

If you are connected to the Internet, there is the potential for people to attack your computer directly. This form of attack is more likely if you have an "always on" connection such as DSL or cable. A dial-up connection is more difficult to attack and is less likely to be attacked. To block these direct attacks, you need something called a *firewall.* This is either part of the computer hardware or a computer software program. If you connect to the Internet indirectly through a network at your workplace, there is probably a hardware firewall in place. If you connect to the Internet through an ISP, you need to install a commercial *personal firewall program* on your computer. Once installed on your computer, the personal firewall program watches every piece of information that attempts to come or go through your Internet connection. Only legitimate activities that are recognized by the firewall program are allowed to succeed. All other activities are blocked. As new methods of attack are discovered, the firewall manufacturer develops new methods to detect and block them and adds these new feature to the firewall program.

Viruses—Indirect Attack

Even if you are never attacked directly, there are always indirect attacks happening through the use of *viruses*. Viruses are small programs hidden inside legitimate files or e-mail messages. The virus-infected files might come as part of an e-mail message or might be given to you on a computer disk. When you access these files or e-mail messages, the viruses start running. They are now on the other side of any personal firewall of your computer. The main way to protect against viruses is to install a commercial antivirus program on your computer. These programs protect your computer from viruses in several ways. They scan your e-mail messages as you access them, looking for telltale signatures of viruses. They constantly monitor certain activities of your computer, looking for actions that may signal a virus starting up. Once a virus detected, the antivirus program alerts you with a message and guides you on how to deal with the virus. As new forms of viruses are discovered, the antivirus program manufacturer develops new methods for detecting and dealing with them and adds these new methods to the antivirus program.

World Wide Web

The *World Wide Web* (variously called WWW, W3, or the Web) was developed in an attempt to make sense of all the Internet resources. The goal of WWW development was to offer a simple, consistent, intuitive interface to the vast resources of the Internet. The WWW provides the intuitive links that humans make between information, rather than forcing people to think like a computer and speculate at possible file names and hidden submenus, as did the previous services. A short history of the development of the WWW may help to understand its services.

In 1989, researchers at CERN (the European Laboratory for Particle Physics) wanted to develop a simpler way of sharing information with a widely dispersed research group. The problems they faced are the same as those you face when using the previous information retrieval systems. Because the researchers were at distant sites, any activity such as reading a shared document or viewing an image required finding the location of the desired information, making a remote connection to the machine containing the information, and then downloading the information to a local machine. Each of these activities required running a variety of applications such as FTP, Telnet, Archie, or an image viewer. The researchers decided to develop a system that would allow them to access all types of information from a common interface without the need for all the steps required previously. Between 1990 and 1993, the CERN researchers developed this type of interface, WWW, and the necessary tools to use it. Since 1993, WWW has become the most popular way to access Internet resources.

Hypertext

To navigate around the World Wide Web, a beginning understanding of *hypertext* is essential. Hypertext is text that contains links to other data. For example, when doing a literature search using the hard copy of CINAHL, the first search term is selected and looked up. After reading through the listings, another idea for a search term becomes apparent. Traditionally, the user marks the first page (to facilitate returning at a later time) and turns to the new term. At the bottom of the listings of the second term is a note that says, "see also" and gives several other words to follow. In a hypertext document, it is unnecessary to wait until the end to find the links; they may be anywhere in the document. Links in hypertext documents are marked either with color bars, underlining, or use of square brackets with numbers so they stand out. Whenever a word is marked as hypertext it can be selected, and immediately the link is made to another document related to the word or phrase. When finished looking at the linked document, simply go back to the previous text with the click of a mouse button, where the program has kept its finger in the page.

This is what makes the Web so powerful. A link may go to any type of Internet resource. For example, the link can go to a text file, a database of information, a video or audio file, a chat room, or a UseNet newsgroup. Another powerful feature of the Web is that hypertext allows the same piece of information to be linked to hundreds of other documents at the same time. The links can also span traditional boundaries. A hypertext document related to a specific professional group may contain links to information in many disciplines.

All Web sites have a welcome page, called a home page, which you see when you first connect to that site. The home page may just give the name of the site but usually contains a list of resources and links available at the site.

Web Browsers

To access the Web, you need a Web browser program on your (or your institution's) computer. A Web browser program knows how to interpret and display the hypertext documents it finds on the Web. There are many browsers on the market. The two most popular graphical user interface (GUI) or windows-based browsers are Microsoft Internet Explorer and Netscape Communicator.

When you first start up your Web browser, you automatically navigate to a Web page that the browser calls its "home" page. This home page is a Web uniform resource locator (URL) that is initially set by the browser manufacturer or your ISP when they connected you to the Internet. You can navigate to the home page of your browser at any time by pressing the browser button called "Home." In addition to the Home button, there are buttons that help you navigate through and display the information you find on the Web.

The World Wide Web project developed a standard way of referencing an item whether it was a graphics file, a document or a link to another computer. This standardized reference is a URL. The URL is a complete description of the item including its location on the Internet. A typical URL is:

http://www.springer-sbm.com

The first part of the URL, which ends with the colon, is the protocol that is being used to retrieve the item. In this example, the protocol is HTTP (hypertext transfer protocol), used for the Web. The next part is the domain name of the computer to which you want to connect (springer-sbm.com). This tells you that the information is on a computer in the commercial top-level domain "(com)." The springer-sbm indicates that the Web site belongs to the publisher Springer in New York (USA). Most Web browsers automatically add the "http://" if you simply type the other part of the URL, www.springer-sbm.com

Searching the Internet

Finding what you need in the sheer volume of information available on the Internet can be daunting. Search sites bring millions of hypertext pages, with their images and multimedia elements into an orderly and searchable structure. Software agents, or "spiders," are sent out by search sites to "crawl" the Web electronically, collecting home pages, keywords, and abstracts that are used to build indexes and directories that can be searched. Search sites use both indexes (www.altavista.com) and directories (www.yahoo.com) to manage Internet information. Other types of search engines include such hybrids as Excite (www.excite.com), which use both indexes and directories, and Google (www.google.com), which uses its own search technology to rank search terms more intelligently. You can go to any search engine or web index by typing the URL in the textbox of your web browser. Once at the site, you begin the search for information by typing a key word or phrase in the textbox. Once you type in the keyword, the search is performed and the results are displayed on your screen. The results are in the form of hypertext links that allow you to click on your choice and be automatically connected with the selected site. Some of the search sites provide a "degree of relevance" for each site found. This gives you a sense of how closely matched the site is to the keyword or phase you used. The more specific the keyword or phrase, the more likely it is that the results will be useful.

Internet Addresses

To look for information or people on the Internet, it is vital to understand Internet addressing. Every person and every computer on the Internet is given a unique address. All Internet addresses follow the same format: the person's User ID (or User Name), followed by the @ symbol, followed by the unique name of the computer. For example, one author's university-based Internet address is

marge@athabascau.ca

In this example, the user ID portion is marge, and the unique computer name is athabascau.ca. That unique computer name is also called the *domain.* The same author also has an Internet account with a service provider. That address is

edwardsc@eybersurf.net

In general, an Internet address has two parts: the user ID and the domain, put together like this:

userid@domain

This combination needs to be unique on the entire Internet so the right person receives the right message.

Internet Applications

Electronic Mail

Electronic mail (or e-mail) was the first Internet application and is still the most popular one. E-mail is a way of sending messages between people or computers through networks of computer connections. Many hospitals and healthcare agencies also have an internal e-mail system.

E-mail on the Internet is analogous to the regular postal system but has faster delivery. E-mail combines a word processor function and a post office function in one program. When an e-mail program is started, a command is used to begin a new message. The message is typed into the computer along with the recipient's e-mail address and the return address. Then the message is "sent," which is something like dropping a letter in the regular postbox. The electronic post office in the personal system takes over and passes the message on. Electronic packets of data carry the message toward its ultimate destination mailbox. The message often must pass through a series of intermediate networks to reach the recipient's address. Because networks can and do use different e-mail formats, a gateway at each network translates the format of the e-mail message into one the next network understands. Each gateway also reads the destination address of the message and sends the message on in the direction of the destination mailbox. The routing choice takes into consideration the size of the message and the amount of traffic on various networks. Because of this routing, it takes varying amounts of time to send messages to the same person. On one occasion, it might be only a few minutes; on others, it might be a few hours.

Anatomy of an E-Mail Message

E-mail messages always have several features in common regardless of the program used to create the e-mail. A typical e-mail message includes a "From" line with the sender's electronic address; a date and time line; a "To" line with the recipient's electronic address; a "Subject" line; and the body of the message. If there are any spelling or punctuation mistakes in the recipient's address, the message is returned from the electronic post office. The "Subject" line is the place to give a clear, one-line description of the message, which is usually displayed when someone checks his or her e-mail. The recipient can decide how quickly to read the message.

If the message has been copied to others, their addresses appear in the "Copies to" line. Copying or forwarding messages to others is easy with most mail programs. For this reason, be prudent about what is said in a message. There is no way to know where it will end up because there is no control over the message once it is sent.

Legal Issues

Privacy, libel, and copyright are legal issues that can affect e-mail users. Understand that privacy is *not* assured with electronic mail. There are no legal requirements that prevent an institution or company from reading incoming and outgoing e-mail messages. For individuals using an employer's equipment, this is especially applicable. In addition, once a message has been sent, there is no control over what the recipient may do. The recipient may send a copy to someone else without the knowledge of the message's originator. Also, do not assume that messages received are private. The sender may have sent that same message to others without using the "Copies to" function. A final note about privacy: even though a mail message has been deleted from a mailbox, do not assume that it has been completely erased. Many institutional and company policies require regular backups of their computer system disks, which generally hold incoming and outgoing mail messages. It is possible that copies of individual users' messages were obtained during a regular system backup. Be aware that e-mail records can be subpoenaed.

A second legal issue for e-mail users is libel. Libel is applicable within e-mail messages and newsgroups. Take care with all comments. What you say can be held against you. Finally, copyright law applies to transferring files and information. It is illegal to distribute copyrighted information by any means, including electronic transfer. It is not uncommon to find material that has been scanned by a user for personal use and then distributed through e-mail. Unless the copyright owner has granted specific permission for the transfer of such material, it is illegal to do so.

Mailing Lists

Mailing lists are an extension of e-mail. When an e-mail message is sent to someone, the address is indicated. When an individual or organization consistently wants to mail to the same group of people, a special recipient name called an *alias* can be set up. For example, a hospital could create an alias called "nursing" that lists the e-mail addresses of all the directors of nursing. To send a message to all the directors of nursing, simply specify "nursing" in the "To" line and the same message will be sent to everyone on that list (alias). The directors of nursing can use this method to have an electronic discussion group. One director sends a message about a certain topic that is distributed to all those users identified by the alias "nursing" (all the other directors of nursing). When another director wants to respond to the topic, a message is sent again to "nursing" and all the directors of nursing receive it.

A mailing list is like an alias that contains hundreds or thousands of users from all over the Internet. Any message sent to the mailing list "alias" is automatically sent to everyone on the mailing list. Everything that anyone says through the mailing list goes to everyone on the mailing list. Mailing lists facilitate electronic discussion groups. Each mailing list resides in a specific computer and is looked after by a human administrator. The host computer is responsible for distributing incoming messages to all mailing list members. The administrator is responsible for maintaining the mailing list. Some mailing lists are also moderated. In these lists, there is a moderator who reviews each incoming message for appropriateness and either passes it through for distribution or rejects it. Some moderators also prepare *digests*, something like an issue of a magazine. The digest is an entire set of messages and articles in one package, making it much easier to keep up with the messages.

Mailing lists are maintained in two ways, either by a person (manually) or by a program. With the manual approach, the list administrator takes care of adding or deleting addresses from the master distribution list. With the program approach, you send messages to the address of a computer that provides this service. The most common mailing list administration program is called *Listserv* (representing *List server*). Mailing lists are scattered across the Web. One place to look for a comprehensive collection of mailing lists is www.liszt.com. This site supports searching and provides some information about the lists.

Newsgroups

Mailing lists and newsgroups enable asynchronous or time-independent discussions on the Internet. Participants can post and read messages at any time. They do not have to be taking part in the discussion at the same time. Although discussions take place on the Internet using both mailing lists and newsgroups, there is a significant difference between the two methods. A mailing list discussion comes directly to an individual's electronic mailbox, just as a letter is delivered by a postal service. However, the messages that form discussions in newsgroups are sent only to the newsgroup administrator, who then sends them to Internet newsgroup system sites (not individual subscribers). Individuals then read the messages in the newsgroup at a particular system site in the same way as walking down the hall to read the messages posted on a bulletin board. In fact, the origin of newsgroups was as a bulletin board service where messages could be posted for all to see.

What Is Usenet?

Usenet (users' network) is made up of all the machines that receive network newsgroups. A machine that receives these newsgroups is called a Usenet Server. Any computer system that wants to carry newsgroups of interest to that site can be a Usenet server.

Instead of forwarding all messages to all users on a mailing list, Usenet forwards all messages (called *articles* to keep up the newspaper analogy) not to individual subscribers but to other Usenet servers, who forward them on until all machines that are part of Usenet have a copy of the article (message). Individuals then use programs called "newsreaders" to access the newsgroup through their own computers. A typical Usenet server receives more than 20,000 articles per day. To organize all these articles, they are assigned to specific newsgroups. Newsgroups are further collected into hierarchies, similar to the domains described in relation to e-mail addresses.

Every Usenet server subscribes to specific newsgroups. Not all newsgroups are available on all Usenet servers. Some newsgroups are moderated. This means that articles cannot be posted directly to the newsgroup. Instead, all messages sent to this newsgroup will be automatically routed to the volunteer moderator. The moderator then decides what articles to send on to the newsgroup. Articles may be edited by the moderator or grouped with other articles before they are forwarded to the newsgroup. In some cases, the moderator may decide not to forward an article at all. Moderators exist to limit the number of low-quality articles in a newsgroup, especially all those "me too" or "I agree" type of articles.

Reading Articles

To read the articles posted to a newsgroup, a program called a newsreader is used. A newsreader is the interface to Usenet that allows individuals to choose the newsgroups to which they wish to belong or to select and display articles. When using a newsreader, articles can be saved to a file, mailed to someone else, or printed. Responding to the article's author or the newsgroup is also done through the newsreader program. There are a number of common newsreader programs: *rn*, *trn*, *nn*, and *tin*.

Newsgroups and mailing lists exemplify the power of the Net. An individual has the ability to call on the resources and creativity of people around the world to help. As well, individuals can contribute their experience and share their knowledge with others.

Internet Chat

Live or synchronous discussion is accomplished through the use of *chat rooms*. Using a Web browser allows you to navigate to a chat room and click on buttons to join the conversations. Chat rooms provide a way for you to "talk" with anyone who is present in the chat room at the same time. Chat rooms (sometimes called channels) generally have a specific theme such as women's health, seniors' health, or endometriosis. There are also chat rooms organized by professional practice discipline or area-of-practice nurse practitioners or oncology nursing. There are no directories of chat rooms. To find a chat room related to a specific topic you would use a Web search engine.

There are two types of chat room: moderated and unmoderated. In the moderated chat room, a person, often a volunteer, acts as host for the chat. This person is responsible for keeping the discussion on track and for removing offensive or unruly participants. Some moderated chat rooms use keyword filtering software to eliminate offensive language from the conversations. Many moderated chat rooms have topics scheduled on a weekly basis so you know what time to join in for a particular topic of interest.

Unmoderated chat rooms have no one monitoring them and so anything can be and often is said. These unmoderated chats are disappointing for people truly seeking information and support for a variety of topics listed under health on some of the more common index sites. Instead of helpful information, they find an unending stream of profanity and pornography. Generally, the most profitable discussions are found in moderated chat rooms. Once you have identified a chat room and have gone to the site, you must sign up and select a user name and sometimes a password. The name you select provides some degree of privacy provided you select a name that does not identify you. Be aware that, because you cannot verify the identity of others in the chat room, participants may take on identities or personas different from their real selves. Many chat rooms post codes of conduct that require appropriate behaviors and respectful conversations.

A chat room is often like being in a room full of people—there are many conversations going on at the same time. If there are many people in a chat room, it is often difficult to follow the simultaneous discussions. Many chat rooms also allow you to send a private message to another person in the chat room, without everyone else seeing it.

Although most of the people you meet in chat rooms are innocuous, there are always some people it is best to avoid. It is almost impossible to distinguish the "reputable" from the "disreputable" based on the information you glean from chatting, so be prudent about disclosing personal identifying information. There have been many tragic stories in the media about unfortunate face-to-face meetings between people who initially met through the Internet. Use extreme caution and lots of common sense if you plan to meet a new "cyberpal" in person.

Intranets and Extranets

As was stated earlier, the real power of the Internet lies in the people and information connected by computers. Many organizations have taken the concepts and tools of the Internet and have applied them within their own structures. The organizations, in effect, create private internets, called *intranets.* Information and people can then be connected in the same easy fashion as on the larger public Internet. Organizations thus have all the advantages for information sharing and communication for their people without the security concerns of using the public Internet. If organizations then selectively allow outside agencies to connect to their intranet, they have now created an *extranet.* This extranet allows several organizations with common purpose to share information on an "extended intranet."

Summary

The integration of telecommunications and health informatics has had a powerful impact on healthcare delivery. We have only begun to see what is possible when telecommunications meets health informatics. Specific applications of the Internet to healthcare (i.e., telehealth) are described in Chapter 8.

Additional Resources

Edwards, M. (2002). *The Internet for Nurses and Allied Health Professionals, 3rd ed.* New York: Springer-Verlag.

Part II
Nursing Use of Information Systems

5
Enterprise Health Information Systems

Healthcare institutions generate massive volumes of information that must be collected, transmitted, recorded, retrieved, and summarized. The problem of managing all these activities for clinical information has become monumental. As a result, computer-based hospital information systems (HISs) were designed, tested, and installed in hospitals of all sizes. The original purpose of HISs was to provide a computer-based framework to facilitate the communication of information within a hospital setting. Essentially, an HIS is a communication network linking terminals and output devices in key patient care or service areas to a central processing unit that coordinates all essential patient care activities. Thus, the HIS provides a communication system between departments (e.g., dietary, nursing units, pharmacy, laboratory); a central information system for receipt, sorting, transmission, storage, and retrieval of information; and a high-speed, data-processing system for fast, economic processing of data to provide information in its most useful form.

The management of information in the hospital setting and its environs is a critical component in the process of healthcare delivery. The problem of information management has been complicated by an exponential increase in the amount of data to be managed, the number of stakeholders in the process, and the requirements for real-time access and response. In the United States, 12% to 15% of the cost of healthcare is attributed to the costs associated with information handling (Office of Technology Assessment, 1995). The cost of information handling in the hospital setting has led to the use of computers in an attempt to provide more data at lower costs. Estimates of the costs of information handling vary between 25% and 39% of the total cost of healthcare (Jackson, 1969). Most health informatics professionals agree that a reasonable expenditure on information systems in healthcare is at least 3% to 5% of the operational budget for a health organization.

This chapter is based in part on previously published material [Hannah, K.J., & Hammond, W.E. (1997). The evolution of clinical information systems. In: Ball, M.J., & Douglas, J. (eds.) *Clinical Information Systems That Support Evolving Delivery Systems.* Redmond: Spacelabs.]

Information systems currently being used in healthcare environments can be broadly categorized into three types. The first type is composed of systems that are limited in objective and scope. They most often exist as a stand-alone module and address a single application area. Examples of such a system are the nursing workload measurement systems currently being used in many hospitals. The Medicus and GRASP systems serve a specific function and therefore fall into this category of systems. In the hospital environment, systems commonly included in this category are dedicated clinical laboratory systems, dedicated financial systems, and dedicated radiology, electrocardiography, pulmonary function, pharmacy, and dietary systems. In a public health setting a stand-alone immunization system is a good example of this category of systems.

The second type of information system is composed of hospital information systems, which usually consist of a communications network, a clinical component, and a financial/administrative component. The overall communications component integrates these three major parts into a cohesive information system. A typical hospital information system in this category may have computer terminals at each nursing station as well as terminals that are in, or accessible to, each ancillary area in the hospital. The terminals are tied together through one or more large central computers, which may be on-site or off-site. Generally such systems are focused on acute care and are organized around departmental functions.

The use of the third type of information system, enterprise health information systems (EHISs), is expanding in health environments. Such systems capture and store comprehensive patient information across the entire continuum of care in health organizations using integrated healthcare delivery models. These records are captured and stored in multiple media including audio, image, animation, and print. The records may be stored centrally, in total or abstracted format, using a data warehouse approach. Alternatively, these records may be physically stored at the point of capture and logically linked to a virtual record that is physically assembled only when required to meet care requirements. These systems are characterized by the fact that they are focused on patients (rather than departments or disciplines) receiving care in multiple integrated settings (e.g., ambulatory care, acute care, long-term care) having one common organizational structure (i.e., a single enterprise). An expanded type of EHIS has emerged recently as the electronic health record (EHR) system. Several countries are moving toward developing nationwide electronic EHRs.

Hospital Information Systems

Early computer applications for hospitals dealt with administration and financial matters. Later applications included task-oriented functions such as admission/discharge/transfer (ADT), order entry, and result reporting. With the availability of minicomputers and finally personal computers, various departmental service-related systems (e.g., laboratory, radiology, pharmacy) were developed. Few if any of these systems were electronically connected. The subsequent development of hospital information systems (HISs) was a combination of factors related to technology (hardware and software), people (developer and user), and economics.

An implicit assumption in the development of HISs is that the ability of complete, accurate, timely data delivered at the point of care to the person providing that care results in a higher quality of care at a more efficient cost. Support for this assumption is provided by simple observation; for example, such systems should eliminate redundant tests, eliminate the need to reestablish diagnoses, increase awareness of drug allergies and adverse events, increase awareness of the medications the patient is taking, and enhance communication among those involved with the patient's care. There are four main functions typical of such hospital information systems.

- Recognize both sending and receiving stations, format all messages, and manage all the message routing (called message switching)
- Validate, check, and edit each message to ensure its quality
- Control all the hardware and software needed to perform the first two functions
- Assemble transaction data and communicate with the accounting system

The first hospital computer systems developed during the late 1960s were geared to batch accounting to meet the complexity of third-party billing, cost statistics, and fiscal needs. The technology of that era was unsuccessfully applied to clinical systems. Terminal devices, such as cathode-ray tubes, were expensive and unreliable. Also, hardware and software were limited, expensive, and highly structured. Database systems that we take for granted today had not appeared. During this period, some hospitals installed stand-alone computers in clinical departments and in business offices to do specific jobs. The most common clinical example is laboratory systems. Most of the hospitals that embarked on these clinical programs for stand-alone systems were large teaching institutions with access to federal funding or other research grants. Usually there was no attempt to integrate the accounting computer with the stand-alone departmental computers—this came much later.

The 200 and 400 bed hospitals that installed computers during the late 1960s for accounting had varied success. During that period accounting needs became more complex, and this trend continues. The result is a constant battle just to maintain and change existing systems to keep pace with regulating agencies. Many hospitals of this size turned to a shared computer service such as Shared Medical Systems. The reason these companies prospered was not only because of their products and services but also because a small hospital simply cannot justify employing and retaining the technical staff and management skills necessary for this complex, conflicting, changing environment.

During the early 1970s, with rampant inflation and restricted cost reimbursement, some large hospitals that had installed their own computers with marginal success changed to the shared service. By this time, the shared companies had better accounting software and audit controls. Most importantly, these companies developed field personnel who understood hospital operations and were able to communicate and translate the use of computer systems into results in their client hospitals. This added dimension of service that is not offered or understood by the hardware vendors increased business opportunities for the service companies. Many of these companies, in turn, increased their scope of services beyond fiscal to clinical and communication applications.

The hardware vendors of the 1960s (e.g., IBM, Burroughs, Honeywell, NCR) committed themselves to large general-purpose computers that attempted to support clinical, communications, and financial systems. During the 1970s, technology such as the minicomputer and personal computer was generally accepted as providing a better alternative to the approach than the large general-purpose computer. In fact, the major hardware companies are moving in this direction. During the same time frame, the service companies began to develop on-site minicomputers to handle data communications and specialized nonfinancial applications. They began to expand their scope of data retention to support clinical applications that required a historical patient database. In other words, hospital information systems vendors and service providers migrated toward a similar concept.

Current hospital information systems grew out of developmental work that took place during the 1970s. Functional specifications, system design, and technology selection were driven by the immediate problem at hand. Hospital information systems were designed to deal primarily with the problem of moving transaction-oriented data throughout an institution. The business functions for which software applications were developed included admission/discharge/transfer (ADT), order entry/result reporting, and charge or cost capture. In most cases, administrative and financial personnel who had responsibility for the accounting systems controlled the systems. Mainframe technology was utilized as the best hardware platform for providing an extensive network.

Gradually, HISs evolved into communication networks linking terminals and output devices in key patient care or service areas to a central processing unit that coordinates all essential patient care activities. The difference among systems that fall into this category is not in their communications but in the complexity of the integration of their application functions. Some systems have more sophisticated provisions for validating, checking, editing, formatting, and documentation than others. Some respond faster and offer a better variety of displays. These variations are differences in the communication and presentation aspects of the system. Other systems provide more complex integration of the application structure and data retention. One example of this is the total integration of information from the laboratory, radiology, pharmacy, and medical records, which then interacts with the nursing stations, providing communication from order entry to result reports. Another difference in hospital information systems is the orientation toward the data content: Some systems are oriented around the financial and administrative data, and others are organized around patient care data. In the latter case, administrative and financial data and functions are derived from patient care information. More patient information, such as history, physical examination, and progress data, is contained in these systems because they emphasize integration of direct clinical information.

Components of HIS

Administrative and Financial Modules

Accounts receivable, accounts payable, general ledger, materiel management, payroll, and human resources applications are the minimum management functions required of the administrative and financial modules of a hospital information system. At a minimum, accounts receivable consists of charge capture for transmission to another system. Other accounts receivable functions include utilization review; professional and technical component billing; proration of revenue; corrections and late charges; adjustments and payments; account aging by method of payment, category of patient and of physician, date of encounter, inpatient/outpatient, and date of payment; and collections, including delinquent accounts reports, collection comments, dunning letters, turnover letters, and collection agency reports. Miscellaneous software applications are required to support other management functions such as environment and energy control, marketing, fund raising, and public relationships.

Departmental management functions include inventory control of supplies, drugs, and perishables; item tracking of such things as specimens, charts, and films; revenue and utilization statistics; word processing; electronic mail; budget and monthly financial statements for use in variance analysis; workload analysis and personnel scheduling; and human resources and payroll.

Admission/Discharge/Transfer Modules

Admission/Discharge/Transfer is the core of any hospital information system. At a minimum, this module must establish a patient record, provide a unique encounter identification number, and document the place of encounter. Other functions include bed availability; call lists; scheduling; collection of demographic data, referral data and reason for admission; precertification; verification of benefit plan and ability to pay; and preadmission orders and presurgery preparation procedures (Fig. 5.1).

The admission process includes updating preadmission/appointment data; creating the hospital account number; collecting admitting diagnosis;

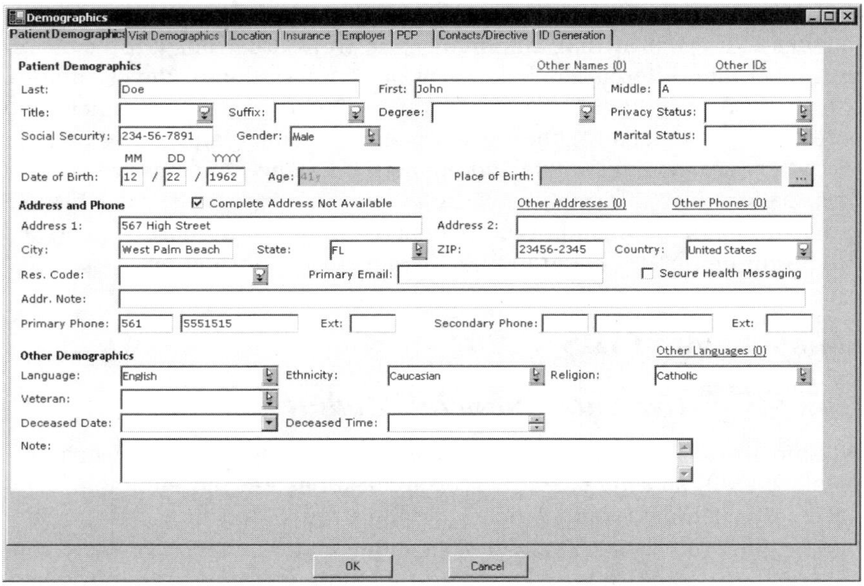

FIGURE 5.1. Admission profile. (Photograph courtesy of Eclipsys.)

initiating concurrent review; notifying dietary, housekeeping, and human services; collecting/initiating orders; notification of orders/requisitions; bed assignment; notification of arrival to all interested parties; census with locators by patient name, identification number, account number, nursing station, physician group (including primary, admitting, referring, and consultant physicians); organizing work flow by data to be reviewed, reports to be completed, and reports to be verified/signed; bed control; room charging including variable services/room and multiple patients/day; concurrent review including utilization, quality assurance, and risk management; transfering the patient including bed control and discontinuing orders.

Pending discharge the process includes notifying the next admission, preparing discharge medications, and contacting the home health provider. At discharge the process includes verifying diagnoses and procedures, and providing a discharge summary, patient instruction, and return appointments, as well as case abstracting, including diagnosis/procedure coding, diagnosis related group statistics, and a retrospective review.

Order Entry Module

The order entry module is a module in a hospital information system (HIS) by which doctors or nurses enter clinical orders or prescriptions using terminals located in patient care areas. Orders are transmitted through the computer system to the recipient for immediate implementation. Using this module, errors at the time of input of the orders are theoretically minimized, and the efficiency of data transmission in hospitals increases. Order entry can occur at either the point of care or at a centrally located terminal. Increasingly, caregivers are seeking systems that allow order entry at the point of care.

Order entry is a function common to almost all service departments in the hospital. At a minimum, orders may be entered in a batch mode as a method of charge capture. The full functionality includes initial order capture of procedure, urgency, frequency, scheduling (beginning date, time, and duration), the performer, the ordering physician, and comments; order verification; order sets; activation of preorders; checking for inappropriate orders including frequency by patient, match to diagnosis, negated by medications, and credential verification. Order follow-up includes looking up the patient by requisition number, listing overdue pending orders and listing continuing orders about to expire; initiating work, including insertion on work-to-be-done list by service department and nursing station, print requisition, queue for scheduling, and print labels; and entering any charge if billing on order entry (Fig. 5.2).

An important capacity of the order entry system is the ability to provide feedback to caregivers at the time they enter orders. For instance, at the University of Tokyo Hospital, when a physician prescribes an inappropriate dosage, the system provides a warning. The system also has the ability to alert

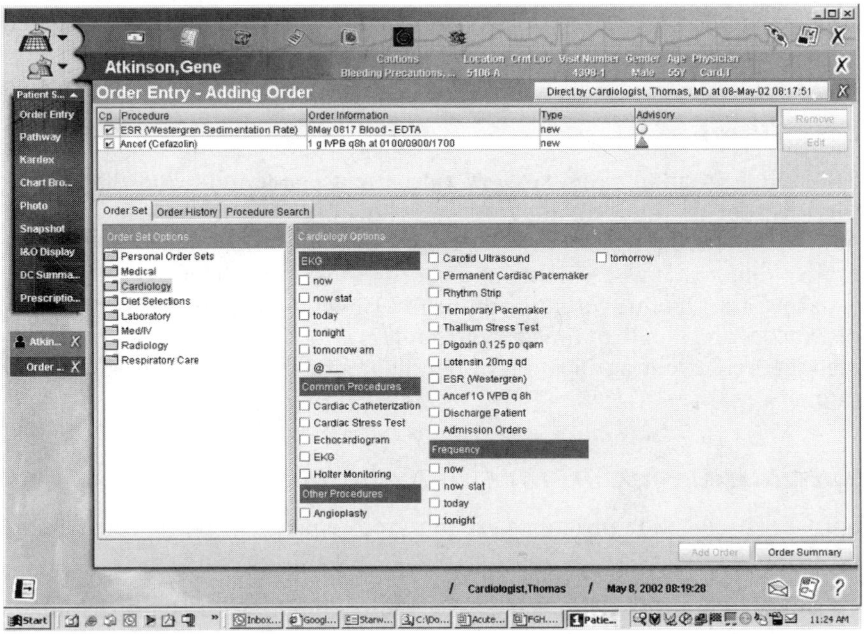

FIGURE 5.2. Order entry. (Photograph courtesy of Misys.)

physicians when they order many clinical tests without sufficient justification. Because the hospital is a teaching hospital, there are many young physicians in training programs. The education and training of physicians are important functions of the hospital. These interns and resident physicians often lack professional self-confidence, are insecure in their clinical judgment, or are excessively curious. Consequently, they tend to order more clinical tests than are required by more experienced physicians. This has been a problem from the financial perspective of the hospital because the insurance body does not provide compensation for these excessive tests. The warning alert on the order entry system had remarkable effects in this hospital, and the number of clinical tests ordered decreased approximately 30% following system implementation. The warning system was evaluated by interviewing the users, and all agreed that the system gave them a chance to reconsider the need for the clinical tests, which had some educational value (Fig. 5.3).

Result Reporting Module

Result reporting requirements vary markedly among departments. Minimum result reporting consists of notification that a procedure is complete. Other functionality includes canceling a procedure; entering a result including flagging a process as complete and billing; entering the normal/abnormal range (numeric, coded, or text); checking data for accuracy through edit tables and internal consistency such as delta checks; and reporting results including immediate result reporting, flow sheets or graphs, related calculated results, and physician prompts (Fig. 5.4).

Scheduling

Scheduling of admissions, surgery, outpatient encounters, and diagnostics is critical for the smooth, integrated working of the healthcare facility. The outpatient scheduling permits the preadmission ordering of tests and preoperative diagnostic assessments and coordinating the performance of those tests and assessments with the admission. Effective management of the mix of patients and length of time for encounters is facilitated by a good scheduling system. Patient notification of pending appointments reduces no-show rates.

Specialized Support for Clinical Functions

Software application programs are required to provide specialized support for departmental services. Some examples are as follows.

- Clinical laboratory tasks include accession numbering, collection list, specimen tracking, specimen logging, automatic capture of results from instruments, and quality control: processing controls, calculation of means and

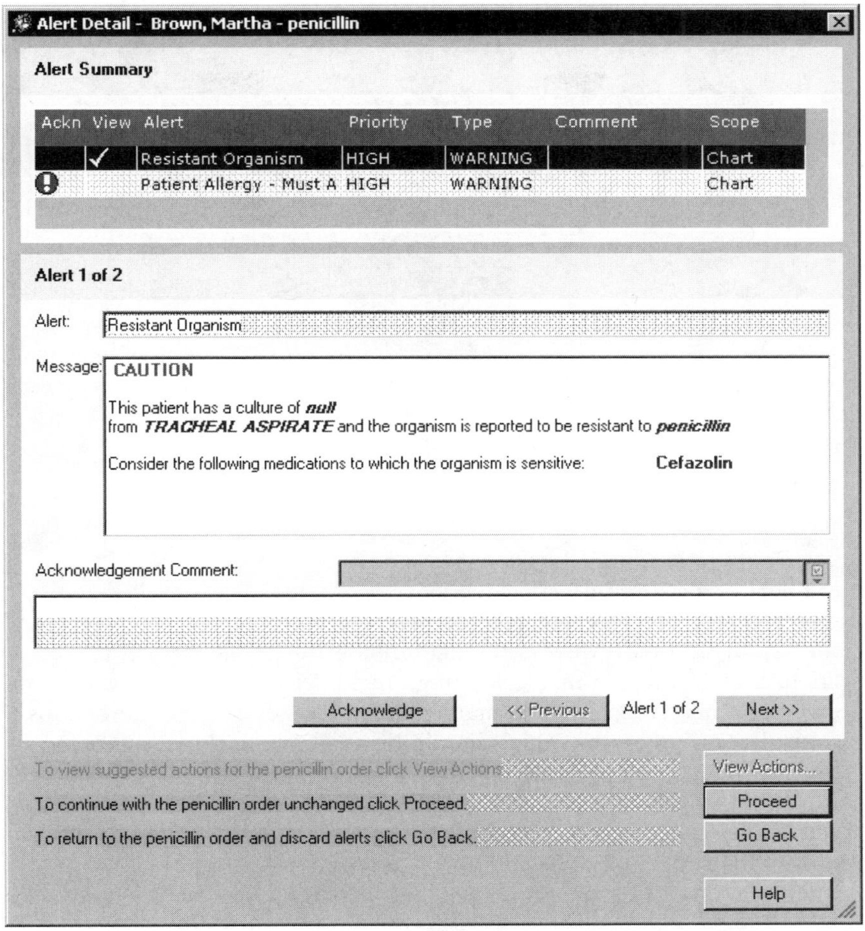

FIGURE 5.3. Order alert. (Photograph courtesy of Misys.)

standard deviation for a test, analysis of patient trends, technologist verification, check for drug/test interactions, and protocols (Fig. 5.5).

- Radiology tasks include result reporting (preliminary, final, amended results), electronic signature, reference file, and images of various types.
- Pharmacy tasks include verification of an order by the pharmacist, dual result reporting by pharmacy (number dispensed) and nurse (number administered), unit dose tracking (fills and returns), intravenous admixture, and chemotherapy protocols.
- Nursing systems must provide nursing assessment, nursing diagnoses, nursing interventions, and care plans (including medication administration records, nursing workload, and nursing note of client outcomes).

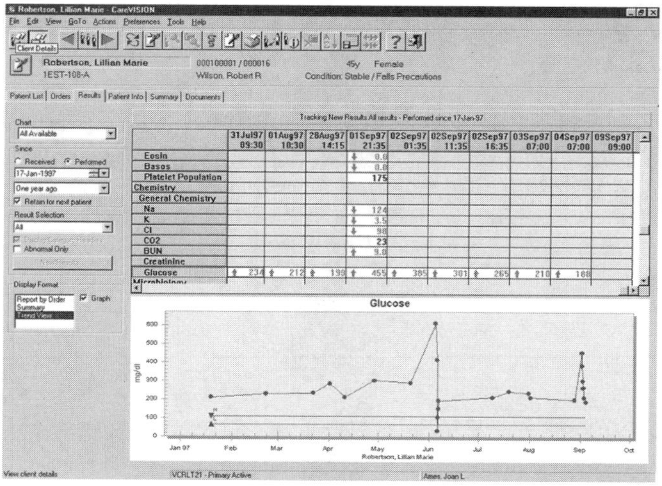

Figure 5.4. Reporting results (Photograph courtesy of Health Vision.)

- Medical records require that the system provide a list of all diagnoses, an encounter-oriented summary abstract, time-oriented summaries (flow sheets), utilization review, and longitudinal studies (Fig. 5.6).
- Dietary tasks include meal planning, menu selection, food distribution, inventory, ordering, nutrition management, and drug–food interactions.
- Consultation programs, which should be available, include bibliographic retrieval, calculations, modeling, decision support systems, protocols, and

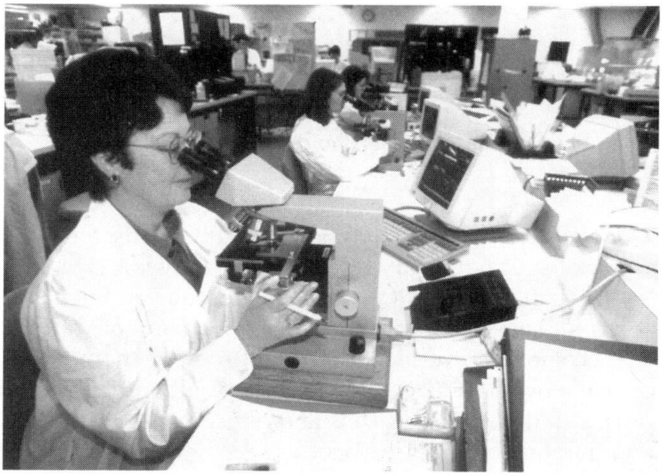

Figure 5.5. Laboratory applications. (Photograph courtesy of Sunquest.)

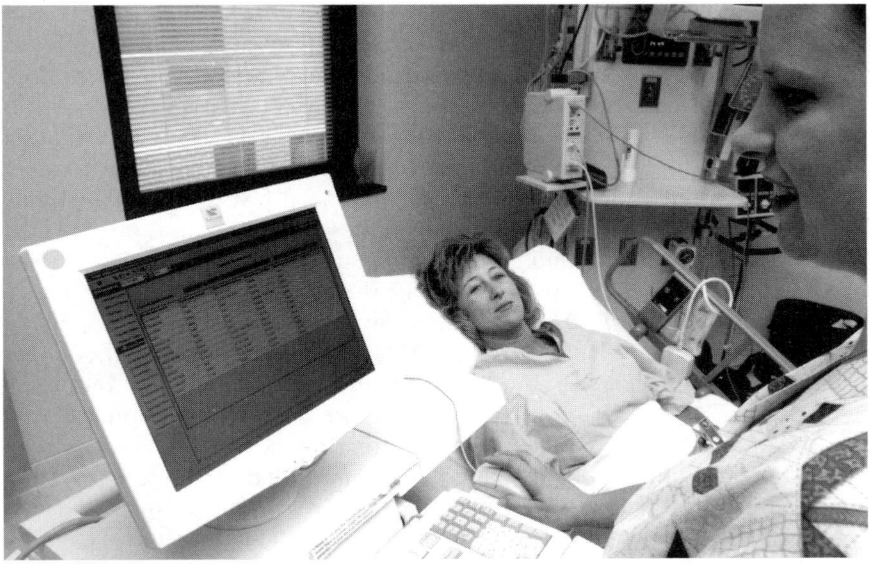

FIGURE 5.6. Medical documentation. (Photograph courtesy of Cerner Corporation.)

health knowledge bases such as the Physicians Desk Reference (PDR), emergency procedures, and poison index.

- Critical care areas have special needs for electronic data capture to facilitate patient monitoring and charting.
- Patient support should include security, privacy, confidentiality of patient data, information sheets for patient education and awareness, concern for general patient welfare, reminders of appointments, admissions, tests, and health maintenance reminders.

Issues Related to HISs

There were many problems encountered during the early implementation efforts. The organizational discipline required to implement hospital information systems was complicated by departmental priority differences and sometimes departmental autonomy. Systems functions that support patient care requirements, when given top priority, most often conflicted with existing administrative systems or at least could not communicate with these legacy systems. Computers traditionally started in accounting, and most hospital applications still have their roots in this area. The operations cycle of patient care is continuous and instantaneous. Fiscal (financial and accounting) methodology and timing are intermittent and historical. To achieve successful utilization of information systems in healthcare, both these disparate needs must be recognized and served.

As indicated previously, currently available, commercial hospital information systems are built primarily around the framework of technologies, design philosophies, and healthcare delivery models of the 1970s. As new concepts and new technology have become available, these classic systems have been modified, most usually on a superficial level, to accommodate these changes. Most of these systems were designed with no thought of an electronic patient record and certainly no concept of a longitudinal, cross-sectoral, multidisciplinary, patient-specific record.

In fact, most of these systems, even today, retain only the data for a single hospitalization and then for only a few months after discharge. The primary orientation of these systems remains financially driven, problem-focused, and task-oriented. These systems use a mainframe computer, a central database, and character-based terminals. Few of these systems support a unified, multidisciplinary patient problem list and complete, integrated studies and therapy data sets. Current systems are primarily an automated form of the manual system for documenting hospital care. The design philosophy reflects the flow of documents as the primary communication. The traditional paper chart still exists in even the most computerized hospitals of today. No major systems are known to exist in which all data and the management of those data are fully computerized.

Major issues in healthcare delivery systems surfaced during the 1980s. Most vendors moved into integrated distributed networking and shared configurations. The initial expectations associated with general purpose computers for developing hospital information systems were not met within the time frame anticipated by early studies. Some of the reasons for this failure to meet expectations are the following.

- The complex information and communication structure, which is required to deliver patient care in hospitals, was grossly underestimated.
- The hardware and software of the 1960s, 1970s, and 1980s were grossly inadequate, rigid, unreliable, and extremely expensive.
- The staffing requirements in terms of systems and data-processing professionals who could manage, define, communicate, and implement systems in hospitals were grossly underestimated.

One more technological advance was necessary. The development of relational database management systems for use in patient care was imperative for nursing to exploit the technology fully. As McHugh and Shultz (1982) suggested:

> Hospital nursing departments have followed the frozen asset path for their data resources. Information contained in existing modular and turnkey systems cannot be easily merged with other computer-stored information.

Experienced users of computers in business abandoned the traditional modular approach to computer file handling that is still being marketed by some vendors to the healthcare industry. Database management systems have long been available that can accomplish the following.

1. Reduce data redundancy
2. Provide quality data
3. Maintain data integrity
4. Protect data security
5. Interface relatively easily with technological advances
6. Facilitate access to a single integrated collection of data for many applications by multiple user groups

Enterprise Health Information Systems

Evolution of Health Enterprises

Most recently, healthcare organizations and health services delivery systems internationally are under enormous pressure from all sides (Fig. 5.7). There is a decrease in the revenue available to fund health services delivery; the explosion of new treatments, new programs, and new technologies is accompanied by citizens' increasing demands and expectations of their health

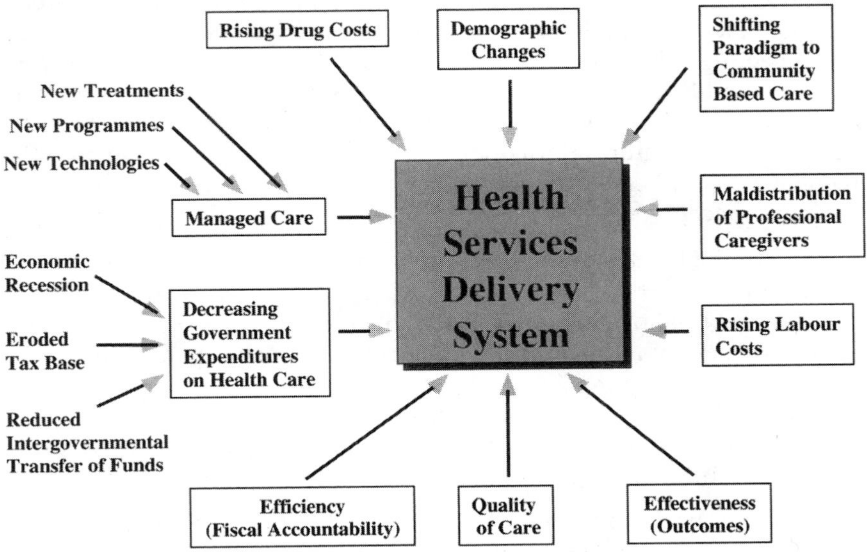

Figure 5.7. Pressures on National Healthcare Systems. (Adapted from Hannah KJ. Transforming information: data management support of healthcare reorganization. *Journal of American Medical Informatics Association* 1995;2:145–155.)

system, reflected in such changing health services delivery modalities as managed care; drug costs are rising; population demographics are characterized by the rising average age; there is a shifting health services delivery paradigm from acute care to community-based care; and employee expectations for remuneration and compensation are resulting in rising labor costs. Simultaneously, there are expectations that the efficiency and effectiveness of health services delivery will improve while the quality of care is maintained or even improved.

For all these reasons, health services delivery systems around the world are under enormous pressure to change. However, decisions about healthcare organizations and healthcare delivery systems must not be based on opinion, emotion, historical precedent, or political expediency. Data and information are essential for rational decision-making and good management of the health services delivery system in any country. The restructuring of health systems worldwide must be based on data and information.

Health services, healthcare delivery systems, and health organizations around the world are undergoing reorganization and reengineering. Rational decision-making about such activities must be based on information. Historically, the field of medical informatics has focused on individual patient care in acute care. Much less attention has been directed toward population-based healthcare. Increasingly, the field is beginning to emphasize health informatics, which has a broader multidisciplinary focus on health services delivery including community needs assessment, population health status indicators, health promotion, and disease prevention in addition to the treatment of illness. Health informatics can and should play a major role in the reengineering and restructuring that is occurring in many healthcare organizations and health services delivery systems. Many of the data presently available are inadequate for these tasks; therefore, current data must be transformed and future information requirements anticipated to support the reengineering of healthcare enterprises and organizations. There are some essential concepts.

- Reconceptualization of health services delivery within a jurisdiction as one enterprise
- Use of information engineering techniques
- Development of a comprehensive information management strategy
- Need to apply information management principles
- Organizational implications of information management
- Conceptual model for achieving added value as a by-product from health service delivery data

Enterprise health information systems (EHISs) can be conceived of as tools intended for use by legislators, policy makers, managers, and caregivers within a health organization to fulfill their responsibilities with regard to the delivery of health services to the population being served. New models for healthcare delivery (e.g., regionalized healthcare delivery enterprises such as those found in the United Kingdom, South Africa, and some Canadian provinces) and managed care such as is developing in the United States have expanded the walls of the hospital and are requiring the development of integrated health services delivery organizations (or enterprises) that involve the hospital, primary care, ambulatory care, extended care facilities, the community, public health, and a multidisciplinary team of caregivers (e.g., traditional healers, physicians, nurses, physiotherapists, nutritionists, dentists, social workers, educators, music therapists, psychologists, speech therapists). This new vision encompasses the concept of the electronic health record (EHR) that is patient-centered and includes all data documenting a person's contact with the healthcare organization. There is an evolution occurring from healthcare systems that treat people only when they are ill to health enterprises that provide integrated services that support people's activities to protect, promote, and maintain their own health in addition to treating people's illnesses. Health service enterprises that provide integrated health services require an electronic health record (EHR). An EHR provides lifelong, multidisciplinary information to document health promotion and protection indicators as well as illnesses. All these changes require an altered approach to information management.

The Future

Future health information systems in jurisdictions responsible for comprehensive integrated health services must take into the account the fundamental principle that the reason a healthcare delivery system exists in any jurisdiction is to provide health services to its citizens. Thus, systems to support the functions of clinical and diagnostic departments as well as administrative and managerial information for use in operating the healthcare delivery enterprise should be a by-product of the care delivery process. The focus is, and must continue, to shift to information management and systems that are centered on the recipient of the care. One can envision a future environment in which current information about health facilities and healthcare delivery systems for use in enterprise planning and policies, as well as resource allocation and utilization, is much more widely available to the professional care providers than in the past.

Responsibilities

The responsibilities related to operating a health services delivery system, that is, a comprehensive health services enterprise, within a jurisdiction (community, state/provincial, national), can be summarized into the following functional categories.

- Assess the health status of the population
- Set health goals and objectives
- Set strategic directions
- Provide programs and services
- Communicate with stakeholders
- Manage resources
- Evaluate the health services delivery system

Such a comprehensive health services delivery enterprise in a jurisdiction requires a health information system that is defined in the broadest and most inclusive fashion possible. It should include the data and the most rudimentary media for gathering the data (e.g., pencil and paper) as well as all possible means of storing, processing, aggregating, and presenting the information. A jurisdictional health information system also should include the people who interface with the system, specifically those who are involved in certain areas.

- Those who generate the data (i.e., the recipients of care and the caregivers)
- Those who use the data in its various forms (i.e., caregivers, health systems managers, policy makers, legislators)
- Those who maintain the data and the means by which it is captured, stored, processed, aggregated, and presented (e.g., data gatherers, filing clerks, forms analysts, data entry clerks, computer operators, network managers)

The decisions facing health services enterprise managers are more complex than decisions faced in the past.

- Decisions are patient-focused rather than discipline focused. The concept of multidisciplinary teams is increasingly being used within healthcare delivery, resulting in data that focus on the recipient of care rather than the provider of care.
- Previously, decisions within the healthcare delivery system have been focused within specific service sectors (acute care, public health mental health, long-term care, insured services) but now are becoming focused within jurisdictions (community, state/provincial, national), geographic areas that require a cross-sectoral perspective.
- Decisions affecting the entire health services enterprise require information about that enterprise.
- Decisions affecting even a part of the health services enterprise still require information about other parts of the health services enterprise because of the impact of interdependence among the sectors; for example, early discharge programs in the acute care sector have a major impact on the home care delivery sector.
- Decisions to reduce expenditures on health services while maintaining the quality and maximizing the benefits to the health of citizens require information about the outcomes of health services. There is a need to know whether what is done for, with, or to a client makes any difference in the health status of that client.

The role of the professional care provider (e.g., physicians, nurses, dentists, physiotherapists) in managing information in healthcare facilities is, of necessity, related to the role of the caregiver in the organization. In most healthcare delivery facilities, it is necessary to manage both patient care and the patient care environment in the organization. Usually, caregivers manage patient care, and managers administer the organization. Therefore, for some time the caregiver's role in the management of information generally has been considered to include the capture and use of the information necessary to manage patient care, and caregivers have also been expected to provide the information necessary for managing the organization (e.g., resource allocation and utilization, personnel management, planning and policymaking, decision support). This dual responsibility has generated an increasing burden on caregivers to provide information because of the redundancy and duplication of information they are expected to provide.

Healthcare delivery is information-intensive. Caregivers handle enormous volumes of patient care information. In fact, caregivers constantly process information mentally, manually, and electronically. In every aspect of patient care, caregivers are continually engaged in problem-solving using clinical judgment and decision-making: assessing; identifying patient problems and diagnoses; determining appropriate action or interventions: evaluating; and reassessing and communicating. Care providers integrate information from many diverse sources throughout the organization to provide patient care and to coordinate the patient's contact with the health system. They manage patient care information for purposes of providing care to patients.

An implicit assumption in the development of Enterprise Health Information Systems is that the ability to deliver complete, accurate, timely data at the point of care to the person providing that care results in a higher quality of care at a more efficient cost. Support for this assumption is provided by simple observation; for example, such systems should eliminate redundant tests, eliminate the need to reestablish diagnoses, increase awareness of drug allergies and adverse events, increase awareness of the medications the patient is taking, and enhance communication among those involved with the patient's care.

Modern healthcare delivery generates massive volumes of information that must be collected, transmitted, recorded, retrieved, and summarized. The problem of managing all these activities for clinical information has become monumental. As a result, computer-based hospital information systems (HISs) were designed, tested, and installed in hospitals of all sizes. The original purpose of HISs was to provide a computer-based framework to facilitate the communication of information in a healthcare setting.

Enterprise-Wide Information Systems

In most countries, the model for healthcare is moving toward integrated delivery systems (Fig. 5.8). This process could be enhanced by developing

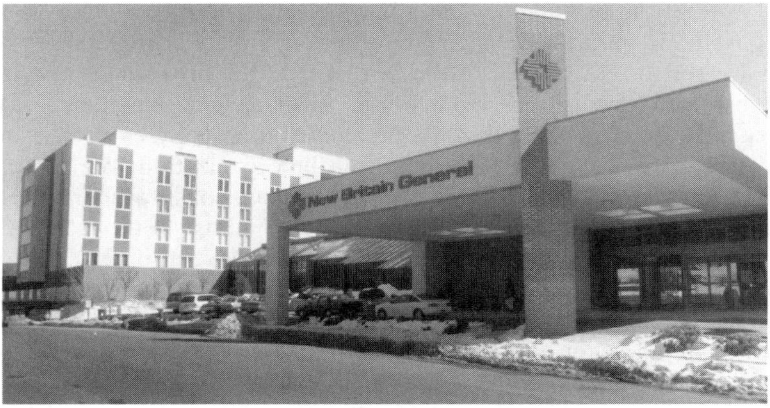

FIGURE 5.8. Enterprise-wide integrated delivery systems service entire hospitals. (Photograph courtesy of Sunquest.)

an electronic health record (EHR) that supports the patient, the primary care provider, physician, nurse, other caregivers, and hospital or other critical care setting. It also supports pharmacies; nursing homes; nursing; home healthcare; payers; federal, state or province, and local authorities; accreditation and quality assurance agencies; and others. All these stakeholders must be integrated into a single, distributed system for maximum return on investments in information management systems. Requirements include the physical network to support such integration; an infrastructure to manage and regulate such a structure; standards for data interchange; a common data model defining the objects to be transmitted; a common, clinically rich vocabulary; and processes (or methodologies) for information gathering and aggregation. Above all, appropriate security must be built into such a system or network to ensure that the confidentiality and privacy of individual records is appropriately respected and protected.

Future systems must reflect the major paradigm shift in health services delivery models. The underlying philosophy must be patient-centered: What are the requirements of a system whose primary purpose is to provide the mechanism for the most effective, efficient, and economical care possible for people receiving health services? Rather than using the computer to improve the current paper-oriented systems, new systems must answer the question: Given the power of modern computation devices with massive storage and ubiquitous network linkages, graphics interfaces, image display capabilities, capacity for vast and instant data analyses, and personalization of function, what can and should the healthcare information system of tomorrow provide? Much of the functionality of current systems is still required. The transmission of orders, processing of orders, and reporting of results remain. Functional requirements of ADT, scheduling, department service management, supply replacement, inventory, materials management, and documentation remain as well. Quality assurance should occur in real time, rather than recognizing days later that something was overlooked or a mistake was made.

As early as an International Medical Informatics Association (IMIA) Working Group 10 workshop on Hospital Information Systems in 1988, Collen stated that the goal of a hospital information system should be to

> ... use computers and communications equipment to collect, store, process, retrieve, and communicate relative patient care and administrative information for all activities and functions within the hospital, its outpatient medical offices, its clinical support services (clinical laboratories, radiology, pharmacy, intensive care unit, etc.), and with its affiliated [health] facilities. Such an integrated, multi-facility, [health] information system should have the capability for communication and integration of all patient data during the patient's service life time, from all of the information subsystems and all facilities in the medical system complex; and to provide administrative and clinical decision support.

This statement is important because it recognizes that clinical information is not the property of a single facility but, rather, is part of a global resource that focuses on the patient-centered record.

Hospital information systems and the concepts underlying them are limited because they focus primarily on operational information and not on a comprehensive patient record. An EHR is one component of a larger EHIS that includes not only hospital functionality but also features of a comprehensive integrated delivery system. The concept of the EHR is just beginning to emerge in some countries, notably Australia, the United Kingdom, and Canada. At the time of this writing, multiple definitions of EHR abound in the international community, and there is no solid consensus on a single definition. The International Standards Organization (ISO) Technical Committee on Health Informatics (TC215) defined EHRs for integrated care environments as (ISO, 2004):

> ... a repository of information regarding the health status of a subject of care in computer processable form, stored and transmitted securely, and accessible by multiple authorized [*sic*] users. It has a standardized [*sic*] or commonly agreed logical information model which is independent of EHR systems. Its primary purpose is the support of continuing, efficient and quality integrated healthcare and it contains information which is retrospective, concurrent, and prospective.

Using anonymized information from an EHR, an EHIS can incorporate the use of aggregated health data for use in the management of the health services delivery system (i.e., assessing population health status, setting health goals and objectives, defining strategic directions, program planning and delivery, and resource allocation).

Health service enterprises in national jurisdictions are able to exploit technological advances because of the networks that have become available. Now the system is the network and the network is the system. Networks are enablers that allow health service enterprises to be virtual organizations. Until recently, the various communication barriers imposed by distance and time made concrete physical organizations essential and dictated management structures partitioned to allow each individual geographic facility to be managed independently. Today, management of virtual health enterprises is possible because the technology ties the various component health facilities together with communication networks. Distance, time, and location all become almost irrelevant.

A patient-centered EHR requires that all data relating to the patient and the patient's well-being must be available at all times and accessible at appropriate locations. Data from all relevant sources must be integrated into a single record including but not limited to demographic data, data related to health determinants, and risk factors, along with diagnostic and treatment data from all contacts with the health enterprise (e.g., primary care providers; all members of the multidisciplinary healthcare team; home care; public or private acute care, long-term care, mental health facilities). This record is likely to take the form of a virtual record and may well be stored in a variety of locations. Initial efforts at exploring such a concept are underway in several countries, although experience with EHRs over large geographic areas and numerous locations across multiple jurisdictions are limited. Initial prototypes or pilot projects are beginning to be reported in Germany, Taiwan, Europe, the United Kingdom, Australia, and Canada.

A common problem list, a complete drug profile, and patient allergies should be centrally stored, maintained, and accessible. Data must be readily shared among all the providers of care. The patient's record must be a lifetime record, extending before birth to after death. The new EHRs eventually will contain character-based data, image data, waveforms, drawings, digital pictures, motion videos, and voice and sound recordings. The networks tying these systems together must have a wide bandwidth to accommodate the volume of data, which must be exchanged in real time among providers at diverse locations. Initially, Internet or electronic mail could provide easy linkage among the providers requesting consultation and discussing a patient's care. A clinically rich common medical and health vocabulary whose major purpose is communication must be developed, accepted, and used by all stakeholders. Confidentiality and privacy issues must be adequately supported with patient consent for the sharing of data.

The new systems must support source data capture, most specifically by primary care providers (e.g., midwives, nurses, physicians, dentists, acupuncturists, traditional caregivers, psychologists, social workers). Ideally, decision support systems would also be available at or near the point of care. Most computer support algorithms are useful only if they are interactive with the person making the clinical decision at the time of decision-making. Workstations customized for physicians, nurses, and other clinical caregivers as well as administrators and researchers are mandatory for tomorrow's systems.

The move toward managed care increases the need for informed, algorithmic driven order sets or regimens. Decision support systems, operating in the background, can save much money as well as improve patient care. As an example, a typical physician session involving ordering tests and prescribing treatment may typically invoke several thousand decision rules. These decision rules must be standardized and shared by the international community.

Prerequisites for EHISs

A prototype for an EHIS incorporating a multimedia, lifelong, multisite computerized patient record was designed and implemented at the University Hospital in Grosshadern, Germany. The following sections describe its essential design elements.

Data Model

The data model describes the medical concepts (e.g., blood pressure) that can be recorded in the electronic patient file and handled by the patient record system. The concepts are based on technical objects (e.g., figures, tests, video) whose properties and relationships are explicitly defined in a data object dictionary.

Presentation Types

Medical items must be modified, displayed, and communicated. A set of basic methods allows the manipulation, presentation, and communication of medical items that are controlled by a large number of parameters. Presentations must be adapted to the specialized needs of individual patient care environments and their corresponding requirements. Examples of presentation types include, but must not be limited to, forms, graphs, images, text, and audio.

Communication

The computerized medical record in an EHIS environment requires standardized protocols (e.g., HL7, EDI, EDIFACT, DICOM) for exchange of data among systems.

Interpreter

An interpreter provides analysis, presentation, and communication of patient data in the computerized patient record system. While global communication techniques make the creation of telemedicine (EHIS) records possible, there are still major barriers, notably the absence of data and communication standards and the lack of public acceptance (see Chapter 8 for more discussion).

Experience in Canada, beginning in 2001 under the auspices of Canada Health Infoway Inc. (Infoway), has seen the foundations laid for a national EHR. The mandate is to provide the necessary national information infrastructure for a pan-Canadian EHR. To that end, Infoway has developed a national EHRS Blueprint (Canada Health Infoway, 2003), conducted a Standards Needs Analysis (Canada Health Infoway, 2004a), and launched a Standards Collaboration Process. It has also initiated six projects that will provide the foundation for the Canada-wide EHRS, specifically Registries, Drug Information Systems, Diagnostic Imaging Systems, Laboratory Information Systems, Public Health Surveillance Systems, and Telehealth (Canada Health Infoway, 2004b).

In the United States, driven by patient safety concerns, a series of reports from a variety of organizations and groups (DHHS, 2004; Institute of Medicine, 1997; PITAC, 2001, 2004) resulted in commitment to the national health information infrastructure (NHII) in the United States in 2002. The NHII has the following features (National Comittee on Vital and Health Statistics, 2001).

- It is an initiative set forth to improve the effectiveness, efficiency, and overall quality of health and healthcare in the United States.
- It is a comprehensive knowledge-based network of interoperable systems of clinical, public health, and personal health information that can improve decision-making by making health information available when and where it is needed.
- It includes a set of technologies, standards, applications, systems, values, and laws that support all facets of individual health, healthcare, and public health.
- It is voluntary.
- It is NOT a centralized database of medical records or a government regulation.

Thus, as illustrated by the preceding examples, EHISs must have a broad multidisciplinary focus on health services delivery, including community needs assessment, population health status indicators, health promotion, and disease prevention, in addition to the treatment of illness. EHISs can and should support the reengineering and restructuring that is occurring in many healthcare organizations and health services delivery systems. Many of the data presently available are inadequate for these tasks; therefore, current data must be transformed and future information requirements anticipated to support the reengineering of healthcare enterprises and organizations using EHIS.

Producing Value-Added Information

Future EHISs must take into the account the fundamental principle that the reason a healthcare delivery system exists in any jurisdiction is to provide health services to its citizens. Thus, administrative and managerial information for use in operating the healthcare delivery enterprise should be a by-product of the care delivery process. One can envision a future environment in which current information about health facilities and healthcare delivery systems for use in enterprise planning and policies as well as resource allocation and utilization must be more widely available to professional care providers than in the past.

As reengineering or restructuring proceeds, information products are of interest to health system decision makers.

- Residents: information about the health needs and health status of the population, their families, and communities
- Recipients: information about residents receiving services from the health services enterprise
- Providers: information about available persons and organizations with health service skills (health workforce)
- Services: information about the range of health-affecting interventions and activities available in the health system
- Programs: information about the objectives, target recipients/populations, resource allocation, and bundling of particular sets of services
- Resources: distribution of fiscal (financial), physical (facilities and equipment), human (people working within the health services enterprise), and information resources
- Utilization: use of resources by the provider of the service, the recipient of the service, the program, and the type of service

Impact of EHISs

The impact of EHISs, which provide healthcare information over wide areas in a secure manner, is profound. Such availability potentially allows data mining of information that are advantageous for both patient and physician.

- Using the information to discover and analyze associations between disease entities and previously unknown risk factors (recorded in the patient history)
- Testing hypotheses regarding putative risk factors or studying disease distribution using demographic data
- Enabling a physician to perform a comparative analysis of a particular patient's symptoms with the symptoms of other patients with similar or different diseases

- Allowing more intelligent video consultations (During these consultation, along with the video, specialists in multiple locations could simultaneously see and annotate a patient's record.)
- Improving the outcome analysis
- Gathering decision support information
- Providing better education of patients to manage their own health

As we move into a new century, the major problems hospitals have experienced with hospital information systems can be resolved if the emerging health enterprises learn from the experiences of others. They must realistically address the following issues.

- The complex information and communication structure related to patient care can be improved by redesigning and reengineering the functions and processes of institutions to capitalize on the efficiencies permitted by modern information management techniques and equipment.
- Involve caregivers (including nursing) in the design and implementation stage.
- Every health enterprise should develop a strategic business plan that provides the foundation for its information management strategic plan. The information management strategic plan is implemented using tactical and operation plans.
- The development of client/server architectures and graphical user interfaces, working with powerful database software and proven application software that is flexible, can now be reasonably implemented.
- Staffing continues to be a major problem. Our academic institutions must address the need for health informatics preparation at all levels of education: undergraduate, graduate, and continuing education.
- With the arrival of reliable software and more graphical user interfaces, the use of information management technology can be expected to benefit the patient.

As we look toward enterprise information systems from the perspective of where health informatics has been, where it is now, what we have learned, and where we are heading in this new century, there is no doubt that the following observations are true.

- Nursing will play a major role in EHIS development.
- Information management, as applied to a wide variety of healthcare disciplines, is a proven reality and will continue to expand during the foreseeable future.
- Financial data processing has been the mainstay in hospital computing but is rapidly being superseded by clinical, administrative, management, and educational applications. In the future, the core of EHISs will be patient care data, with all other uses being value-added reprocessing of these data.

- The introduction of client/server architectures and networks to the health arena is revolutionizing the older concepts of centralized data processing.
- Real-time distributed use, in conjunction with central data storage, data warehousing, or infomart technology, will continue as a rapidly growing trend.
- Cost of hardware has decreased, making new options for the user increasingly feasible. Indeed, major technological changes will influence the entire medical and health science professions.
- Advances in technology will enable the use of multiple media to capture, store, and retrieve data and information
- Government policy statements will lead to further growth and support of health informatics. This has further implications for information management regarding rural medicine.
- A final prediction is that during the coming decade, caregivers, including nurses, will have portable, handheld, personal, digital telecommunications devices that enhance productivity by their capacity to access information and navigate through databases in remote geographic locations.

Advantages for nurses accruing from the use of an EHIS include the following.

- It is time-saving by reducing clerical activities, telephone calls between departments, and hand-written information transfer.
- Continuity of care through the current and status documentation is available on the system for the nurse.
- There is elimination of duplicate effort and more effective use of personnel, providing financial savings for the patient and time-saving for the nurse.
- Patient records and data for patient care, quality assurance, and research are more complete.
- Evidence-based nursing practice is enhanced because of the greater accuracy and speed of information transfer.
- The scope of nursing practice is expanded.

Time saved from manual information-processing tasks provides more time for the nursing process. More complete patient records, greater accuracy, and the increased speed of transferring information facilitate the nursing assessment and enhance patient safety by reducing communication errors. More effective use of personnel, continuity of care, support for evidence-based nursing practice, and the expanded scope of nursing practice can only result in better quality care for patients.

Summary

Countries around the globe are searching for ways to improve the delivery of healthcare and reduce the costs connected with providing this care simultaneously. The ultimate goal of sustaining and improving the health status of the population of a local state, national, or even international community purportedly guides all such efforts. An interesting phenomenon associated with the changes being undertaken in a number of healthcare systems emerges when even cursory comparisons of various attempts are drawn. Various countries demonstrate remarkable differences in approach, sometimes even adopting strategies that seem to move their healthcare systems in opposite directions (e.g., health reform initiatives in the British National Health Services, Canadian provincial healthcare systems, and the United States are striking examples). Yet these initiatives and many others claim to support improved healthcare and health status among their respective populations. The common goal is "health for all." However, if health systems are changing in different ways for the same reasons, can all the strategies for change be effective? How can they be evaluated? How can the outcomes of the health systems and health services be evaluated? Previous concepts of the scope of a hospital information system must change along with changes in the healthcare process and the restructuring of national and regional health systems. The functionality presently provided by such systems merely provides a base for beginning the development of the health information systems of the future. Information is key, and information systems are essential for enabling and informing the delivery of health services and for the effectiveness of national health systems.

References

Canada Health Infoway. (2003). *EHRS Blueprint*. http://www.canadahealthinfoway.ca/resourcecentre/index.php?lang=en (accessed December 15, 2004).

Canada Health Infoway. (2004a). *Standards Needs Analysis*. http://www.canadahealthinfoway.ca/home.php?lang=en (accessed December 15, 2004).

Canada Health Infoway. (2004b). *Coming Together 2003–2004 Annual Report*. http://www.canadahealthinfoway.ca/home.php?lang=en (accessed December 15, 2004).

Collen, M.F. (1998). HIS Concepts, Goals, Objectives. In Bakker, A.R., Ball, M.J., Scherrer, J.R., & Willems, J.L. Towards new hospital information systems. Amsterdam: North Holland. p. 3

International Standards Organization. (2004). *Health Informatics—Electronic Health Record—Definition, Scope, and Context*. TR 20514.

Institute of Medicine. (1997). To Err Is Human. Washington, D.C.: National Academy Press.

Jackson, G.G. (1969). Information handling costs in hospitals. Datamation 15:56.

McHugh, M., & Schultz, S. (1982). Computer technology in hospital nursing departments: future applications and implications. In: Blum BI (ed.) *Proceedings, Sixth Annual Symposium on Computer Applications in Medical Care*. Los Angeles: IEEE, pp. 557–561.

National Committee on Vital and Health Statistics. (2001). *A Strategy for Building the National Health Information Infrastructure*. Washington, D.C.: U.S. Department of

Health and Human Services. http://aspe.hhs.gov/sp/nhii/Documents/NHIIReport 2001/ (accessed December 16, 2004).

National Health Information Infrastructure. Washington D.C.: U.S. Department of Health and Human Services. http://aspe.hhs.gov/sp/nhii/ (accessed December 16, 2004).

Office of Technology Assessment, Congress of the United States. (1995). *HealthCare Online: The Role of Information Technologies*. OTA-ITC-624. Washington, D.C.: US Government Printing Office.

President's Information Technology Advisory Committee (PITAC). (2001). *Transforming HealthCare Through Information Technology*. Arlington, VA: National Coordination Office for Information Technology Research and Development.

President's Information Technology Advisory Committee (PITAC). (2004). *Revolutionizing HealthCare Through Information Technology*. Arlington, VA: National Coordination Office for Information Technology Research and Development.

Additional Resources

Adelhard, K., Eckel, R., Holzel, D., & Tretter, W. (1996). Design elements of a telemedical medical record. In: Cimino, J.J. (ed.) *Proceedings, AMIA Fall Symposium*, pp. 473–477.

Alvarez, R.C., Curry, J., Hodge, T., Chatwin, B.J., & Hannah, K.J. (1992). A provincial health information processing strategy: a case study. In: Lunn, K.C., Degoulet, P., Piemme, T.E., Reinhoff, O. (eds.) *Medinfo '92 Proceedings.* Amsterdam: North-Holland.

Ballardini, L., Mazzoleni, M.C., Tramarin R., & Caprotti, M. (1996). Remote management of a cardiac magnetic resonance imaging session by a low cost teleconsulting system. In: Cimino, J.J. (ed.) *Proceedings, AMIA Fall Symposium*, p. 825.

Chang, I.F., Suarez, H.H., Ho, L.C., Cheung, P.S., & Ke, J.S. (1996). Nationwide implementation of telemedicine and CPR systems in Taiwan. In: Cimino, J.J. (ed.) *Proceedings, AMIA Fall Symposium*, p. 878.

Donsez, D., Tiers, G., Modjeddi, B., & Beuscart, R. (1996). Improving the continuity of care: The ISAR–Telematics European Project. In: Cimino, J.J. (ed.) *Proceedings, AMIA Fall Symposium*, p. 890.

Forslund, D.W., Phillips, R.L., Kilman, D.G., & Cook, J.L. (1996). Experiences with a distributed virtual patient record system. In: Cimino, J.J. (ed). *Proceedings, AMIA Fall Symposium*, pp. 483–487.

Hannah, K.J. (1995). Transforming information: data management support of health-care reorganization. *Journal of the American Medical Informatics Association 2*:147–155.

6
Nursing Aspects of Health Information Systems

Motivation for the development and implementation of computerized hospital information systems has been financial and administrative (i.e., driven by the need to capture charges, reduce costs, and document patient care for legal reasons). Most of the systems marketed today have been motivated by those two factors. Historically, such systems have required a major investment in hardware (typically a mainframe and networks); and even though they have demonstrated significant improvement in hospital communications (with a corresponding reduction in paper flow), they have been characteristically weak in supporting professional nursing practice. These factors have prevented the level of acceptance by nurses that was originally foreseen. Only recently have developers and vendors begun to consider the nature of modern nursing practice and its information-processing requirements (Fig. 6.1).

If one considers the original principles that Campbell (1978) identified when observing the activities nurses perform when caring for patients, nursing roles fall into three global categories. The first is managerial roles or coordinating activities that involve the gathering and transmission of patient information, such as order entry, results reporting, requisition generation, and telephone booking of appointments. Although many of these activities have been delegated to unit clerks (at least on day shifts), current hospital information systems can help nurses with those activities. The second category is physician-delegated tasks. Current systems can capture these tasks from the physicians' order entry set and then incorporate them into the patient care plan. The third category is autonomous nursing function, characteristic of professional nursing practice, when knowledge unique to nursing is applied to patient care. Current systems are beginning to support nurses in fulfilling their responsibilities in this category. All three categories—managerial/coordinating, physician-delegated, autonomous nursing function—must fit together to create a fully operational system. Current systems, although they release nurses to focus on professional nursing practice, fail to provide the appropriate support essential to professional nursing practice. The future requires decision-making

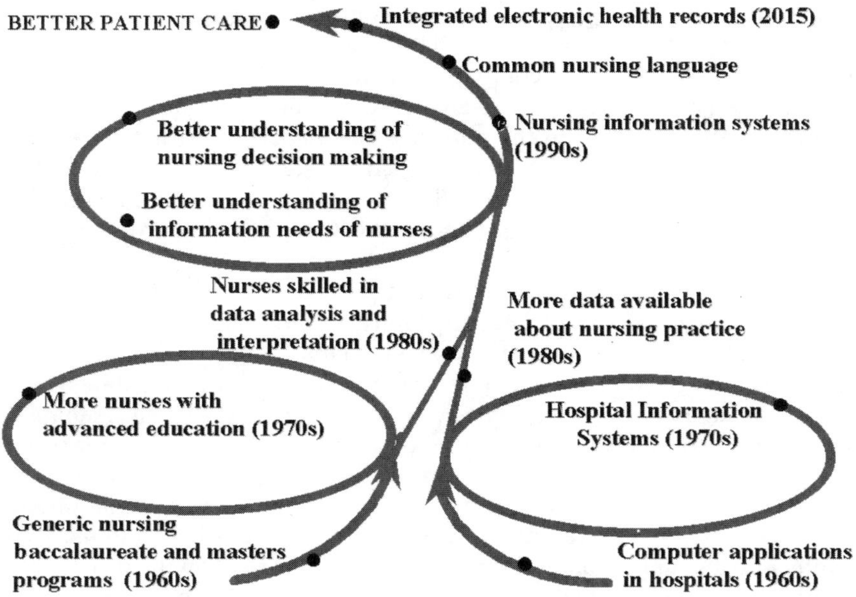

FIGURE 6.1. Evolution of nursing information systems.

support for professional nursing practice and the capture of information from the patient care plan for nursing administration decision-making related to nursing resource allocation.

Nursing Management Information Systems

From an economic point of view, the combination of the shrinking healthcare dollar and escalating healthcare costs makes it imperative that the productivity issues associated with nursing dollars spent be considered. To that end, nurse managers must ensure that appropriate nursing information is incorporated into any management information system. The major objective of such systems is the provision of information on which decisions can be based that effectively and efficiently allocate nursing resources for the highest quality of patient care. Nursing management information needs to integrate the clinical data about patients that ultimately affect the cost of providing patient care. Historically, nursing costs have never been reliably projected because they did not incorporate fluctuating patient acuity levels and the associated needs for nursing care. Based on the integration of patient clinical data, some current systems now have the capacity to ascertain costs of nursing care for individual patients. This costing must incorporate multiple components such as quality and workload measurements, financial considerations (payroll and general ledger), and staff utilization as well as educational and professional qualifications, contractual obligations, and costs. Such a nursing management system enables the development of productivity standards by which one can compare patient care outcomes as well as variance analysis, which enables the manager to rationalize deviations from the budget. Furthermore, when the nursing costs associated with patient type are accurately and reliably quantified, such a system has great potential in forecasting and long-range planning. This ability has potential for healthcare planning that incorporates costs associated with patient care groupings. On an operational level, the nursing management information system includes human resource capabilities such as staff profiles, educational credentials, professional licensure status, and scheduling, all of which facilitate effective development and deployment of nursing resources.

The overall goal must be the development of comprehensive, integrated nursing management information. Such information may reside in a separate system or be contained in an integrated management information system. In any case, it must clearly identify, sort, and analyze uniquely nursing information. Such a system must have the capacity to integrate with, and build upon, a variety of hospital information systems. In addition, systems generating nursing management information must capitalize on the distributed processing concepts as well as the communication capacity of networks and the power of client-server architecture to provide clinical workstations for decision support. Achieving such a goal requires the application and use of existing technology in an innovative manner. These concepts are elaborated in Chapter 9.

Clinical Nursing Documentation

Clinical documentation is an essential part of the healthcare delivery system, with a wealth of information residing in the documentation compiled at each patient encounter. The current process of gathering and using this information is such that documentation is fragmented rather than synergistic, and its potential to improve the delivery of healthcare and clinical outcomes is not being realized. The application of information technologies in healthcare has the potential to transform clinical documentation into an integrated, multidisciplinary tool with the prospect of improving clinical outcomes and enhancing the overall healthcare environment. Several healthcare institutions have begun to implement technology-enabled clinical documentation solutions and are experiencing positive outcomes. Building on these experiences, the approach to clinical documentation that holds the greatest promise lies in the implementation of an integrated, multidisciplinary, patient-centered electronic health record, with provider order entry and a problem-driven approach at its core.

Developments in nursing informatics must assist nurses in the gathering and aggregating of clinical nursing data to make decisions related to the nursing care of patients. Modern nursing practice no longer focuses on the assessment and labeling phase of the nursing process (i.e., defining the nursing diagnosis, nursing problem, or nursing phenomenon). Instead, it emphasizes decision-making and exercising clinical nursing judgment in patient care. Because of the growing complexity of patient care and the rising acuity level of patients in hospitals today, nurses have acquired an expanded repertoire of intervention skills. These skills reflect the autonomous aspects of nursing practice that are based on the body of nursing knowledge and the nurse's professional judgment. Autonomous nursing interventions are complementary to, not competitive with, physician-prescribed treatments. The major objective in this section is to discuss the evolving role of clinical documentation and to show how the application of information technologies can lead to a new paradigm, integrated and multidisciplinary in nature, that can ultimately transform the quality and continuity of patient care.

...nentation in Clinical Care

...nglish Dictionary (Second Edition) ...roof; give evidence. Clinical docu... ...e of the following.

...althcare team

...ocedures, treatments, and patient

...onse to diagnostic tests and inter-

...patient's interaction with, and as

...highly complex healthcare en- ...unmanageable challenge and has be- ...use of many patient safety issues and other problems. Busy physicians may not view and access nurses' notes as critical data. Busy nurses may not have time to read the physicians' notes. Moveover, information entered into the patient record by other healthcare professionals is seldom integrated into the physician and/or nursing documentation. This lack of integration of multidisciplinary documentation leads to a less-than-perfect care plan for the patient. Data generated by one group of healthcare providers—especially nurses—that is of significant interest to another group of providers—especially physicians—needs to be made easily accessible. Areas of common interest to a number of clinicians regarding patient care include vital signs, intake/output, Kardex/care plan data, and the medication administration record. Narrative notes, which capture patient information essential for decision-making, still comprise most of the patient record and is the area most seriously in need of improvement.

One of the challenges of healthcare documentation is that the primary purpose or intention behind documentation is the clinicians' need to fullfill explicit requirements about what and when items should be documented to show that a standard of care was met. The patient's clinical record is the best defense against litigation involving malpractice or negligence. Nurses, physicians, and the rest of the healthcare team contribute significantly to meeting the regulatory requirements of federal and state regulatory agencies, payers, accreditation organizations, healthcare consumer groups, and legal entities. Utilizing documentation as a tool that promotes patient-centric communication and care coordination at the same time one is documenting to protect the hospital, physicians, and nurses makes it difficult to keep the patient's immediate needs in mind. A computerized, longitudinal patient record enables clinicians to meet both purposes (see Chapter 5).

In the current, fragmented, fast-paced, healthcare environment, the electronic patient record (EPR) takes on primary importance as a communication tool among members of the healthcare team. To be effective in this environment, the record must be easily completed and organized. It should facilitate teamwork and integration of clinical care workflow among all disciplines involved and allow real-time entries so diagnosis and treatment happen in a safe and timely manner.

Most attempts to computerize clinical documentation have done little more than mimic paper documentation on a computer. In the information age, documentation ought to be driven by the nature and content of the information itself and to best support a patient-centric work process. In the information age, the only limitations to moving from documentation as a burdensome, redundant task to documentation as a tool that enables clinical judgment and decision-making for quality care are lack of imagination and practicality.

Knowledge-based documentation contains content that enables clinicians to utilize current or best practice clinical research as part of their documentation work process. When one documents, one uses critical thinking skills to review information that is in the record and to analyze data and arrive at conclusions. Many times the output of this analysis is an order for assessment or interventions or the decision to monitor for signs and symptoms of a potential complication. Clinical documentation is embedded in the clinician's work process. Expert practitioners can always tell what information they need to care for patients. They also know how they would like to see that information and what reference material or reminders would be best to assist them in ensuring that the standard of care is met. Clinical information is, in fact, distinct from the medium through which it is recorded and can truly serve the patient's—and the healthcare worker's—best interest only when it is treated as such.

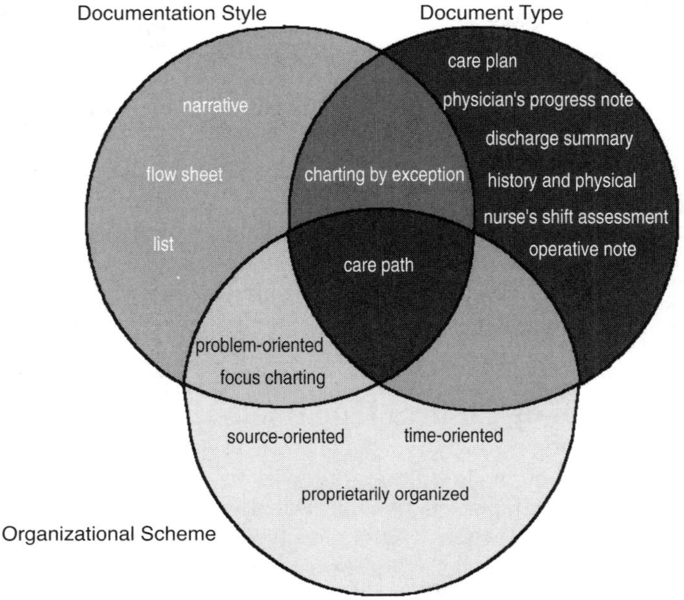

Figure 6.2. Forms of documentation according to their function.

Documentation Approaches

Some document approaches are document types, some are documentation styles, and some are combinations thereof, as illustrated in Figure 6.2 (Ball et al., 2004).

Popular documentation approaches include the following.

- Charting by exception
- Narrative
- Flow sheets
- Source of origination (e.g., laboratory, respiratory therapy)
- Problem-oriented
- Focus charting
- Care plan
- Critical pathways, protocols, collaborative problems

There are overlaps in documentation styles and organizational schema between and among nurses.

Nursing Orders as Documentation

Orders perform the function of clinical documentation, and they should be considered as such. They initiate the treatments carried out by nurses, pharmacists, respiratory therapists, and other healthcare providers. Frequently nursing orders are used interchangeably with nursing interventions. Nursing interventions describe the activities and behaviors used to deliver nursing treatments (McCloskey and Bulechek, 1996). As previously indicated, some of these respond to a physician's order but many do not. Reimbursement systems are heavily focused on physician services, which has contributed to fragmentation of the patient record. The computerized patient record does not have to be limited by this reality. Overly focusing on care as being driven by the order workflow alone limits the degree to which the clinical information system becomes a tool that is useful to all disciplines caring for the patient.

Characteristics of Clinical Documentation

In some situations, clinical documentation is an endpoint, whereas in others it is not. From one perspective, clinical documentation can be considered an endpoint only when it is not utilized after it has been recorded. Although one cannot predict whether a document will be consulted after it has been created, certain documents have a greater likelihood of being accessed. Clinical documentation is surely not an endpoint when the documents influence future clinical decision making by members of the healthcare team, whether in the short or long term. The repeatability aspect of information is a key benefit of implementing an integrated computerized patient record. Without integration the ability to view current and past key patient information is impeded by needing to access disparate systems for viewing results.

From another perspective, clinical documentation can be considered an endpoint when it does not serve as the direct basis for future documentation. When there is no required continuity between serial notes (as is currently the case for most clinical documentation), each note can stand by itself without reference to issues raised in previous notes and without any assurance of consistency, continuity, or closure. The lengthy history and physicals (H+P) document is often an endpoint. The H+P is an especially poignant example in which smart information technology can create major efficiency gains by distinguishing between the document and the information that it conveys. Nurses, physicians, and other disciplines utilize similar document types for H+P. A case can be made for the creation of an integrated H+P format that allows users to filter their views to see all the information they want: all disciplines, all history or some disciplines, some history. This process closely follows the clinician's clinical decision-making process. Technology can enable evolution and acceleration of clinical decision-making and knowledge through an integrated world view of information, contributing to decisions made regarding patient care. Currently, an integrated computerized patient record best facilitates this.

Informatics Approaches to Clinical Documentation Issues

Nurses are utilizing informatics to address clinical documentation issues on a continuum from the most primitive to the most advanced. On the most primitive end of the continuum, hospitals continue to provide nurses with plenty of paper and writing instruments. Stepping up the evolutionary ladder, some institutions have skeletal paper forms or templates available for many highly detailed forms for nursing documentation.

Some hospitals have begun to "pave the cow path" by introducing electronic health records (EHRs), which allow nurses to word-process free-text notes and even eliminate new paper notes. The more savvy users soon learn to copy, paste, and edit old notes to be able to write new notes quickly and efficiently (Hier, 2002). Many EHRs also offer boilerplate template functionality. Even though they tend to be static, they are still useful in prompting the nurse for information. Some EHRs support automatic import of laboratory results, medications given, and so on (e.g., the Veterans Administration's EHRs) into free-text notes, although people who know how to do this are the exception. (This speaks to the importance of interface design and training.) The VA system, especially, makes document retrieval easier by requiring users to assign a formal a coded document type (Brown et al., 2001).

Enabling clinical documentation and results viewing via interfacing different information systems can produce a less than elegant information flow. Well designed information retrieval and viewing, with ease of data entry, speeds up the clinical decision-making process, innovates current research content into practice, and can improve care. To the extent that any piece of documentation can be used for legal defense, one can assuredly say that documentation is never an endpoint.

Belmont et al. (2003) identified four key guiding principles to be followed to strike a new path for clinical documentation systems.

1. "Build a Coherent Patient Story . . . a story unique to one patient—across the continuum of care. Instead of being a collection of dissociated forms, clinical documentation must build a story in partnership with the patient that includes the evidence-based, patient-specific care given as the patient moves through the system.
2. "Empower Interdisciplinary Care . . . keep the members of the interdisciplinary clinical team informed of the care other members are providing . . . Because no one clinician has all the expertise a patient might need, clinical documentation must empower the interdisciplinary team to provide care as a team, not a separate and distinct disciplines and caregivers.
3. "Support Integrated Scopes of Practice for All Clinicians . . . support defined scopes of practice that clarify the responsibilities, competencies, and evidence-based knowledge for which each member of the interdisciplinary team is accountable.

4. "Provide Evidence Based Information at Point of Care... Clinical practice guidelines take evidenced based information, combine it with individual patient data, and relate it to individual patients."

Characteristics of Electronic Clinical Nursing Documentation

As aspects of a plan for informatics-enabled clinical documentation are developed, the following areas of focus and issues need to be addressed.

- Understanding the distinction between content and form (or data and display)
- Standardization of the clinical data and content, given the above diversity of methods used at present
- Content in conjunction with workflow process through the system
- Data gathering and recording
- Data and information retrieval and review
- Handling inter- and intrashift and interdepartmental communications

The objectives for standard interdisciplinary documentation might be the following.

- Eliminate redundancies and duplication in documentation
- Enhance the quality and reporting of clinical care from a multidisciplinary perspective through standardization
- Define and standardize common clinical documentation data element needs for all patients
- Develop an approach for standardizing clinical documentation practices for both automated and manual (paper) settings
- Automate an ideal clinical documentation workflow

The overarching goal is to transform care. The complexities and transformation processes resulting in new innovative actions begin to unravel. The greatest challenge is to determine how to integrate the documentation generated by each healthcare provider, so each can then benefit from the work done by his or her colleagues. There is no doubt that nursing documentation, in and of itself, serves a valuable purpose. As we move into a multidisciplinary environment, if the goal is to have all caregivers, including nurses, perform their documentation in an integrated fashion at the point of entry, as currently called for by the computerized provider order entry initiative in the United States, the end-product is similar in nature to the problem-driven medical record this chapter has described. System developers, however, have been remiss in capitalizing on where these functions intersect on the Venn diagram (see Fig. 6.2) and in providing relevant, useful information to the various healthcare professionals involved in the care of the patient.

How can technology help nurses care for patients? The ideal nursing system requires the technology for source data capture and considerable work by nurses on the development of the nursing knowledge base. Until relatively recently, it was not possible to even consider such a system because the technology did not exist. Now that it does, the onus is on nursing to develop effective means to use the technology.

From the nursing perspective, there are three major areas related to health information systems that must be addressed in the immediate future. To provide information management assistance to nurses, the areas of (1) source data capture, (2) nursing data standards, and (3) decision support systems must be addressed. These three areas are crucial to providing computer support for nurses in the delivery of patient care.

Source Data Capture

In this context, source data capture means gathering data and information about patients where it originates, that is, with the patient. The concept of "terminals by the bedside" was introduced during the mid-1980s. Most experts agree that bringing the computer access closer to the patient (i.e., locating it at the "point of care") is a valid premise, and clinicians appear to favor the bedside terminal as a means to reduce much of the clerical workload and improve access to clinical data.

Point of care systems are still not in widespread use. Their potential has yet to be fully realized. As more facilities and organizations implement source data capture systems, including bedside terminals, the concept will gain acceptance in the industry and, in fact, become the standard for nursing systems. This conclusion is based also on the fact that significant funds are presently being channeled toward research and development of bedside and other point of care devices in Canada, the United States, and around the world.

Criteria for Source Data Capture

Such technology must meet specific criteria. Specifically, it must permit nurses at the patient's bedside, be it in the patient's home or in the hospital, to interact with the main patient database and the main care planning system or hospital information system. It must have the capacity to interact with existing hospital information systems or regional EHRs so effort already expended in developing hospital and health information systems is not wasted. Such technology must be small and compact so as to occupy the minimum amount of space at the patient's bedside or the nurse's bag and, therefore, not interfere with the use of other important equipment necessary to the care of the patient. This technology must be rugged and durable.

In addition, it must be constructed so it can be disinfected between patients. Also, it must be easy and uncomplicated to use and have high-resolution screens with graphics capability that can be read in the dark. Provision must be made for a variety of means of data entry (e.g., bar code reader, physiological probe, digital camera, natural language, or keyboard). A volume control is necessary to mute any keyboard sounds. Moreover, because patients do not always stay in hospitals or beds or even at home, this type of technology must allow nurses the maximum degree of mobility to enter data wherever the patient may be. Wireless transmission of encrypted data can now be configured to provide an acceptable level of security and confidentiality for patient information. Much work remains to be done before a satisfactory system for source data capture is fully developed.

"Point of Care" Devices

Three "point of care" devices are presently available. The first is the standard stationary terminal. The most expedient approach to the concept of source data capture was simply to place a standard keyboard and monitor (i.e., a CRT) at the bedside; Misys CPR (formerly Ulticare) has used this approach (Misys Healthcare, 2005). The second type of terminal is specially designed for the purpose of source data capture. One variety of special-purpose terminal is a small footprint terminal, fixed at the bedside and having special function keys for data input. The systems used in critical care usually are of this type; Spacelabs (2005) and GE Healthcare (2005) patient monitoring systems are both examples of this type of system. The third device is a handheld portable terminal, not restricted to a particular space such as the patient's room in a hospital.

Overall, there is still far too little experience in the healthcare field with point of care, or source data capture, devices to allow a consensus as to whether a fixed bedside terminal or a portable handheld terminal is best suited for both patient care and optimum system utilization. However, there is an emerging consensus that the choice should be made based the purpose for which the device is to be used. For example, fixed, small footprint terminals are likely the best choice in critical care environments where space is at a premium, whereas portable wireless hand held devices are most useful to nurses providing care in patients' homes.

Uses of Source Data Capture in Healthcare

Sensmeier et al. carefully and succinctly show that "Documenting at the point of care gets nursing back into the 'chart as you go' workflow, eliminating long hours of overtime charting at the end of the shift, struggling to remember what was done hours earlier"(Sensmeier et al., 2003). The capacity for source data capture could be more greatly exploited by nurses if assessment guidelines and interview instruments were developed with a view to remote access and downloading to the point of care device. Data input of responses in an interactive fashion at the patient's bedside would permit source data capture. More accurate documentation of patient care would be the first outcome. Ultimately, it should be possible to develop and deliver decision support systems or knowledge bases for nursing use in evidence-based practice at the patient's bedside. The initial uses of such technology will likely be in acute care facilities. Eventually, extended-care and long-term care facilities, the occupational health field, outpatient clinics, community health, and home care are prime areas for development of software for use with this technology. The latter areas have been sorely underserved by the healthcare computing industry primarily because until now the technology was unable to serve the highly mobile and geographically dispersed nature of practice in these fields of healthcare.

With the convergence that is occurring among wireless technologies [personal digital assistants (PDAs), PC-compatible productivity tools, cellphones, text mail, the Web], there is almost unlimited opportunity (Blackberry, 2005; PalmOne, 2005). With these advances, point of care technology has exceeded, at least temporarily, nurses' capacity to develop clinical uses and applications for it.

Nursing Data Standards

Nurses continually use mental processes, often unconsciously, to organize information systematically by grouping data according to common features. We do this to make sense of the massive amounts of information with which we are daily bombarded. The problem arises because nurses do not have a common system or language with which to communicate precisely, even with each other. Lang has well described the situation: "If we cannot name it, we cannot control it, finance it, teach it, search it or put it into public policy" (Clark and Lang, 1992, p. 109). Because nursing has not had universally accepted methods for defining and collecting nursing data, nursing data have not been collected. For example, the patient discharge abstracts prepared by medical records departments in hospitals contain no nursing care delivery information. The abstracts therefore fail to acknowledge the contribution of nursing during the patient's stay in the hospital. The abstracts are used by many agencies for a variety of statistical and funding purposes. Patient discharge summaries need to include nursing workload data that recognize the personnel providing the care in addition to the substance of that care (i.e., the nursing components of patient care, the type of nursing care provided, and the impact of that care on patient outcome). Presently, much valuable information is being lost.

Information about and for nursing is essential not only for funding purposes but also for nurses to be able to develop evidence-based practice. Data to support evidence-based practice is required not only for clinical practice but also to inform evidence-based decision-making by nurse managers. Therefore, as the development of nationwide health databases increases, it is vital that a minimum number of essential nursing elements be included in local and national databases.

A variety of concepts interlink when considering the capture of nursing practice data. They include the derivation from nursing practice of nomenclature, terminologies, language, classification systems, reference terminology model and minimum data set, and the resulting feedback loop (Clark and Lang, 1992, p. 11).

> The practicing nurse finds word (labels) for the elements of her/his practice. When these words are standardized among nurses, they can be called a nursing nomenclature. These word-labels can then be combined within a defined structure and systematic management to form a language system for nursing. From this point onward, the data that are labeled according to a nursing nomenclature, structured into a nursing language, and classified by means of common features, can be collated for inclusion in a nursing minimum data set which in turn can be fed back into nursing practice at the center of the spiral; and the continuous process of development, refinement and modification in response to external change begins again.

Chapter 12 describes the interaction of these concepts in detail and the ways that various countries have addressed the need for nursing data standards.

Issues in the Development and Use of Nursing Data

As nurses embark on the development of nursing data standards, several issues emerge. Attention must be directed to the coordination and linkage of data. Three aspects of data linkage demand attention. First, the computer hardware must support database linkage. Second, the content of the nursing data standard must be developed in a way that lends itself to integration with other information. Finally, the ethics of data linkage with respect to patient information, including security confidentiality and privacy of data, must be addressed. Integration is a key consideration as the developments in various countries converge. Once nursing data standards are developed, three more issues emerge: (1) promoting the idea to ensure widespread use, (2) educating the users to ensure the quality of the data that are collected, and (3) establishing mechanisms for review and revision of the data elements.

Evidence-Based Nursing

Increasingly, nursing, like other health professions, is moving toward evidence-based practice. This means that no longer are nursing judgments based on intuition, ritual, or tradition. Nurses increasingly are basing their practice on knowledge that has been developed through empirical research. However, because of the rapid increase in the volume of information in the body of nursing knowledge, it is no longer possible to expect nurses to retain the entire knowledge base of the profession in their heads. Consequently, nurses require access to the resources that contain empirically developed nursing knowledge.

Decision Support Systems

The nursing literature regarding decision support systems exhibits confusion and lack of clarity because of the various definitions and conceptualizations. It is characterized by authors who use the same term to refer to different concepts or who use different terms for the same concept. A broad definition that has some professional consensus is that computerized decision support systems (CDS or DSS) include "any computer software employing a knowledge base (facts and/or rules) designed for use by a clinician involved in patient care, as a direct aid to clinical decision-making" (Langton et al., 1992, p. 626). There is a consensus among authors that decision support systems should be used to extend the nurse's decision-making capacity rather than to replace it. Most care planning systems now in use are not decision support systems. Standardized care plans, whether manual or computer-based, provide care only for standardized patients. Standardized care plans neither enhance nor support nursing decision-making; on the contrary, their "cookbook" approach discourages active decision-making by nurses. Therefore, they are not congruent with a professional practice model of nursing.

A decision support system for nursing practice is intended to support nurses by providing them with information to facilitate rational decision-making about patients' care. In other words, decision support systems help nurses maintain and maximize their decision-making responsibilities and focus on the highest priority aspects of patient care. The major caveat that must be considered in a professional practice model of nursing is that clinical judgment that considers contextual factors as well as the recommendations of decision support systems must be exercised. In addition, because the current status of computer technology and understanding human cognition restricts the performance of such systems, nurses must be discriminating users of these systems and ensure that the systems are providing appropriate recommendations before acting on the output of such systems.

Eddy (1990) believed that the complexity of modern healthcare has now exceeded the limitations of the unaided human mind. Decision support systems offer great potential to help nurses handle the volumes of data and information required. Pryor (1994, p. 300) has identified six major uses of decision support.

1. *Alerting*: Alerting systems are those that notify the clinician of an immediate problem that calls for a prompt action or decision. These alerts are commonly clinician alerts that appear on the screen at the time of entry of orders, assessments, or laboratory values. These systems may also provide management alerts based on problems with an individual patient (DRG cost overrun) or an individual clinician (use of expensive resources not generally warranted).
2. *Interpretation*: This type of CDS system is one that works to interpret particular data such as from the electrocardiogram or blood gas assays. A system such as this works by assimilating the data and transforming it into a conceptual understanding or interpretation. The interpretation is then presented to the clinician for use in decision-making.
3. *Assisting*: A system that is used to speed or simplify clinician interactions with the computer is classified as an assisting system. These systems usually assist in the ordering or charting process by offering the clinician such things as standing order lists, patient-specific drug dosing, or appropriate parameters for charting based on earlier identified patient problems.
4. *Critiquing*: Systems that provide critiques are primarily in the research stage and not yet available for implementation. This type of system is designed to critique a set of orders for particular problems. For example, a clinician might enter orders for a change in respirator settings, which the system would then critique in light of the most recently entered blood gas results. The clinician would be presented with an alternate set of orders and the rationale for changes made. The clinician would have the option of accepting or rejecting the changes suggested by the computer.
5. *Diagnosing*: This type of decision support system uses general assessment data to generate suggested diagnoses. These systems may then ask for additional data to rule out, rule in, or otherwise refine the list of diagnostic possibilities. Other systems that can be considered in this category are those that provide predictive scoring of mortality, estimation of treatment benefits based on effects of competing risks, or prediction of specific risks (pressure ulcers, falls).
6. *Managing*: The computer automatically generates the treatment or plan of care from assessment data and/or diagnostic categories, and the nurse or physician then critiques the computer and its logic. Although those systems with fixed protocols are easy to program and implement, the lack of individualization leaves the clinician with the job of extensive critiquing. This type of system can be used in a developmental manner, however, so the clinician gives a rationale for changing the plan or the protocol; this rationale is then used to determine further data needs and decision rules so the protocols are further refined. The variation in intervention and the rationale offered can be combined with data of outcomes of care to determine which interventions are most effective in producing the desired outcome. Thus, the refined protocols result in a progressively higher quality of care.

Knowledge-Based Systems

All six types of decision support systems outlined have been combined in a knowledge-based or expert system. For the sake of simplicity, the term "expert system" is used here to encompass advisory systems and knowledge-based systems. The purpose of expert systems is to recommend solutions to nursing problems that reflect the judgment of nurse experts regarding the most expedient response to nursing situations. Expert systems capture or encapsulate, in a computer system, the knowledge of a human expert within a particular domain of practice. Their function is to mimic the clinical reasoning and judgment of one specific human expert in the aggregation and interpretation of data in a precisely defined area of practice. Expert systems are characterized by using artificial intelligence principles, specifically the symbolic representation of specialist knowledge to make decisions within a specified domain; the capacity to interrogate the user sensibly; and explanation of reasoning (rationale) underlying a decision on request by the user; and incorporation into the knowledge base of systematic feedback about the effects of decisions.

General approaches used as the basis for expert systems are knowledge engineering elicitation of a knowledge base and decision rules from an expert; actuarial data based on multiple observations of patient encounters; and objective probability based on the subjective judgment of multiple experts using heuristics to determine what a reasonable professional nurse would decide in a particular situation. The components of an expert system include a knowledge base, an inference engine, a patient database, and a user interface. The knowledge base may incorporate that which constitutes empirically validated research; clinical experience-based heuristics; and authority, tradition, and textbooks. An inference engine deals with the interpretation of knowledge using such techniques as logical deduction (decision rules), semantic networks, and logical relationships (Bayesian, probabilistic, or "fuzzy" logic). The patient database is composed of the data gathered from the patient who is the subject of the decisions. The user interface provides the capacity for natural language communication with the system to enable the user to pose questions and to enter and receive information. Nursing decision support systems and nursing expert systems are reported in the literature (Caelli et al., 2003; Carter and Cox, 2000; Harris et al., 2000; Jovic et al., 2002; Lyons and Richardson, 2003; New 2000; Reilly et al., 2000; Ruland, 1999), but none has progressed much beyond research, development, or testing to widespread incorporation into production systems incorporated into software marketed by vendors of hospital/health information systems and EHRs.

There is still much work to be done, both when considering the implications of expert systems in a care-giving environment and when developing and implementing expert systems—to say nothing of their content. Issues that remain outstanding relate to legal liability; ethical concerns such as privacy, confidentiality, and data integrity when using electronic patient records, and professional practice. Expert systems integrated into nursing information systems and hospital/health information systems informed by source data capture and made possible through nursing data standards offer the potential to affect significantly the evidence-based practice of nurses for the purpose of enhancing patient care.

Summary

There is no doubt that the problem-driven approach can eliminate redundancies between and among the various providers, will eventually create major operational improvements, and will lead to a much more effective, efficient way to document patient care. It is high time that some of these new innovative solutions be put to work to assist nurses in their work environments. Healthcare providers, administrators, and patients can work together to transform our patient care delivery system in a way that not only reduces the risks of medical error but provides health professionals with a better-quality work environment and the satisfaction that comes from providing the best possible care to patients. As hospital information systems move beyond the developmental stage and are marketed and installed on a wide scale, they provide nurses with access to a great deal of information about their practice and increase the time needed to analyze and consider this information.

Simultaneously, the level of educational preparation of nurses began to rise with the proliferation of master's and doctoral programs that produced a cadre of nurses with much greater appreciation for, as well as sophistication and skill at, data analysis and research. We believe that the consequence of this concurrent evolution of both technology and the nursing profession will be advances of astronomic proportions in nursing practice. We are just beginning to initiate the cycle whereby information availability promotes greater understanding of nursing decision-making and diagnosis. This, in turn, not only facilitates higher level functioning of nurses but generates additional information and further stimulates the cycle.

References

Ball, M.J., Rothschild, A., Dietrich, L., Wurtz, H., & Farish-Hunt, H. (2004). Clinical documentation in the digital age: IT as the agent of transformation. Unpublished.

Belmont, C., Jesse, H., Wesorick, B., & Troseth, M. (2003). *The Clinician Perspective Special Section: Clinical Documentation*. www.HCTProject.com (accessed February 24, 2005).

Blackberry (2005). http://www.blackberry.com (accessed February 8, 2005).

Brown, S.H., Lincoln, M., & Hardenbrook, S., et al. (2001). Derivation and evaluation of a document-naming nomenclature. *Journal of the American Medical Informatics Association 8*(4):379–390.

Caelli, K., Downie, J., & Caelli, T. (2003). Towards a decision support system for health promotion in nursing. *Journal of Advanced Nursing* 43(2):170–180.

Campbell, C. (1978). *Nursing Diagnosis and Nursing Intervention.* New York: Wiley.

Carter, M., & Cox, R. (2000). Nurse managers' use of a computer decision support system: Differences in nursing labor costs per patient day. *Nursing Leadership Forum 5*(2):57–64.

Clark, J., & Lang, N. (1992). Nursing's next advance: An international classification for nursing practice. *International Journal of Nursing 39*(4):102–112, 128.

Eddy, D.M. (1990). Practice policies: where do they come from. In: Clinical decision-making: From theory to practice (series). *Journal of the American Medical Association 263*:1265–1275.

GE HealthCare (2005). http://www.gehealthcare.com (accessed February 8, 2005).

Harris, M.R., Graves, J.R., Solbrig, H.R., Elkin, P.L., & Chute, C.G. (2000). Embedded structures and representation of nursing knowledge. *Journal of the American Medical Informatics Association 7*(6):539–549.

Hier, D.B. (2002). Physician buy-in for an EMR. *Healthcare Informatics 19*(10):37–40.

Johnson, M., Maas, M., & Moorhead, S. (1997). *Nursing Outcomes Classification(NOC).* St. Louis: Mosby.

Jovic, L., Compagnon, A., & Fabre, F. (2002). [Best practice tools and decision support aids for nursing care.] *Rech Soins Infirm* 69:30–40.

Langton, K.B., Johnston, M.E., Haynes, R.B., & Mathieu, A. (1992). A critical appraisal of the literature on the effects of computer-based clinical decision support systems on clinician performance and patient outcomes. *In:Proceedings of the Annual Symposium on Computer Applications in Medical Care (SCAMC),* pp. 626–630.

Lyons, A., & Richardson, S. (2003). Clinical decision support in critical care nursing. *AACN Clinical Issues 14*(3):295–301.

McCloskey, J.C., & Bulechek, G.M. (1996). *Nursing Interventions Classification (NIC)*, 2nd ed. St. Louis: Mosby.

Misys HealthCare (2005). http://www.misyshealthcare.com (accessed February 8, 2005).

New, T.D. (2000). Clinical decision support tools in A&E nursing: a preliminary study. *Nursing Standard, 14*(34):32–39.

PalmOne (2005). http://www.palmone.com (accessed February 8, 2005).

Pryor, T.A. (1994). Development of decision support systems. In: Shabot, M.M., & Gardner, R.M. (eds) *Decision Support Systems in Critical Care.* New York: Springer-Verlag, pp. 61–72. Cited in Braden, B.J., Corritore, C., & McNees, P. (1994). Computerized decision support systems: Implications for practice. In: Gerdin, U., Tallberg, M., & Wainwright, P. (eds.) *The Impact of Nursing Knowledge on HealthCare Informatics.* Amsterdam: IOS Press, pp. 300–304.

Reilly, C.A., Zielstorff, R.D., & Fox, R.L., et al. (2000). A knowledge-based patient assessment system: conceptual and technical design. *Proceedings of AMIA Symposium*, pp. 680–684.

Ruland, C.M. (1999). Decision support for patient preference-based care planning: Effects on nursing care and patient outcomes. *Journal of the American Medical Informatics Association 6*(4):304–312.

Sensmeier, J., Raiford, R., Taylor, S., & Weaver, C. (2003). Improved operational efficiency through elimination of waste and redundancy. *Nursing Outlook 51*(3):S30–S32.

SpaceLabs (2005). http://www.spacelabs.com (accessed February 8, 2005).

The Compact Oxford English Dictionary (Second Edition) (1993). Oxford: Oxford University Press.

Additional Resources

Urden, L.D. (1996). Development of a nurse executive decision support database: A model for outcomes evaluation. Journal of Nursing Administration *26*(10):15–21.

Zielstorff, R.D., Estey, G., & Vickery, A., et al. (1997). Evaluation of a decision support system for pressure ulcer prevention and management: preliminary findings. *Journal of the American Medical Informatics Association, Symposium Supplement.* Nashville: Hanley & Belfus, pp. 248–252.

Part III
Applications of Nursing Informatics

7 Clinical Practice Applications: Facility Based

New applications for facility-based clinical practice continue to be the fastest growing area of interest in nursing informatics (Fig. 7.1). Although there are many technological advances discussed here, the areas of greatest interest are conceptual. Source data capture, the development and use of decision support and expert systems, and the development of a nursing minimum data set as they relate to facility-based care are the most important issues (see Chapter 12 for a full discussion). Although none of these concepts is easily categorized, the nursing process provides the structure for this chapter. Clinical applications of nursing informatics are related to assessment, planning, implementation, and evaluation.

Assessment

Computerization helps when gathering and storing data about each patient. For example, assessment data can be physiological measures automatically charted through a patient monitoring system (Newbold, 2003; Varon and Marik, 2002; Wong et al., 2003). Other assessment data are added to the electronic patient record by departments such as the laboratory and radiology. The largest source of assessment data is the ongoing nursing assessment. The following sections briefly describe these sources of assessment data.

Patient Monitoring

The major area of development for automated patient monitoring originally was coronary care. In coronary care units and pacemaker clinics, computers were initially used to monitor electrocardiograms, analyze the information, and reduce former volumes of data to manageable proportions, generally some type of graph. The computers were also programmed to recognize deviations from accepted norms and to alert attending personnel to the deviation by some indication (e.g., an alarm or light).

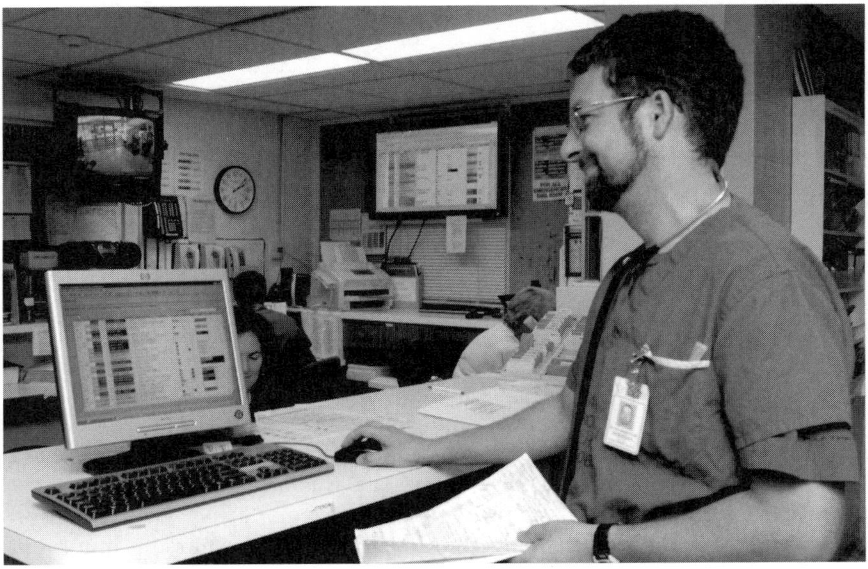

FIGURE 7.1. Facility-based nursing informatics. (Photograph courtesy of Cerner Corporation and St. Joseph's Health Care, London.)

In addition to arrhythmia monitoring, computers in acute care areas, such as emergency departments and intensive care (ICU), coronary care (CCU), and neonatal intensive care units, are now widely used for hemodynamic and vital sign monitoring, calculation of physiological indices such as peripheral vascular resistance and cardiac output, and environmental regulation of isolets. Sophisticated computerized ICU monitoring systems for management of patient data, including patients' heart rates, arterial blood pressure, temperature, respiratory rate, central venous pressure, intracranial pressure, and pulmonary artery pressures, are used around the world (Varon and Marik, 2002; Wong et al., 2003). Automated approaches to patient monitoring free the nurses from the technician role of watching machinery and allow them to focus their attention on the patient, the family, and the nursing process. It is now widely accepted that computerized cardiac monitoring of patients dramatically increases the early detection of arrhythmias and contributes to decreased mortality of CCU patients. Additionally, many of these monitoring systems are integrated into decision support systems (Staggers, 2003).

Assessment Data from Other Departments

Detailed discussion of computer systems designed for use in special diagnoses (e.g., laboratory, radiography), support (e.g., pharmacy, dietary), or special treatment (e.g., radiation therapy, dialysis) is beyond the scope of this book. However, patient data from many departments forms the basis for computerized patient care plans and many decision support systems. Nurses must be able to retrieve and use these data to provide quality patient care.

Nursing-Generated Assessment Data

Source data capture is the key to useful nursing generation of patient data. Source data capture means gathering data and information about patients where it originates, that is, with the patient. By entering data wherever the patient is, the reliability of the data is increased. There is less chance of transcription errors than if the nurses copy data they have written on their hands (or on pieces of paper towel) into the patient chart.

For source data capture to be feasible, nurses must be able to enter patient data from many places other than the nursing station. This need has required a revolution in computer hardware. The local nursing station terminal of the hospital mainframe computer is no longer adequate. Computer data entry must occur wherever patients are found. This is called a "point of care" information system. Goals for moving to point of care systems are identified as follows (Hughes, 1995).

- To minimize the time spent documenting patient information
- To eliminate redundancies and inaccuracies of charted information
- To improve the timeliness of data communication
- To optimize access to information
- To provide information required by the clinician to make the best possible patient care decisions

Source data capture is the first step reducing the time nurses spend charting and eliminating redundancies and inaccuracies. When information can be entered directly into the patient's electronic health record at the point of care by the healthcare professional or a medical device such as hemodynamic monitors, infusion pumps, or ventilators and it is made immediately available to others involved in the patient's care, time is saved and data have been accurately transformed into usable information (Hughes, 1995). Point of care systems use a variety of computer hardware. Ideally, a portable, real-time communication device with many input options (e.g., touch, pen, voice) able to display patient information as needed, including graphics, an easy documentation method, and long battery life, is preferred. Technology is fast moving toward this ideal. However, most point of care systems in existence rely on full-sized personal computers, workstations, bedside terminals, and some portable terminals (Figs. 7.2–7.4).

When considering the adoption of point of care systems, the following points should be evaluated.

1. Point of care systems must allow the nurse to interact with the main information system. Systems that do not allow information to be extracted, as well as entered, are not useful to nurses.

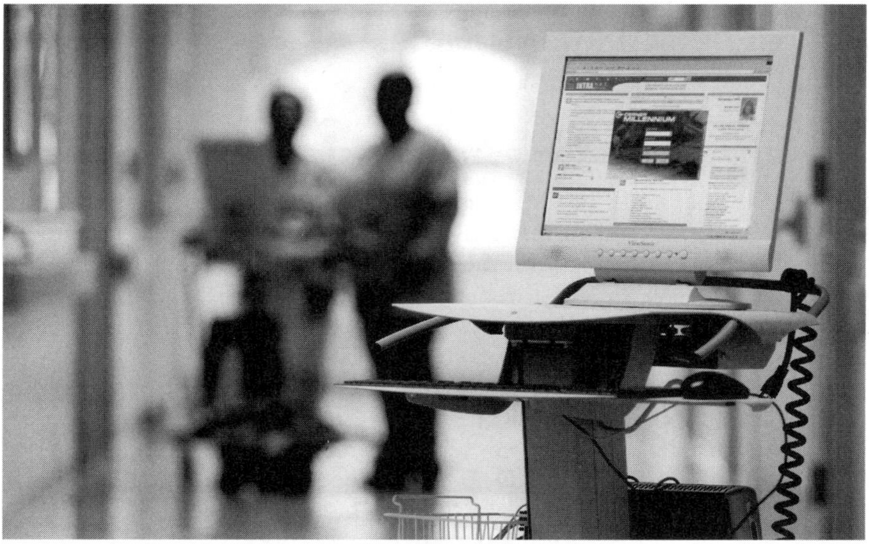

FIGURE 7.2. Portable terminal. (Photograph courtesy of Cerner Corporation.)

2. Point of care systems must interface with the existing hospital information system. The nurse at the patient's bedside must be able to access data that has been generated by the laboratory, or radiology, or pharmacy.
3. The open systems concept is valuable to nurses considering point of care systems. This concept allows machines from all vendors to communicate. Open systems allow the most appropriate type of machine to be selected for each nursing environment.
4. Point of care systems must have a small footprint (take up a small amount of floor space). Not all hospitals have the opportunity to configure a new building from the ground up. Most hospitals are trying to fit new technology into "old skin." Early examples of bedside terminals took up a large amount of space in patient rooms. With limited electrical outlets and no piped-in oxygen or suction, a patient room that had all the equipment necessary to care for seriously ill patients left no room for the nurse.
5. Point of care systems must be easy to use and must adapt to a variety of nursing environments. Patient contact occurs 24 hours a day. For example, bedside terminals must allow the nurse to access and input data without turning on the lights or disturbing the patient. The annoying little "beeps" a computer makes when you have made a mistake in data entry have no place in bedside terminals.
6. Point of care systems must be easily disinfected and cleaned between patients. Bedside keyboards should have a membrane keyboard or a protective "skin" over the keyboard to protect it from liquids.

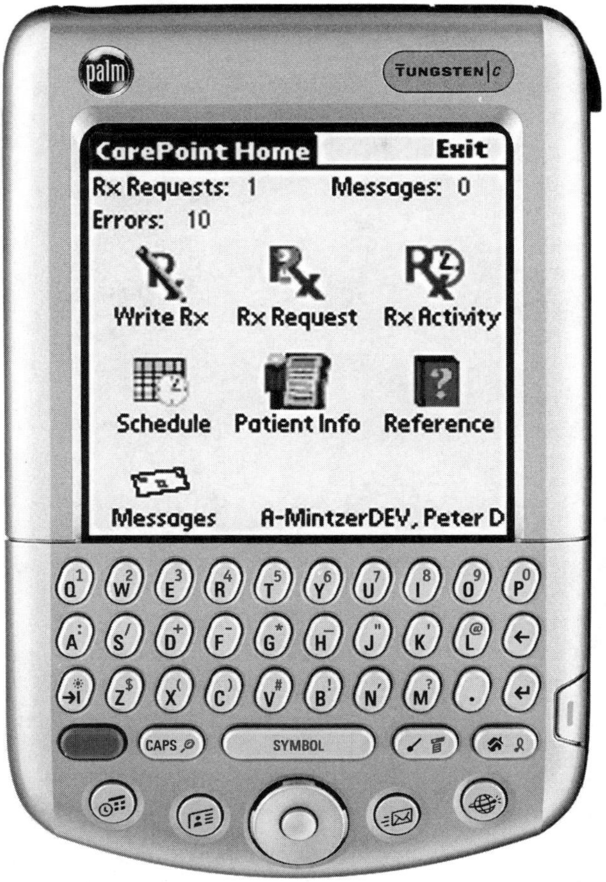

FIGURE 7.3. Portable terminal. (Photograph courtesy of palmOne.)

7. For source data capture to be easily accomplished, nurses require a variety of ways for entering data. Keyboards require some typing skills. Other devices include bar code readers (Fig. 7.5) for scanning identification bands and medications, physiological probes, microphones for voice input, light pens and touch screens, digital cameras, and natural speech input devices. The touch screen illustrated in Chapter 2 uses icons (pictures) rather than words. Icon menus are easier to use, especially if the exact key word is not known.
8. For effective source data capture, the nurse must go wherever the patient is. If that is the visiting lounge or the coffee shop or the outside deck, a fixed bedside terminal is not appropriate. Notebook technology and pen-based portable systems offer the best choice for mobility.

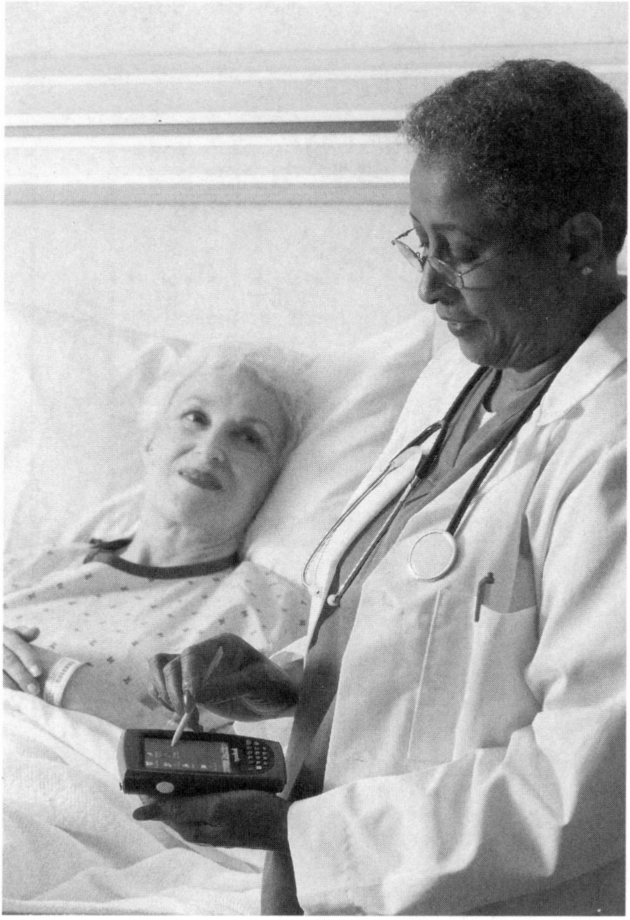

Figure 7.4. Portable terminal. (Photograph courtesy of Misys.)

9. Information to be retrieved using the point of care system must be represented in ways that can be quickly used and easily understood by nurses. Traditional nursing notes are voluminous. Trying to find key data in a narrative is too time-consuming when the information is urgently needed. Figure 7.6 illustrates a cardiac risk assessment tool. At a glance, the nurse can tell which factors must be addressed.

We have talked about the advantages of using source data capture through point of care systems. Alternatives to traditional charting have also been mentioned. However, a brief discussion of computer-mediated documentation is necessary because it is the primary application of nursing informatics in many institutions.

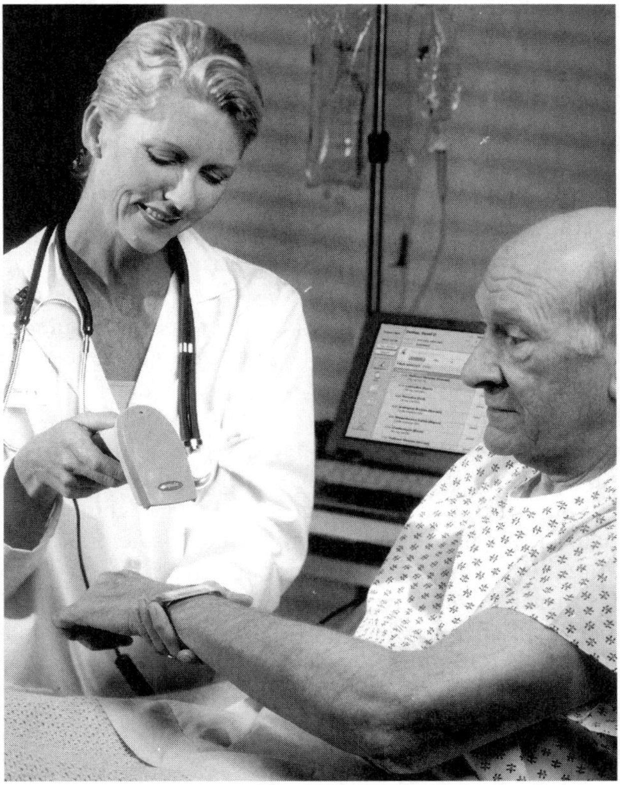

FIGURE 7.5. Bar code reader. (Photograph courtesy of Bridge Medical.)

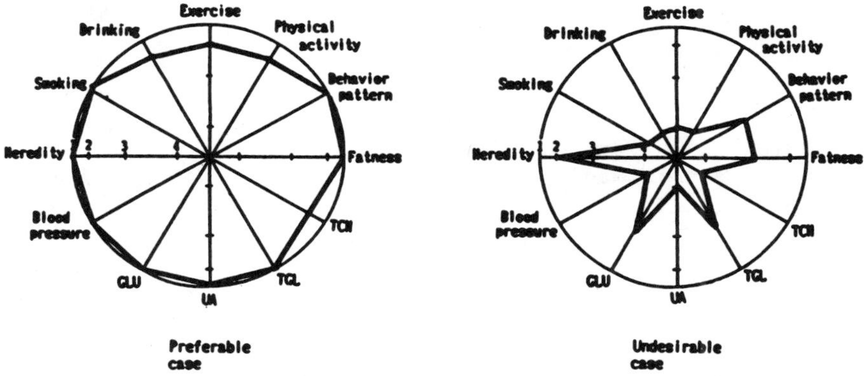

FIGURE 7.6. Cardiac risk assessment. (From Bakker AR, Ball MJ, Scherver JR, Willems JL (eds). Towards New Hospital Information Systems. New York: Elsevier-North Holland, 1988, with permission.)

Documentation

Good nurses' notes are generally lengthy, narrative, handwritten, and unbiased observations. At their worst, they are inaccurate, inconsistent, incomplete, or consist of such trivia as, "Had a good day." Automated methods for recording nursing observations are some of the most readily available nursing informatics applications. Two approaches predominate. With the first approach, a computerized library of frequently used phrases is arranged in subject categories. The nurse chooses the phrase or combination of phrases that best describes the patient's condition. For example, by selecting a primary subject such as "sleeping habits," a screen menu of standard descriptions appear, allowing for additionally selected comments such as "slept through breakfast—voluntarily" or "awoke early at a.m." When completed, the nursing station printer immediately prints a standard, easy-to-read, complete narrative that could then be attached to the patient's chart. An example of an assessment screen is shown in Figure 7.7.

The second approach has been to develop a "branching questionnaire." The terminal displays a list of choices, and the nurse selects her choice and indicates it by pressing the corresponding number on the keyboard or touching the terminal with a light-sensitive input device (called a light pen). The terminal then displays a further list of choices appropriate to the original selection. Thus, the nurse is led through a series of questions that can be "customized"

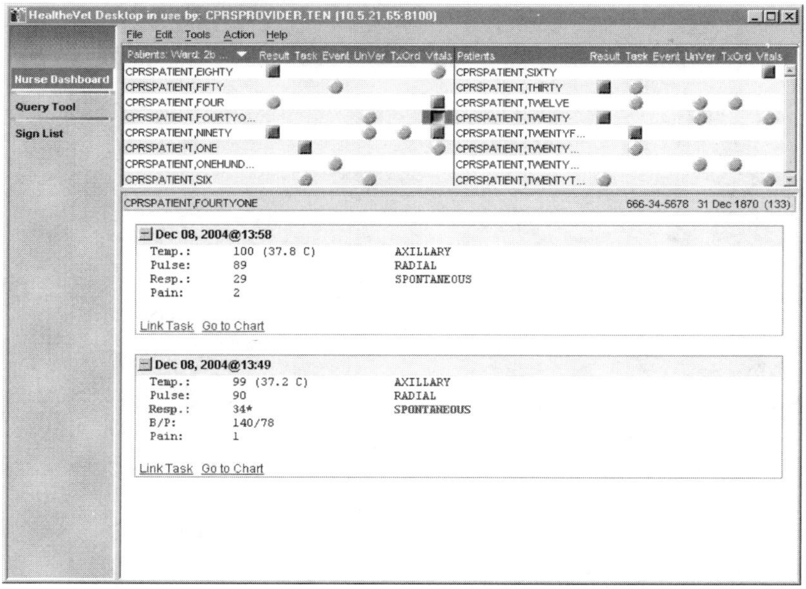

FIGURE 7.7. Example of an assessment screen. (Photograph courtesy of Department of Veterans Affairs, Office of Information.)

for each patient. For example, a question might be "Skin intact—yes, no." If "yes" was selected, no further questions in that set would be necessary. If "no" was selected, other choices might appear such as a choice between "wounds," "pressure ulcers," and so on. The option of free-form input is usually available via the terminal's keyboard. At the user's signal that the entry has been completed, the computer processes the information and provides a narrative printout for the patient's chart. In both approaches, the option of free-form narrative text input, using the keyboard, is usually also available.

Many advantages that have been claimed for automated documentation of nursing observations include the following (Husting and Cintron, 2003; Moody et al., 2004).

- Content standardization: increased charting completeness including increased numbers of observations because of prompting or forced recall and increased standardization, accuracy, and reliability of observations
- Improved standards compliance
- Increased efficiency: legible notes, which decrease reading time and increase accuracy of interpretation and elimination of repetitive data recording and resulting transcription errors
- Enhanced timeliness: less time spent writing notes, specifically end-of-shift charting
- Expanded accessibility: data available on-line immediately and access not limited to one person at a time as with paper record
- Augmented data archive: ready statistical analysis and easier nursing audit because of the use of standard terminology

Better observations—that is, increased number, accuracy, and reliability of observations—facilitate better assessment, planning, and evaluation of nursing care. Less time spent writing notes provides more time for assessment, planning, implementing, and evaluating care. Increased use and accuracy when interpreting notes facilitates consistency and continuity of care. Statistical analysis facilitates research that ultimately leads to refinements in the nursing process and improved patient care.

Data Issues

Nurses spend a great deal of time and energy gathering data. Unfortunately, many of these data are probably for someone else's use (e.g., administrative or government statistics). Often these same data are duplicated by the data-gathering activities of other healthcare professionals (e.g., how many times are patients who are being admitted to your institution asked by different categories of staff why these patients have presented themselves). Similarly, data are gathered ostensibly for nursing use but are never looked at again (e.g., the voluminous nursing histories gathered in many institutions). Nurses should only be gathering data that are essential for nursing decisions about patient care. The principle involved is to gather essential information while avoiding replication and duplication of data that waste resources such as manpower, storage space, and memory. Although much research remains to be done in this aspect of nursing practice, the foundation work has been done that defines that essential information (see Chapter 12 for a detailed discussion of minimum data sets and nursing classification systems).

Planning

Automated Care Planning

In most healthcare settings, the kardex or some similar tool has been the repository of nursing care plans. This tool has had drawbacks similar to those encountered with nursing notes as well as other drawbacks that are unique to the kardex. Nursing care plans, if they are ever entered in the kardex at all, are usually outdated, illegible, inconsistent, and incomplete. Notations are made by all levels of nursing personnel from nursing aides to head nurses. Written patient care assignments are usually accompanied by verbal explanations that are often forgotten.

Alternate approaches to the automation of nursing care plans is to design care maps or pathways for meeting patient needs, store them in the computer memory banks, and then adapt them to individual patients (Catt et al., 1997; Renholm et al., 2002). The resulting printout is unique for each patient's assessed needs for daily care. In all cases, it is the nurse who assesses, plans, and evaluates the plan for care, although auxiliary personnel might be involved in implementing the plan. The evolving approach to care planning is the development of decision support systems for nursing practice.

The following list summarizes the advantages of automated care plans or pathways over traditional nursing care plans.

- Time is saved by eliminating the need for daily handwriting of patient assignments and by decreasing the amount of verbal explanation required.
- Accountability is increased because personnel have printouts of care plans for each of their patients.
- Errors and omissions are decreased.
- Consistency of care from shift to shift and day to day is increased; quality of patient care improves.
- Judgments for nursing care are no longer delegated to whoever walks into a room to care for the patient; they are the responsibility of the professional nurse who now has tools available to help make nursing judgments.

There are many implications of these advantages for nursing practice (DeLuc, 2000). Time saved during the preparation and communication of care plans means more time available for the nursing process. Increased accountability for care improves nursing practice because documentation is available to evaluate the quality of care and thus the quality of practice.

Benefits to patient care of decreased errors and omissions and increased consistency of care include more rapid diagnosis, more valid assessment, and more rapid recovery. These factors all reduce the cost of healthcare for the patient and open the system to more patients. Placing the responsibility for nursing judgments clearly on the shoulders of the professional nurse helps define nursing practice and helps the profession in its search for a clearly delineated identity.

Decision Support Systems

Decision support systems help nurses maintain and maximize their decision-making responsibilities and focus on the highest priority aspects of patient care. The care planning systems previously described are not decision support systems. Standardized care plans, whether manual or computer-based, provide care only for standardized patients. Standardized care plans do not enhance nursing decision-making; on the contrary, their "cook-book" approach discourages active decision-making by nurses.

A true decision support system allows nurses to enter their assessments at the bedside using source data capture technology (discussed earlier) and then use the computer to analyze those assessments and recommend nursing diagnoses. The nurse then accepts or rejects the recommendations. Having accepted a particular diagnosis, the range of interventions acceptable in that agency or institution can be retrieved and presented by the computer. The nurse can then choose the nursing interventions appropriate for the patient (Wong et al., 2000).

Decision support systems are being developed for a variety of care settings and situations. Decision support systems are useful because each nurse's repertoire of interventions is based solely on previous professional experience. The nurse's repertoire is also influenced by a "forgetting" curve. If the nurse has not encountered a specific nursing diagnosis for a long time, the remembered interventions may not reflect the whole repertoire. The advisory or expert system not only accumulates the experience of *all* nurses in the organization but also serves as a "reminding" function. Decision support systems have been developed for a variety of settings, including critical care (Lyons and Richardson, 2003), cancer pain management (Im and Chee, 2003), and pediatric fever (Lambell et al., 2003).

As you may have noted, decision support systems are not appropriate for all patient care settings or at all times. Emergencies such as cardiac arrest do not allow time for the nurse to scroll through suggested actions. Highly complex patient problems may also prove too great a challenge for the current types of decision support systems. In addition, decision support systems are usually designed to address nursing diagnoses one at a time, not in combination.

Decision support systems can never replace the need for nurses with expert clinical and decision-making skills. Brennan and McHugh (1988, p. 93) stated that the "complexity and/or detail necessary in the decision making process are beyond human capacities, yet some human judgment is necessary either because all the information needed to make a decision is not available to the computer, or because the decision making process is too poorly understood to specify the steps in such a way that the computer can be programmed to make the decision." Therefore, the nurse is still required to exercise clinical judgment, regardless of whether a decision-modeling or expert system has been used. The fundamental idea that must be stressed is that decision support tools should *add* to the nurse's decision-making capacity, not attempt to replace it.

Implementation

Computers rarely help the nurse in the giving of care or nursing service. Generally, computers are used more in other phases of the nursing process. One example of how computers are used in intervention is the programmed administration of preloaded drugs in the ICU.

Evaluation

Computers can be used to evaluate nursing care through real-time auditing and quality management activities. These uses are discussed in detail in Chapter 9.

Summary

Nurses must respond to the challenge to identify the data essential for decisions about patient care; "Nurses cannot leave the decision making about nursing's essential retrievable data to vendors and other healthcare professionals; those decisions are part of the responsibilities that members of an autonomous profession must assume" (Werley, 1988, p. 431). Nurses must also evaluate technology so it better serves their needs and the needs of their patients. Finally, now is the time to capture the immense collective knowledge of nurses to create the decision support systems that will lead to consistent, high-quality patient care and acknowledgment of our nursing expertise.

References

Brennan, P.F., & McHugh, M. (1988). Clinical decision-making and computer support. *Applied Nursing Research 1*(2):89–93.

Catt, M.A., Nagle, L.M., & Shamian, J.S. (1997). The patient care process: Pathways in transition. In: Gerdin, U., Talberg, M., & Wainwright, P. (eds.) *Nursing Informatics: The Impact of Nursing Knowledge on HealthCare Informatics*. Amsterdam: IOS Press, pp. 318–329.

De Luc, K. (2000). Care pathways: an evaluation of their effectiveness. *Journal of Advanced Nursing 32*(2):485–496.

Hughes, S.J. (1995). Point-of-care information systems: state of the art. In: Ball, M.J., Hannah, K.J., Newbold, S.K., & Douglas, J.V. (eds.) *Nursing Informatics: Where Caring and Technology Meet*, 2nd ed. New York: Springer, pp. 144–154.

Husting, P.M., & Cintron, L. (2003). Healthcare information systems: education lessons learned. *Journal for Nurses in Staff Development 19*(5):249–253.

Im, E.O., Chee, W. (2003). Decision support computer program for cancer pain management. *CIN: Computers, Informatics, Nursing 21*(1):12–21.

Lambell, P., Coopers, A., Hoyles, S., Pygall, S.A., & O'Cathain, A. (2003). An audit of paediatric fever in MHS Direct: consistency of advice by nurses using computerized decision support software systems. *Clinical Governance 8*(3):222–227.

Lyons, A., & Richardson, S. (2003). Clinical decision support in critical care nursing. *AACN Clinical Issues: Advanced Practice in Acute Critical Care 14*(3):295–301.

Moody, L.E., Slocumb, E., Berg, B., & Jackson, D. (2004). Electronic health records documentation in nursing: nurses' perceptions, attitudes, and preferences. *CIN: Computers, Informatics, Nursing 22*(6):337–344.

Newbold, S.K. (2003). New uses for wireless technology. *Nursing Management* October: 22–27, Special edition: IT Solutions.

Renholm, M., Leino-Kilpi, H., & Suominen, T. (2002). Critical pathways: a systematic review. *Journal of Nursing Administration 32*(4):196–202.

Staggers, N. (2003). Human factors: imperative concepts for information systems in critical care. *AACN Clinical Issues: Advanced Practice in Acute & Critical Care 14*(3):310–319.

Varon, J., & Marik, P. (2002). Clinical information systems and the electronic medical record in the intensive care unit. *Current Opinion in Critical Care 8*(6):616–624.

Werley, H.H. (1988). Research directions. In: Werley, H.H., Lang, N.M. (eds.) *Identification of the Nursing Minimum Data Set.* New York: Springer, pp. 427–431.

Wong, D.H., Gallegos, Y., Weinger, M.B., Clock, S., Slagle, J. & Anderson, C.T. (2003). Changes in intensive care unit nurse task activity after installation of a third-generation intensive care unit information system. *Critical Care Medicine 31*(10):2488–2494.

Wong, H.J., Legnini, M.W., & Whitmore, H.H. (2000). The diffusion of decision support systems in healthcare: are we there yet? *Journal of Healthcare Management 45*(4):240–249.

8 Clinical Practice Applications: Community Based

Community-based care is the fastest growing segment of healthcare. Health reform in all parts of the world has meant a decrease in the number of hospital beds and an increase in home care. Community-based health promotion and illness prevention programs are also increasing. Surveillance programs must also be maintained. Informatics are playing an integral role in facilitating community-based care. Many community-based organizations have information systems that mirror those of hospital facilities. Systems are typically used for tracking, scheduling, billing, and human resources functions. Because of health reform reorganization, many community-based care providers and organizations are now incorporated into regional health systems. Often the information systems are also combined.

Patient appointment-identification systems are found in many community-based settings. At this level of computer support for nursing, three functions are performed by the automated system. The patient appointment system helps the scheduling of a patient's clinic visits to minimize waiting time, smooth the clinic load, and establish patient priorities for appointments along carefully delineated guidelines. The second function is to maintain the patient registry and determine the extent to which the patient must pay for services and establish billing procedures for third-party liability for each individual patient. The third function of this system is to maintain security and guarantee the privacy and confidentiality of the remainder of the patient record. Access is limited to authorized personnel: Nurses and physicians have total access, secretaries and laboratory technicians have limited access. This type of system frees the nurse from many tedious clerical chores. By restricting access to the patient record, this system maintains the confidentiality of the patient record and thus increases the credibility of the professional staff by assuring patients that their confidences are truly confidential. This fact is particularly important in such areas of distributive nursing as mental health clinics and venereal disease clinics, where the risk of social stigma is a significant factor in an individual's decision to seek care.

The greatest gains in applying informatics to the community setting have come from the linkage with telecommunications. This chapter describes the concepts of telehealth and provides examples of applications in a variety of settings.

Telehealth

The nurse in the community and the hospital-based nurse require similar information to deliver the required patient care. Both practitioners require patient demographic data, past medical history, diagnosis, laboratory, and radiology test results, and a treatment and/or care plan. Additionally, whether in the hospital or community setting, delivery of patient care is facilitated by the availability of patient teaching materials, policies and procedures, drug and treatment information, technical data, community services listings, and current contact directions. The point of care is in the community or the patient's home. Traditionally, however, the patient's medical record, policy and procedure manuals, teaching materials, and clinical reference books are inaccessible because they are kept in the agency offices. Another key missing link in community-based care, yet traditional in the hospital setting, is collaboration with a multidisciplinary health team during delivery of patient care. Telehealth offers technological and information systems solutions to many of the challenges of community-based nursing practice.

There have been many definitions of telemedicine in the literature, but few definitions to aptly define telehealth, an integrating and more holistic term encompassing all the telematics applications in health and healthcare. In Europe, the field is referred to as *healthcare telematics*. Also in Europe, Telenursing is not related to telecommunications applications specifically but is the name of the European Community (EC) classification and nomenclature project. *Telehealth* is defined as "the use of communications and information technology to deliver health and healthcare services and information over large and small distances" (Picot, 1997). Telehealth is born of the confluence of information technology and telecommunications (IT&T), healthcare, and medical technology. Each of these three sectors is undergoing transformation although in quite different directions. The first, IT&T, is enjoying accelerated growth with rapid technological and regulatory changes. Healthcare and medical technology, however, have lately been subject to downsizing and restructuring in many parts of the world. Several factors are influencing the development of telehealth.

- *Aging population*: The needs of aging healthcare consumers have initiated efforts to develop and adopt better telehealth systems outside institutional walls, systems that would be better geared for home-based applications.
- *Cost containment*: Telehealth systems are facilitating redistribution of healthcare services, reducing duplication, reducing numbers of drug interactions and inappropriate prescriptions, and reducing patient and professional travel.

- *Access*: Demand is increasing for equitable access to healthcare services for inhabitants of isolated geographic areas (e.g., in sparsely populated areas of Canada's north and in many parts of Latin America, China, and Africa).
- *Technology*: Ever more powerful technologies and communications bandwidths are becoming available at decreasing costs.
- *Demand*: The increasing consumer demand for wellness and health information of all kinds has fueled increased access to the Internet and the World Wide Web.
- *Information explosion*: The exponential increase in medical and health information has given rise to demands for better information management systems, faster and more efficient electronic access, and better on-line research networks.

Telehealth encompasses practices, products, and services bringing healthcare and health information to remote locations. Remote can mean across the street or across the globe. Telehealth extends the arm of the healthcare system for people at home and provides health services direct to consumers. It offers continuing medical, nursing, and health education and assists consumers in obtaining emergency assistance wherever they may be. Health informatics and telematics applications are incorporated, using communications technologies in association with monitoring and medical devices; emergency systems; health, medical, and computer systems to transform and transfer health content and deliver health services; education; and assistance at a distance. An overview of possible applications is found in Table 8.1 (Picot, 1997, p. 8). Specific applications are described later in the chapter.

Nursing telepractice is nursing-specific application of telehealth that includes all client-centered forms of nursing practice and the provision of information, conferences, and courses for health professionals occurring through, or facilitated by, the use of telecommunications or electronic means (CNA, 2001). A nursing role in telehealth is found in a variety of applications including call centers (Omery, 2003; Valanis et al., 2003), specific disease management (Hill et al., 2004; Pierce et al., 2002; Roupe, 2004; Wilbright et al., 2004), and community health (Hill and Weinert, 2004; Johnston, et al., 2000; Young and Ireson, 2003). The remainder of the chapter describes a variety of telehealth applications used by nurses in nursing telepractice.

The technologies and systems used for telehealth vary greatly from one application to another. However, each application, even the simplest, contains at least three components.

1. A device or means to capture, process, and store content (*input*)—whether sound only, electronic or digital images, tracings, alpha-numeric data, or a combination
2. Content and a means to transfer or exchange the content (*throughput*)—communications, telecommunications, or network technologies of all kinds and their associated software

Table 8.1. Telehealth applications that can facilitate healthcare procedures

Healthcare procedure, process	Possible telehealth application
Telephone-based or face-to-face consultation between specialists and general practitioner	Videoconferencing, IATV, computer-based e-mail
Physical transfer of medical image for specialist opinion on radiographs, ultrasound, CT scans, pathology slides	Electronic transfer of images to specialists via any number of networks Comparison of images against banks of stored electronic slides and images for comparison
Handwritten, paper-based patient files and charts	Palmtop pen-based computer tablets, desktop workstations, computerized patient records
Handwritten, paper-based prescriptions	Electronic ordering of the prescription using a CHIN, HIN, or pharmanet
Consulting CPS for information regarding drug being prescribed	Drug interaction software, drug information database on line
Home visits unassisted by technology	Laptop or portable computer with modern to communicate with physician or healthcare institution
Home care, elder care	Telemonitoring from the home; assisted devices and technologies
Visits to the emergency room of the local hospital	Telecare, tele-assisted triage, 1–900 telephone calls to obtain assistance, video visits
Referrals from general practitioner	Appointments by e-mail, by electronic scheduling from general practitioner's office
Patient traveling from remote location if requiring specialized counselling, diagnosis, or treatment	Videoconsultation with specialist from afar
Literature search in medical library for current literature on new procedures, clinical trials, etc.	Electronic search from home or office using Medline or other medical information management and database retrieval service
Travel to another location for grand rounds, CME, conference, meetings, seminars	Attendance from home or office via audio, video, or computer conferencing, or IATV
Clinical trials	Clinical trial management systems, expert advice on line

CT, computed tomography; CPS, Compendium of Pharmaceutical Specialties;
CME, Continuing medical education; IATV, interactive television;
CHIN, community health information network; HIN, health information network.

3. A means for receiving, storing, and displaying the content (*output*)—possibly a video monitor, a computer file server, or a recorder of some kind

The various technological systems are used to transfer different kinds of information, such as epidemiological, clinical, research, or educational. Users range from healthcare professionals and administrators to patients and consumers. Settings for telehealth include pharmacies, hospitals, clinics, physician's offices, remote nursing stations, and private homes. Table 8.2

Table 8.2. Categorization of telehealth applications and users

Category	User
1. All forms of healthcare at a distance: teleconsultations, telepathology, teleradiology, telepsychiatrty, teledermatology, telecardiology	Physicians Nurses Psychologists Other healthcare professionals Healthcare institutions
2. Interinstitutional patient and clinical records and information systems: electronic health and clinical records and databases accessible by network	Healthcare institutions and organizations Healthcare professionals Researchers Physicians offices and community health centers
3. Public Health and Community Health Information Networks (CHINs) and multiple-use health information networks	Government (including policy makers) Epidemiologists Public health professionals Pharmacies Healthcare providers' offices and clinics
4. Tele-education and multimedia applications for health professionals, and patients, and networked research databases. Internet services	Healthcare professionals Patients and consumers Universities and colleges
5. Telemonitoring, telecare networks, telephone triage, remote home care and emergency networks	Consumers Elderly Chronically ill Telenurses Call center users and operators

categorizes telehealth applications and users (Picot, 1997). This categorization is used to structure the following discussion of more specific telehealth applications.

1. *All forms of healthcare at a distance: teleconsultations, telepathology, teleradiology, telepsychiatry, teledermatology, telecardiology.* The Telemedicine Exchange Database (http://tie.telemed.org) reports more than 200 telemedicine projects worldwide, including those concerned with dermatology, oncology, radiology, pathology, surgery, cardiology, and psychiatry. Echocardiograms, frozen sections, ultrasound seans, computed tomography (CT) scans, and mammograms are routinely sent by telemedicine applications between remote centers and receiving institutions and between researchers requiring more than the written word. Many of these applications have implications for nurses in both remote and urban areas. In remote areas, videophones, digital medical imaging (X-rays), and electrocardiography (ECG) monitors transmitting over a regular telephone line can be used to provide information for a consultation with a physician or hospital (Artinian, 2004; Halstead et al., 2003). In the same way, in urban areas it is often the nurse who uses the technology to gather the patient information that is transmitted to medical facilities.

The U.S. military operates one of the largest telemedicine organizations and is especially active in researching new applications and technologies (Zajchuk and Zajchuk, 1996). With its military personnel located in 70 geographic locations worldwide, telemedicine provides medical personnel in the field with 24-hour tertiary care capability. The MERMAID (medical emergency aid through telematics) system uses the full range of telecommunications technology, including two-way transfer of live images to maximize the effectiveness of medical assistance to sailors at sea (Anogianakis and Maglavera, 1997). Several areas use telemedicine in correctional facilities to decrease transfers of inmates, thereby improving the safety of healthcare personnel and the public (Picot, 1997; TRC, 1997).

2. *Interinstitutional patient and clinical records and information systems: electronic health and clinical records and databases accessible by network.* Telehealth covers the use of networks to link care providers and their institutions. Regional health networks and community health information networks (CHINs) often include pharmanets, which link clinics and physicians' offices to pharmacies for the transmission of information regarding prescriptions. At the basis of the CHIN and the community health management information system (CHMIS) is the electronical health information system (EHIS) or electronic health record (EHR) (see Chapter 5 for more detail). A major trend in telehealth applications is the integration of health networks, including institution-based and community-based systems. The major benefits are realized from avoiding duplication, timely provision of information, reducing unnecessary multiple diagnostical procedures, and optimizing resources.

3. *Public health and community health information networks (CHINs) and multiple-use health information networks.* Surveillance systems and registries are being used increasingly by policy makers and funders to measure progress and compare delivery systems. Population health networks permit epidemiologists, health policy makers, and governments as well as public health officials to exchange information regarding the health status of entire populations. This type of information has become all the more valuable in recent times because of the prevalence of certain diseases believed to have environmental causes. The WHO makes increasing use of the Internet to disseminate population health information widely (http://www.who.org).

Disease surveillance networks are designed to identify epidemics and emerging diseases. National governments have supported such networks to support disease prevention efforts and to monitor and control risks to health. It will be some years before fully operational global emergency and disease prevention networks become a reality. There is a growing realization that such networks are essential in light of the high volume of travel and exchange between countries and the growing number of senior and frail travelers.

4. *Tele-education and multimedia applications for health professionals and patients; networked research databases, and Internet services.* Tele-education, not telemedicine, constitutes the principal content in many telehealth

networks. Mediated distance education for health professionals has been ongoing since the 1930s, when radio was the main communication medium. Many universities and colleges worldwide offer credit and noncredit courses by distance using all forms of telecommunications, from videoconferencing to the Internet. Virtual nursing education for postbasic degree programs is available across North America and Europe from a variety of universities. Continuing medical education (CME) and continuing nursing education (CNE) are increasingly offered via telecommunications and computer-based networks. In many institutional settings, the teleconferencing facilities used for telemedicine applications are also used for tele-educational purposes.

Patient education remains a growing field. The advent of the Internet and the World Wide Web (WWW) have had a substantial impact on tele-education for consumers (Dauz et al., 2004). Consumers now have access to health information that previously was unavailable to them, even in public libraries. Web sites offering medical advice are popular, as are newsgroups, electronic medical forums, virtual hospital, and even disease support networks, such as Global Health Network (www.globalhealthnetwork.org). The WWW is also a source of wellness information, although with quackery as a potential hazard there is rising demand for guarantors granting legitimate status to the content published by various information providers.

5. *Telemonitoring, telecare networks, telephone triage, remote home care, and emergency networks*. It is difficult to discuss each of these applications separately as many overlaps occur in reality. The rise of ambulatory care, shorter hospital stays, and the care of the elderly and chronically ill in the home setting have all generated community care needs that can be effectively met, in part, with video visits or telemonitoring devices. New products such as cardiac monitoring and hemodialysis systems complete with telephone coupling mechanisms have been developed to serve this need. Videoconferencing systems, including the use of videophones for home care video visits, are gaining in popularity. Examples include the use of videophones to monitor persons with congestive heart failure (Jenkins and McSweeney, 2001; Johnston et al., 2000), home-ventilated children (Miyasaka, 1997), and cystic fibrosis patients (Adachi, 1997) and to provide stroke rehabilitation (Clark et al., 2002). Videophones are becoming widely available and, as the cost decreases, will be used increasingly in healthcare. Videophones do not require a computer; they use standard telephone lines; and the technology is as simple as making a phone call. Videophones include a wide range of features to facilitate telehealth applications including electronic pan, tilt, zoom, self-view, and autoanswer.

Telecounseling using videoconferencing or videophone technology has been reported as having high user satisfaction and reducing travel costs to both patient and professional. Some patients prefer the television monitor or videophone to the face-to-face experience (Elford and House, 1997; Johnston et al., 2000; Strecher et al., 2002). Telepyschiatry and telecounseling applications are expected to rise, as practitioners are increasingly located in large urban areas where most patients are located. Relocating psychiatrical and mental health professionals to rural areas may not be feasible because of the lower numbers of patients in rural or remote areas.

Another outgrowth of the telecounseling application is the advent of on-line support groups, either sponsored by an organization specifically for its patients (Hill and Weinert, 2004; Pierce et al. 2002) or open to the general public. ComputerLink projects serving persons living with acquired immuno-deficiency syndrome (AIDS) and caregivers of persons with Alzheimer's disease provide information organized in an electronic encyclopedia, electronic communication including public bulletin boards and private mail, and a decision support service. Comments from users have indicated that the ComputerLink serves as a "support system without walls" (Brennan, 1997, p. 522).

In-home monitoring is available for ECG, blood pressure, heart rate, and peak-flow spirometer readings (Artinian, 2004; Johnston et al., 2000). In many instances the facility receiving the transmissions speaks directly to the patient while the information is being transmitted. Immediate feedback can be given to the patient; and if necessary, ambulance services or mobile intensive care units can be summoned. This approach removes the intervention of third parties who have traditionally taken the ECG and transmitted it to the physician and reduces the number of unnecessary visits to emergency departments. Natori et al. (1997) has reported on a program for low risk pregnant women to transmit their own cardiotocograms via e-mail and thus reduce routine physician visits.

Video and telecommunications technology, sometimes but not always coupled with telemonitoring, has spawned the development of many remote home care programs for the elderly (Clark, 2002; Johnston et al., 2000). The benefits of this type of program are identified as follows (Roman, 1997, p. 79).

- Empowerment and independence of the elderly patient
- Return to the comfort of home with the security of flexible healthcare for an estimated 5% of those currently in nursing homes
- Great savings to nations

Some additional home care services that can be teleassisted, partly replacing and augmenting home care visits, include the following: wound management; oncology patient management via home infusion; electronic and tele-house calls; remote programmable infusion; blood glucose meters with telecommunication capabilities; telemonitoring of hemodialysis; use of laptop computers by home care nurses to note and check the medication and progress on patients' electronic health records and to communicate electronically with home care teams; and emergency or alert systems linking homes to clinics or hospitals (Picot, 1997) (Fig. 8.1).

The healthcare sector is increasingly using the concept of call centers in the delivery of services. Many jurisdictions and managed care organizations have implemented toll-free numbers and call centers to handle healthcare queries and problems. Nurses are providing emergency or first level information and triage and advice over the telephone (Omery, 2003; Valanis et al., 2003).

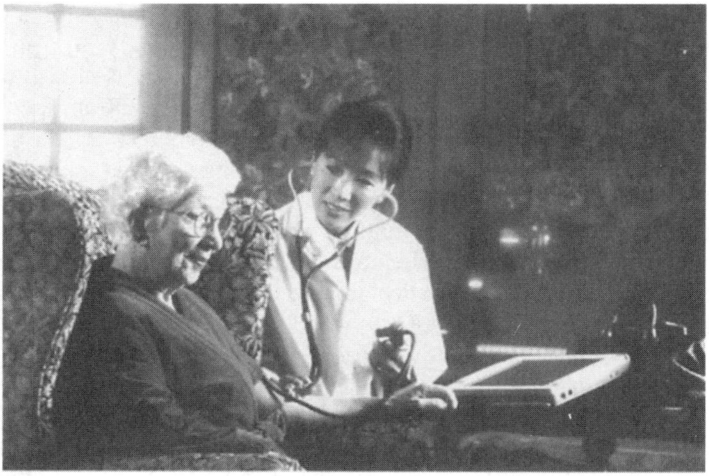

FIGURE 8.1. Community-based nursing informatics. (Courtesy of Prologix.)

Challenges Related to Telehealth

Although the potential for telehealth applications to contribute to healthcare is unlimited, several challenges remain to be addressed.

- *Obsolescence*: Many of the technologies have a short shelf life. Rapid obsolescence is a major concern for managers and administrators because most information technologies come in 18- to 36-month cycles, each bringing significant increases in processing speeds, flexibility, and storage capacity and decreases in price.
- *Access*: Even with user acceptance and available funding, telehealth is not accessible to any and all who need it. Technical infrastructure dictates at least in part the if, how, where, when, and what of telehealth technologies that can be implemented.
- *Health information infrastructures*: The creation of a health information infrastructure requires integration of existing and new architectures and application systems and services. A core element of this infrastructure includes patient-centered care facilitated by computer-based patient record systems (electronic patient record).
- *Provider reimbursement*: The issue of physician and other provider compensation for telehealth services has yet to be resolved in most jurisdictions.
- *Interdisciplinary and interinstitutional collaboration*: Jurisdictional conflicts between institutions and among physicians, nurses, pharmacists, radiologists, and nuclear medicine specialists must be resolved.
- *Documentation standards*: Telehealth documentation standards must be developed for use by all providers to ensure a useful and usable patient record.

- *Data security*: Confidentiality, privacy, and security issues related to the collection, storage, and transmission of patient information must be resolved to the satisfaction of professionals and consumers alike.
- Liability issues: Medical and nursing responsibility issues related to continuing responsibility for a patient's care, liability of consultants' opinions, and licensing for cross-jurisdictional consultation must be resolved.

Summary

The development of inexpensive, reliable telecommunications technology enables health professionals, patients, and consumers to access health information, healthcare resources, and health service delivery directly from and in their homes. Telehealth applications exist as discrete nursing interventions and provide pathways for nurses to reach patients and provide nursing interventions. Nurses can use technology to assist them in providing home care and in-home monitoring. Networks serve as educational vehicles whereby nurses can reach patients and clients with health promotion, disease and prevention, information, and illness management nursing interventions. Telehealth applications hold, great promise for extending the ability of nurses to reach individuals in communities and the communities themselves.

References

Adachi, T. (1997). How videophones affect patient's families. In: *Proceedings of the 3rd International Conference on the Medical Aspects of Telemedicine*, Kobe, Japan, p. 58.

Anogianakis, G., & Maglavera, S. (1997). MERMAID—medical emergency aid through telematics. In: *Proceedings of the 3rd International Conference on the Medical Aspects of Telemedicine*, Kobe, Japan, p. 154.

Artinian, N.T. (2004). Innovations in blood pressure monitoring: New, automated devices provide in-home or around-the-clock readings. *American Journal of Nursing 104*(8):52–58.

Brennan, P.F. (1997). The ComputerLink projects: A decade of experience. In: Gerdin, U., Tallberg, M., Wainwright, P. (eds.) *Nursing Informatics: The Impact of Nursing Knowledge on HealthCare Informatics*. Amsterdam: IOS Press, pp. 521–525.

Canadian Nurses Association. (2001). The role of the nurse in telepractice. Ottawa: Canada.

Clark, D. (2002). Older adults living through and with their computers. *CIN: Computers, Informatics, Nursing 20*(3):117–124.

Clark, P.G., Dawson, S.J., Scheideman-Miller, C., Post, M.L. (2002). TeleRehab: Stroke teletherapy and management using two-way interactive video. *Neurology Report 26*(2):87–94.

Dauz, E., Moore, J., Smith, C., Puno, F., & Schaag, H. (2004). Installing computers in older adults' homes and teaching them to access a patient education web site: A systematic approach. *CIN: Computers, Informatics, Nursing 22*(5):266–272.

Elford, D.R., & House, A.M. (1997). Telemedicine experience in Canada 1956–1996. Presented at Medicine 2001 Conference, Montreal, 1996. Cited in Picot J. (1997) *The Telehealth Industry in Canada.* Ottawa: Industry Canada.

Halstead, L.S., Dang, T., Elrod, M., & Convit, R.J. (2003). Teleassessment compared with live assessment of pressure ulcers in a wound clinic: A pilot study. *Advances in Skin and Wound Care 16*(2):91–98.

Hill, W., Schillo, L., & Weinert, C. (2004). Effect of computer-based intervention on social support for chronically ill rural women. *Rehabilitation Nursing 29*(5):169–174.

Hill, W., & Weinert, C. (2004). An evaluation of an online intervention to provide social support and health education. *CIN: Computers, Informatics, Nursing 22*(5):282–288.

Jenkins, R.L., & McSweeney, M. (2001). Assessing elderly patients with congestive heart failure via in-home interactive telecommunications. *Journal of Gerontological Nursing 27*(1):21–28.

Johnston, B., Weeler, L., Deuser, J., & Sousa, K. (2000). Outcomes of the Kaiser Permanente tele-home health research project. *Archives of Family Medicine 9*(1):40–45.

Miyasaka, K. (1997). Videophone system for pediatric home care. In: *Proceedings of the 3rd International Conference on the Medical Aspects of Telemedicine.* Kobe, Japan, p. 56.

Natori, M., Kitagawa, M., & Akiyama, Y. (1997). A preliminary study of home nursing for low risk pregnancy. In: *Proceedings of the 3rd International Conference on the Medical Aspects of Telemedicine*, Kobe, Japan, p. 81.

Omery, A. (2003). Advice Nursing Practice: On the Quality of the Evidence. *Journal of Nursing Administration. 33*(6):353–360.

Picot, J. (1997). *The Telehealth Industry in Canada.* Ottawa: Industry Canada.

Pierce, L.L., Steiner, V., & Govoni, A.L. (2002). In-home online support for caregivers of survivors of stroke: a feasibility study. *CIN: Computers, Informatics, Nursing 20*(4):157–164.

Roman, L.I. (1997). Caring for the elderly at home. In: *Proceedings of the 3rd International Conference on the Medical Aspects of Telemedicine*, Kobe, Japan, p. 79.

Roupe, M.Y. (2004). Interactive home telehealth: a vital component of disease management programs. *CIN: Computers, Informatics, Nursing 9*(1):47–49.

Strecher, V., Wang, C., Derry, H., Wildenhaus, K., & Johnson, C. (2002). Tailored interventions for multiple risk behaviors. *Health Education Research 17*(5):619–627.

Telemedicine Research Center (TRC), (1997). What Is telemedicine? (http://tie.telemed.org).

Valanis, B., Moscato, S., Tanner, C., Shapiro, S., Izumi, S. D., & Mayo, A. (2003). Making It Work: Organization and Processes of Telephone Nursing Advice Services. *Journal of Nursing Administration. 33*(4):216–223.

Wilbright, W.A., Birke, J.A., Patout, C.A., Varnado, M., & Horswell, R. (2004). The use of telemedicine in the management of diabetes-related foot ulceration: a pilot study. *Advances in Skin and Wound Care 17*(5):232–239.

Yoshio, M., Kunihiko, D., Masayuki, N., & Eisuke, F. (1997). A report of telecare for the aged at home via ISDN. In: *Proceedings of the 3rd International Conference on the Medical Aspects of Telemedicine*, Kobe, Japan, p. 80.

Young, T.L., & Ireson, C. (2003). Effectiveness of school-based telehealth care in urban and rural elementary schools. *Pediatrics 112*(5):1088–1096.

Zajchuk, J.T., & Zajchuk, R. (1996). Strategy for medical readiness: transition to the digital age. *Telemedicine Journal (Special Issue on Telemedicine and the Military)* 2:3.

9
Administration Applications

WITH CONTRIBUTIONS BY HÉLÈNE CLÉMENT

Managers and caregivers throughout the healthcare system are being asked to increase the efficiency and effectiveness of patient care while simultaneously reducing or at least maintaining levels of resource consumption. A principal strategy being used to achieve these goals is to consider information as a corporate strategic resource and provide enhanced information management methods and tools to caregivers and managers across the health sector. The idea is to use information to help managers utilize available resources most effectively.

Administrative uses of information systems in nursing can be classified in two ways: those that provide nurse managers with information for decision making and those that help nurse managers communicate the decisions. In this chapter, the administrative uses of information systems that help nurse managers with decision making are called "management information systems." Those applications of information systems in nursing administration that help nurse managers communicate their decisions are called "nursing office automation systems." This chapter defines management information systems and describes the nursing information needs related to the management of nursing units. The chapter concludes with the nursing role in the management of information and obstacles and issues in management information systems.

Definition of Management Information Systems

The idea of management information systems was developed in the business and industrial sectors. It has been studied, analyzed, and evaluated in detail by management scientists for a considerable time. In those sectors, there are many definitions of the concept of management information systems (MISs). Some definitions place an emphasis on the physical elements and design of the system, and others focus on the function of an MIS in an organization. In this book, MIS refers to the classic notion of "a method of collecting, storing, retrieving, and processing information that is used or

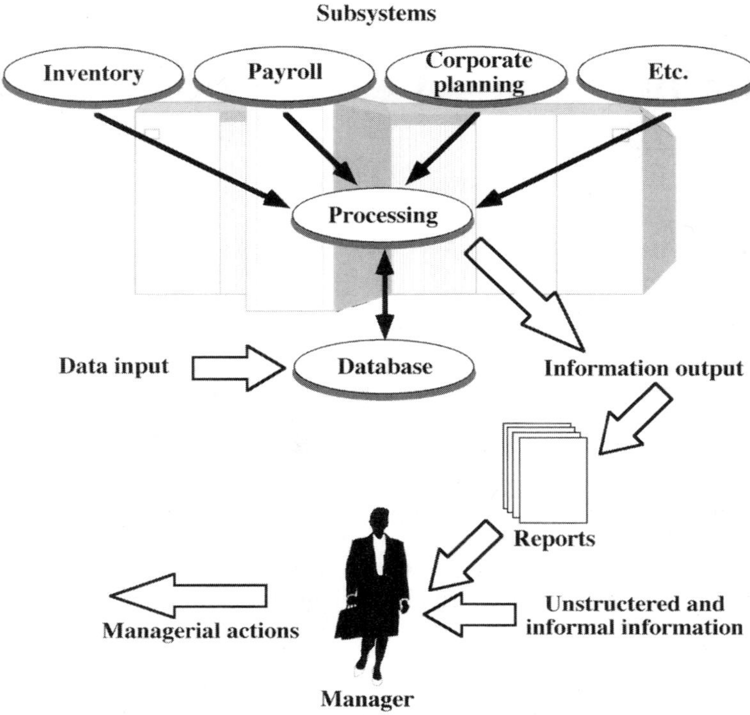

FIGURE 9.1. Management information system.

desired by one or more managers in the performance of their duties" (Ein-Dor and Segev, 1978). Although this definition could include both manual and computerized systems, we discuss only computerized MISs in this book. Figure 9.1 illustrates a simplified management information system.

Nursing Information Needs for the Management of Nursing Units

This aspect of information need focuses on the information that the organization (as represented by its nurse managers) needs to fulfill that aspect of its mission related to providing patient or client care. Management information systems help nursing in the areas of quality management, unit staffing, and ongoing reporting. Such systems also support nurse managers in their responsibilities for allocation and utilization of the following resources necessary to accomplish the nursing function in the patient/client care environments: human resources, fiscal resources (including payroll, supplies, and materiel), and physical resources (including physical facilities, equipment, and furniture).

Quality Management

Total quality management (TQM) and continuous quality improvement (CQI) continue to be commonly encountered approaches to quality management and improvement (Shojania and Grimshaw, 2005). TQM is an important process for staff nurses and administrators alike. It is useful to staff nurses in two ways: It provides them with feedback about the nature of their individual practice and provides them with opportunity to influence patient care in their organization. Nurse administrators use it to assess the general quality of patient care provided within their institutions and as a process to receive and communicate opportunities to enhance patient care and organizational effectiveness.

A process of establishing and maintaining organizational effectiveness (i.e., the quality of care provided to patients), TQM is an institutional plan of action to establish a process for empowering staff to influence corporate achievement of the highest possible standards for patient care. The delivery of patient care is monitored by all staff to ensure that these standards are met or surpassed. Implicit in the concept of TQM is the ongoing evaluation of the standards themselves, thus ensuring that they reflect current norms and practices in healthcare. Institutions use a variety of formal and informal means to gather information to evaluate the quality of care provided to patients. The formal means are encompassed in a quality assurance program. Information needs associated with quality assurance might include patient care databases, patient evaluations of care received, nurses' notes on the chart, patient care plans, performance appraisals, and incident reports. These sources of information are reviewed by either a concurrent or retrospective audit. Concurrent nursing audits occur during the patient's stay in the hospital, whereas retrospective nursing audits occur after the patient leaves the hospital. Audit reviews are a major tool for any TQM program.

Originally, the impetus for the establishment of quality assurance programs came during the 1970s as the result of rising consumer awareness, increasing healthcare costs, and the growing professionalism of nursing. An additional factor was the desire of the U.S. government to monitor the cost and quality of care associated with its Medicaid program. Almost simultaneously, three things happened: Professional standards review organizations were established in the United States, the American Nurses Association published its standards for practice, and the American Joint Commission on Accreditation for Hospitals established the requirement for medical and nursing audits. These events added pressure to the entire quality assurance process. The established quality assurance programs were dependent on reviewing and evaluating massive amounts of data. These reviews and audits consumed enormous amounts of nursing time. As these audits were done, nurses gained an increased awareness of their professional accountability. This greater awareness, in turn, prompted nurses to produce more documentation in the form of nursing care plans and patient records. This further increased the volume of information to be reviewed and evaluated in the nursing audits.

As the pressure from nursing audits was building, integrated hospital information systems made their timely entry into the healthcare delivery system. Quality assurance programs in nursing needed two things to succeed: standardized terminology and standardized care plans. These two things were also required if information systems were to be any help to nurses. The standardization of terminology required for computerized documentation of nurses' notes, and the development of standardized care plans for use in generating computerized patient care plans, coincided with the need for standardized terminology (see Chapter 13) and quality assurance standards.

The ability of a computer to retrieve, summarize, and compare large volumes of information rapidly has proven useful for nurse administrators charged with the responsibility of implementing quality assurance programs. The first obstacle to using computers for this purpose is the lack of widespread availability of integrated hospital information systems. The second obstacle is the lack of a widely implemented common nursing vocabulary and method of coding nursing diagnoses and interventions (see Chapter 12).

Both obstacles are on the verge of being overcome. The lack of widely available integrated hospital information systems is being resolved by the decreasing cost of such systems and their greater sophistication. Taxonomies for nursing diagnoses, interventions, and contributions to patient care outcomes have been developed (Lunney et al., 2005). Unfortunately, much of this work has not yet received widespread implementation in the nursing profession and has not yet been incorporated as a framework for the organization of nursing databases by developers of information systems. Figure 9.2 attempts to summarize the interrelationships between clinical practice, informatics, and computer technology.

Another problem associated with computerized quality assurance programs is the quality of the tools used to provide input to the program. The validity of even the most widely used audit tools and criteria is largely unsubstantiated. Consequently, much effort has been focused on the process aspects incorporated in the TQM concept. Unfortunately, the vendors of computer software have not given high priority to the information needs related to TQM or the development of clinical software packages for healthcare institutions. This situation has created a major barrier to the effective, widespread use of information systems for quality monitoring in hospitals. Several institutions have developed sophisticated TQM programs that incorporate procedures for conducting concurrent chart audits. These institutions use a manual concurrent audit conducted by staff nurses (with special training in concurrent auditing) on the nursing units. The data from the completed audit forms are then put into the computer for tabulation, analysis, and summarizing. This combination of manual and computer methods

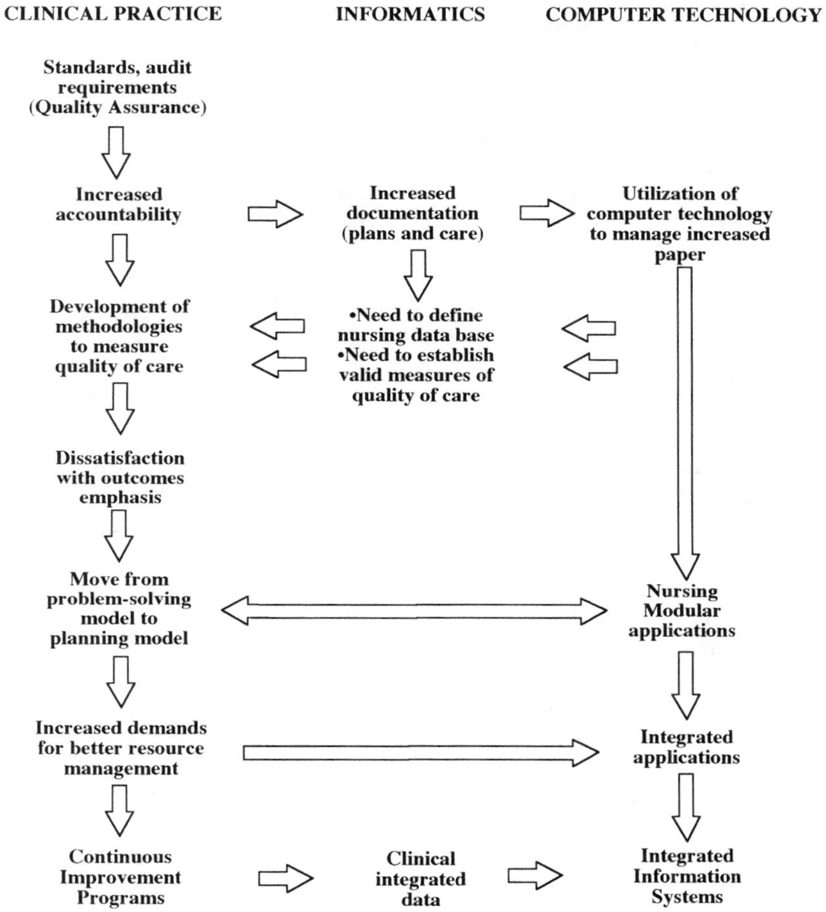

FIGURE 9.2. Relationships between clinical practice, informatics, and computer technology.

partially reduces the labor-intensive process associated with totally manual audits.

There is a growing emphasis on patient care outcomes as the major focus of nursing TQM programs. Similarly, there is a growing trend away from the problem resolution model to a planning model as the major criterion for measuring quality assurance. Simultaneously, there is an increasing demand from the public for better resource management in the healthcare sector, and the public has an increasing awareness of quality as a cost component of healthcare. These factors are creating a demand for the most sophisticated computerized information handling in the form of relational database software.

Patient Classification, Nursing Workload, and Unit Staffing

In the past, innumerable head nurses and supervisors in healthcare institutions and agencies around the world spent countless hours each day "doing the time." Even when master rotation plans were used, manual scheduling of personnel work rotations could not eliminate all the problems, such as vulnerability to accusations of bias when assigning days off or shift rotation, difficulty establishing minimum staffing to avoid wasting manpower, and depending on an individual's memory in the nursing administrative structure. Consequently, automated staff scheduling is a highly desired component of a management information system for nursing administration. Frequently, when an institution has limited resources and no other computerized nursing management information system, it mobilizes resources to set up a computerized staffing system.

Researchers at many healthcare institutions have developed diverse systems for personnel time assignment. The complexity of these systems varies greatly. Some merely use the computer to print names into what was formerly a manual master rotation schedule; others adjust staffing interactively and dynamically on a shift-to-shift basis by considering patient acuity, nursing workload levels, and the expertise of available personnel. To develop complex, sophisticated systems for automated personnel scheduling, a great deal of planning and data gathering is required: The nursing workload must be identified in the institution; the various levels of expertise of staff members must be categorized and documented; criteria for determining patient acuity and nursing workload must be established; personnel policies must be clearly defined; and the elements of union contracts must be summarized. When all this information is available, a computer program is designed to schedule nursing staff on nursing units. The capacity of the computer to manipulate large numbers of variables consistently and quickly makes personnel time assignment an excellent use of this technology.

Documented advantages of automated scheduling of personnel include the following.

- Easier recruitment and increased job satisfaction because schedules are known well in advance
- Less time spent on manual scheduling, thereby providing more time for nurse managers to carry out other duties
- Advance notice of staff shortages requiring temporary replacements
- Unbiased assignment of days off and shift rotation
- More effective utilization and distribution of personnel throughout the institution or agency
- Capacity to document the effect of staff size on quality of care
- Ability to relate quantity and quality of nursing staff to patient acuity

Workload measurement systems function with automated scheduling. Nursing workload measurement systems (NWMSs), sometimes called patient classification systems (PCSs) are tools that measure the number of direct, indirect, and nonclinical patient care hours by patient acuity on a daily basis (Hall et al., 2003; Seago, 2002). PCSs and NWMSs have evolved to focus on providing uniform, reliable productivity information to help with staffing, budgeting, planning, and quality assurance. NWMS have become a valuable management tool for nursing unit managers, nursing department heads, hospital administrators, and governments alike. As healthcare costs and demands continue to escalate, the appropriate and effective utilization of scarce human resources becomes increasingly onerous. There are many PCSs and NWMSs on the market. All differ in one or many respects, and the criteria used to choose such a system ultimately depend on the specific institution's needs.

Increased job satisfaction, easier recruitment of staff, unbiased rotation assignment, workstation printouts, and advance notice of temporary shortages—all contribute to improved staff morale and thus indirectly result in better patient care. Administrative time saved and more effective utilization and distribution of personnel have also been suggested as factors influencing quality of patient care within the agency or institution. Documentation of the relation between staffing and quality of patient care gives the nurse manager strong data to justify staffing requests and decisions to senior hospital management.

Reporting

In most hospitals, nursing costs represent upward of 40% of the entire hospital budget. Management information systems collect, summarize, and format data for use in administrative decision making related to the nursing component of the hospital budget. Nurse managers are familiar with periodically produced budget summaries that allow monitoring of the budget, adjustments between overcommitted and undercommitted categories, and help when planning next year's budget. A variety of retrieval modules have been designed and are being refined to provide similar decision-making support in areas ranging from the nosocomial infection rate to sickness and absentee abuses by staff members. The emphasis in these reports is on graphic displays (e.g., histograms, time series charts, map plots). The advantages for nurse managers with this level of support lie mainly in the speed with which data can be retrieved, compiled, summarized, and presented in a meaningful and comprehensive form. Another major advantage is the ability to tailor reports to each nurse manager's information needs. Furthermore, sharing data and developing knowledge of clinical staff at all levels not only improve data quality but also assist in a more effective and efficient use of the data included in reports for decision-making. This facilitates the ongoing monitoring of activities within the institution and the preparation of reports by the nurse manager to superiors or outside agencies.

Human Resource Management

Management of people on a nursing unit is a complex, time-consuming task. In the increasingly decentralized administrative structures that characterize hospitals, nurse managers need information related to all aspects of the allocation and utilization of staff on nursing units. For example, the nurse manager must have immediate access to such information as the following.

- Skills and education of all nursing employees
- Job classification and salary level for all staff on the unit
- Dates for performance reviews
- Dates for recertification of medically delegated and transferred functions
- Dates for annual inservice education sessions, whether required by contract, by organizational policy, or by accreditation standards (e.g., back care, cardiopulmonary resuscitation, fire and disaster response, restraints)
- Annual vacation schedule summary for the unit
- Statutory holiday schedules
- Labor relationships contracts for all collective bargaining units representing employees employed on the unit, including grievance procedures
- Sick time records for each employee

Through access to hospital information systems from a personal computer or terminal, including human resources databases, the nurse manager is quickly able to obtain the necessary information without the need to maintain duplicate records.

Fiscal Resources

Hospitals are gradually moving toward the implementation of business-oriented management information systems. These systems identify, define, collect, process, and report the information necessary for the planning, budgeting, operating, and controlling aspects of the management function. The current demands for fiscal responsibility in hospitals exceed all previous experience in the healthcare sector. Increasingly, nursing managers are expected to understand the contextual challenges of their organizational environment. To respond to internal and external factors influencing the corporate environment in which they function, nurse managers must do many things.

- Understand their fiscal responsibilities and situation
- Identify the issues and opportunities
- Generate solutions
- Monitor progress toward unit and organization goals
- Evaluate the effectiveness of the solutions or the achievement of goals and objectives
- Link data with process improvement and best practice in a cost-efficient model.

These activities require the management of financial and statistical data. The ultimate objective is to relate the cost of resources consumed to patient outcomes. To manage effectively the information related to their responsibilities for fiscal accountability, nurse managers require financial information (including payroll, supplies/materiel, and services) and statistical information (e.g., patient length of stay, nursing hours per patient-day). This information must be timely, accurate, relevant, comprehensive, complete, consistent, concise, sensitive, and comparable.

Physical Resources

Nursing managers are also responsible for overseeing the care and maintenance of the physical facilities of their patient care unit. They are responsible for equipment and furniture on their units and ensuring that it is in good working order. Although the actual inventory may be conducted by another department (such as materiel management), nursing managers are accountable for budgeting, ordering, and retaining capital assets on their units and for initiating maintenance or replacement procedures. Consequently, nursing managers need access to capital asset inventory for their unit. In addition, they should conduct regular systematic inspection of the workplace for physical hazards such as faulty electrical equipment or loose floor tiles. These inspections must document identified hazards, the date on which corrective action was requested or initiated, and the date that the hazard was repaired or removed from the workplace. Such information must be stored on the nursing unit in an easily retrievable format with a calendar to bring forward reminders of follow-up items.

Office Automation

Nursing office automation is the integrated electronic technology distributed throughout the nursing administrative office. The purposes of nursing office automation are to improve effectiveness, efficiency, and control of nursing office operations. This technology can have application in nursing administration, nursing education, continuing nursing education, and nursing research. Office automation affects the filing and retrieval of documents, text processing, telephone communications, and informal meetings. Nursing office requirements demand more skills in transcription, word processing, spreadsheets, and electronic filing. Offices have special printers, teleconferencing and video conferencing, voice response systems, voice mail, and e-mail systems.

Nursing's Role in Managing Information in Healthcare Facilities

Nursing's role in managing information in healthcare facilities is, of necessity, related to the role of nursing in the organization. In most hospitals, nurses manage both patient care and patient care units in the organization. Usually, nurse clinicians manage patient care and nurse managers administer the patient care units in the organization. Therefore, for some time, nursing's role in the management of information generally has been considered to include the information necessary to manage nursing care using the nursing process (see Chapter 6) and the information necessary for managing patient care units in the organization (e.g., resource allocation and utilization, personnel management, planning and policymaking, decision support).

As the role of staff nurses in organizational governance and decision-making diversifies, their role and responsibility for information management to support these decision-making responsibilities will also change. Information related to organizational planning and policies, as well as resource allocation and utilization, widely available to nursing staff, supports these roles and responsibilities.

Obstacles to Effective Nursing Management of Information

In most hospitals, the major obstacles to more effective nursing management of information are the sheer volume of information, the lack of access to information-handling techniques and equipment, and the inadequate information management infrastructure. As the reader must have noted from reading Chapter 6 and the preceding sections, the volume of information that nurses manage on a daily basis, for patient care purposes or organizational management purposes, is enormous and continues to grow. Nurses continue to respond to this growth with incredible mental agility. However, humans do have limits, and one of the major sources of job dissatisfaction among nurses is information overload, resulting in information-induced job stress.

Manual information systems (e.g., handwriting an order, a requisition, a medication card, and a kardex entry for each medication) and outdated information transfer facilities (e.g., nurses hand-carrying requisitions and specimens for stat blood work to the laboratory on nights because the pneumatic

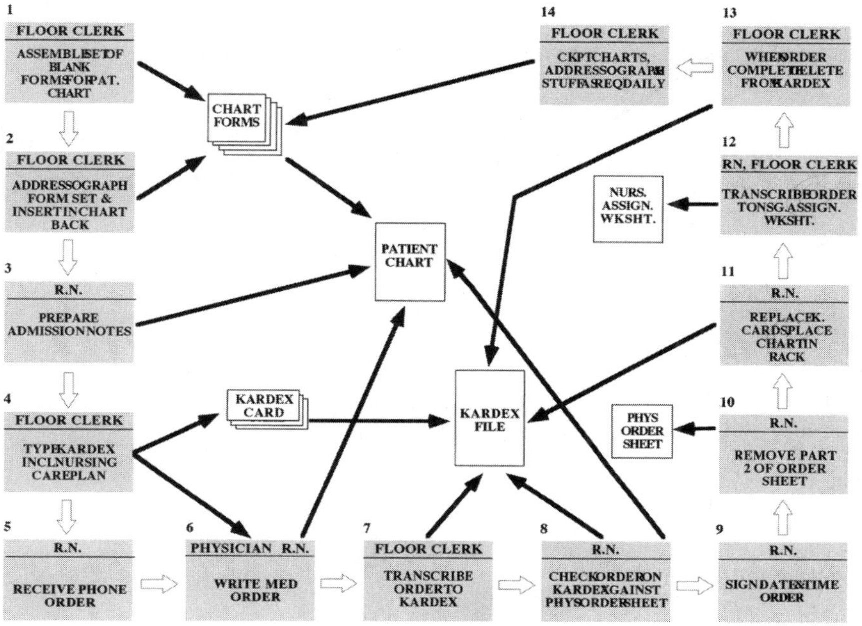

FIGURE 9.3. Manual preparation of new chart and processing of new medical order.

tube system and the portering system are not available between the hours of 2400 and 0700) are information-redundant and labor-intensive processes, to say nothing of an inappropriate use of an expensive human resource. Electronic information transfer and communication systems allow rapid, accurate transfer of information along electronic communication networks (Figs. 9.3 and 9.4).

The lack of the software and hardware for electronic communication networks is only one aspect inhibiting the development of an information infrastructure. The other major aspect lacking in most hospitals is appropriate support staff to facilitate information management. Information systems support staff require preparation in health information science to gain expertise in both information systems and a solid understanding of the functioning of the healthcare system, its organizations, and its institutions. Similarly, financial and statistical support staff are necessary to help nursing managers appropriately interpret information.

Issues Related to Effective Nursing Management of Information

Primary among the nursing issues regarding information management is the lack of adequate educational programs in information management techniques and strategies for nursing managers. Presently, there are only a few

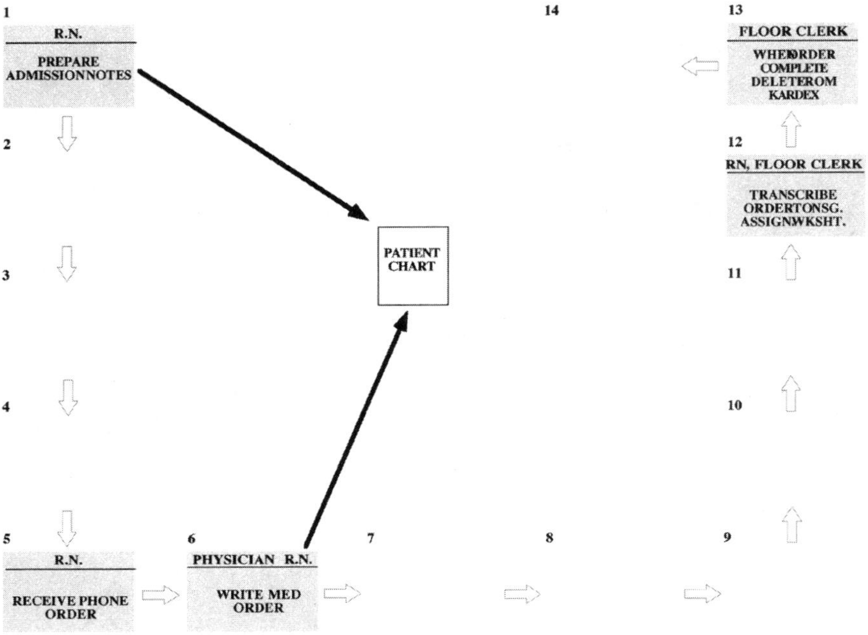

FIGURE 9.4. Electronic preparation of new chart and processing of new medical order.

programs in prelicensure nursing education programs offering a course in electronic information management techniques and strategies related to nursing. At a minimum, such a course must include advanced study of information management techniques and strategies such as information flow analysis, the use of spreadsheets, databases, and word-processing packages. Ideally, such courses would also introduce concepts and provide hands-on experience related to the use of patient care information systems.

Nursing involvement and participation in the selection and installation of patient care information systems and financial management systems is imperative. Regrettably, many senior nurse managers fail to recognize the importance of this activity and opt out of the process. They then complain when the systems do not meet the needs of nursing. Senior nursing executives must recognize the importance of allocating staff and money to participate in the strategic planning process for information systems in their organizations. Other senior management personnel must also recognize the importance of nursing input into the strategic planning process for information systems. In any hospital, nurses are the single largest group of professionals using a patient care system, and nursing represents the largest part of the budget requiring financial management. Nursing, therefore, represents the single largest stakeholder group related to either a patient care information system or an enterprise health information system.

The final major issue that nursing must address regarding information management in hospitals is the patient discharge abstract. The patient discharge abstracts prepared by medical records departments across Canada and the United States currently contain little if any nursing care delivery information. Therefore, the abstracts fail to acknowledge the contribution of nursing during the patient's stay in the hospital. This is important because the abstracts are used by many agencies for a variety of statistical purposes including funding allocation. Presently, much valuable information is being lost. This information is important for determining hospitalization costs and the effectiveness of nursing care. As the importance of national health databases increases, it is imperative that a minimum number of essential nursing elements be included in that database. Such a set of data elements would be similar to the nursing minimum data set (see Chapter 6). Such data are essential to allow description of the health status of populations with relation to nursing care needs, establish outcome measures for nursing care, and investigate the use and cost of nursing resources. The nursing profession must provide leadership when defining appropriate nursing data elements that must be included in the patient discharge abstract.

Summary

Management information systems and nursing office automation systems enable the nurse manager to contribute to organizational efforts to increase the efficiency and effectiveness of patient care while simultaneously reducing or at least maintaining levels of resource consumption. This can be accomplished in part by considering *information* as a corporate strategic resource and thinking of nurse managers' *use* of information as a management method and tool, thereby empowering nurse managers to utilize available resources most effectively.

References

Ein-Dor, P., & Segev, E. (1978). *Managing Management Information Systems.* Toronto: Lexington Books.

Hall, L.M., Doran, D., & Laschinger, H.S., et al. (2003). A balanced scorecard approach for nursing report card development. *Outcomes Management* 7(1):17–22.

Lunney, M., Delaney, C., Duffy, M., Moorhead, S., & Welton, J. (2005). Advocating for standardized nursing languages in electronic health records. *Journal of Nursing Administration 35*(1):1–3.

Seago, J.A. (2002). A comparison of two patient classification instruments in an acute care hospital. *Journal of Nursing Administration 32*(5):243–249.

Shojania, K.G., & Grimshaw, J.M. (2005). Evidence-based quality improvement: The state of the science. *Health Affairs 24*(1):138–151.

10
Education Applications

RICHARD S. HANNAH

Impact of Computers on Education

Technological change has placed a strain on the educational system. In trying to keep pace with the information explosion associated with the technology revolution, educators have had to devote more time and energy to simple information transfer, leaving little time to help beginners apply information.

Historically, three eras, or "waves," of education can be identified. The "first wave" of education preceded the printed word. Education was a controlled, tutorial process that was available for the few under special circumstances. It was reserved for the literate elite: the clergy and nobility. The Gutenberg press ushered in the "second wave." With the printed word, a centralized education process evolved. Colleges and universities multiplied and became the focal points of learning. Their libraries served as the repositories of existing knowledge. The first two waves of education relied on approaches to learning that remain the cornerstones of today's educational system. These two traditional approaches are academic education and training. Academic education encompasses the conceptual learning process. It is subject-driven. Credit is given for learning achievement, and the application of knowledge gained is usually deferred. Achievement is decided by examination. Training is task- and skills-oriented. Application of knowledge is immediate, and achievement is demonstrated by performance and behavior.

Computer-based multimedia is the "third wave" in education. Computer-based multimedia aids in the knowledge and information transfer process, provides feedback to students about the efficiency of their learning processes, provides access to a vast warehouse of electronic databases, and enables students to problem solve and apply their learning. Ultimately, computer-based multimedia frees the teaching staff to concentrate on helping students with their individual learning needs, with emphasis on the "art" rather than the "science" of nursing. The computer applications in this chapter can be applied to the initial entry into practice education of nursing students, to staff development (continuing education), and to patient education.

When educating healthcare professionals, as in all areas of education, the traditional modes of learning are straining under the requirements of technological change. The good news is that although technology has created problems in the traditional educational system, it has also provided the solutions for resolving them. Computer-based multimedia has the potential to help educators create a new order from confusion and chaos. With computer-based multimedia, education can move from an era of scarce resources into an era of abundant learning resources. Computer technology and information management have moved faster than the ability of educational and healthcare systems to assimilate it. The integration of technology-assisted information gathering and learning into the educational system will take time. Three basic stages of assimilating technology can be described as follows.

- *Stage 1: Replacement.* New technology replaces old technology, but outcomes are not altered. An example is the use of computers to perform accounting functions. Stage 1 data-processing functions such as automated record-keeping, drill and practice, and machine-scored multiple-choice examinations have been successfully introduced into healthcare education. Universities use search systems and software for cataloguing, accessing, and retrieving library information, student records, and other types of data.
- *Stage 2: Innovation.* The capabilities of technologies are combined with traditional functions to create new tasks. For example, increased computing speed and the establishment of wide area networks have created new home learning opportunities including literature searches and data gathering over the internet. CD-ROM technology, which allows storage and retrieval of vast amounts of information, makes literature searches fast, feasible, and complete.
- *Stage 3: Transformation.* Innovations accumulate, transforming the way we live. For example, telecommunications and computers have transformed the life and work of radiologists to provide services that would have been impossible, at any cost, a decade ago. Computed tomography (CT) and magnetic resonance imaging (MRI) scanning have transformed X-ray departments into diagnostic imaging departments, and radiologists now read and interpret images from their homes.

Current applications of computer technology in the education system are concentrated during stages 1 and 2 of development. In many areas, computer technology has been adapted to the established approaches of academic education and training. Stage 3 transformations are beginning to be seen in education of nurses after entry into practice. There are now numerous distance education programs for nurses to pursue studies at the post-RN baccalaureate and graduate level.

The remainder of this chapter focuses on the use of computer technology in health education. This is not to imply that other technologies (e.g., television, two-way audiovisual communication, videotext) are unimportant, merely that they are beyond the scope of this book. Large central computer systems, minicomputers, personal computers, digital video disks, and other modes of interactive learning provide a means for individualizing learning even within a centralized learning system. The traditional modes of academic instruction and training will always have their place. However, they will be augmented by the power of individualized learning systems to act as information and knowledge transfer vehicles, freeing faculty members to do what only people can do: develop understanding, skill, judgment, and wisdom (Jenkins et al., 1983).

The use of computers in nursing education dates back to 1966 when Bitzer and Bitzer (1973) reported using computer assisted instruction (CAI) via the PLATO system to teach nursing courses. In 1971, the earliest forms of simulated patient management problems were instituted (Harless et al., 1971). There has been a trend during the intervening period since these developments toward the increasing use of technology in nursing education. This is the result of the need to individualize instruction in nursing education and the availability of the technology to do so. Many factors have contributed to the development of this trend: among them are influences arising from general education and nursing practice factors.

General Education

- Tremendous growth in human knowledge and the resulting increase in the amount of information to be learned
- Increased understanding of the teaching-learning process and greater sophistication in identifying the learning styles of individual students with diverse abilities and rates of learning
- Financial retrenchment and budgetary restraint internationally in postsecondary educational institutions, which has produced a need to maximize effective use of limited human and financial resources. Increased widescale availability and affordability of educational hardware (e.g., microcomputers, personal computers, television, video players, CD ROM/DVD players, videotext).

Nursing Practice

- Increased diversity in the settings where nursing is practiced. The focus of nursing practice ranges from the highly technical and largely physical nursing care required by individuals in acute critical care areas (e.g., emergency departments and intensive care, coronary care, and neonatal intensive care units) to the predominantly psychosocial nursing care provided to families in communities (e.g., family counseling, health maintenance, and health promotion)
- Need for nurses to have greater skills in independent decision-making
- Need for nurses to have skills that allow them to continue learning throughout their professional careers

What's in a Name?

The term computer-assisted learning (CAL) and its subdivisions, computer-assisted instruction (CAI) and computer-managed instruction (CMI), have been in existence for some time. Initially, CAI involved using video display terminals (monitors) linked to mainframe computers where the student was asked a series of questions and the computer responded with statements like "Yes that is correct" and suitable feedback for wrong answers such as "No that is incorrect because ... try again." Students quickly learned to answer incorrectly to view all the feedback responses placed in the program by the instructor. When personal computers became available they were still primitive by today's standards, and CAI slowly evolved to include text-based lessons with a few images and colors added but was still referred to as CAI. Because the computer has become a much more multipurpose tool since these terms were defined, how do we rationalize this older terminology with what the computer is capable of today? During a past number of years, the addition of words such as interactive and multimedia to the existing terminology has resulted in a taxonomic nightmare. A brief survey of the literature resulted in the following list of synonymous terms, which is by no means all-inclusive.

- Computer-mediated multimedia
- Interactive multimedia instruction
- Interactive multimedia
- Learner-controlled instruction
- Learner-controlled computer-assisted instruction
- Interactive computer-assisted instruction
- Multimedia computer-assisted instruction
- Multimedia computer-based training
- e-Learning

This inconsistent terminology is confusing to the novice and expert alike.

What Is Multimedia?

In general, multimedia refers to computer-based technologies that permit an integration of traditional forms of communication to allow seamless access or interaction by users. It also implies that the computer-based technologies go beyond a single computer to include national and international networks such as the Internet. Because the field is evolving so fast, with so many diverse interest groups, a more concise definition is not possible at this time. The primary advantage of a multimedia approach over more traditional forms of communication is based in the freedom it allows for the creative and innovative expression of ideas and the opportunity it provides for interactive

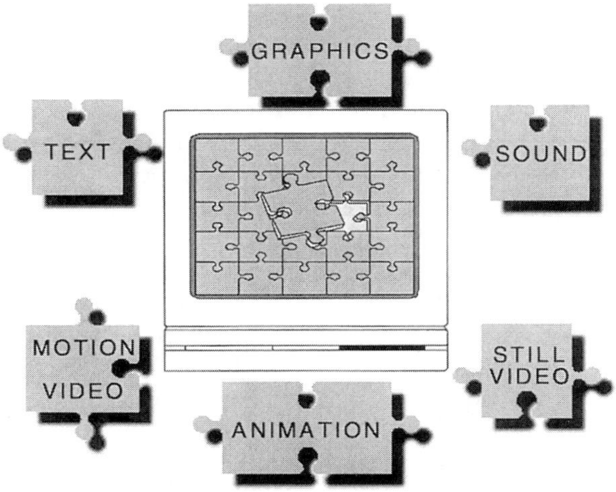

FIGURE 10.1. "Pieces" of the multimedia puzzle.

student–teacher dialogue through a common tool—the computer. How well multimedia will be able to fulfill its enormous potential remains to be seen.

The many traditional forms of communication that form the "pieces" comprising multimedia are summarized in Figure 10.1. They include textual material, graphics, video (both still and motion), animation, and sound; and most recently virtual reality capabilities have been added to this list. Who knows when the senses of taste and smell will also be accommodated?

Just as there are many diverse tools that come together to make up a multimedia program, so there are many ways in which this thing called multimedia can be used. The major hurdle to overcome lies in making sense of the multiplicity of terms and categories that abound in the literature. As demonstrated in Figure 10.2, there are many flavors of multimedia but only two basic or primary goals.

- Information-gathering activities: Information gathering programs provide the user with information and are controlled by the user.
- Learning activities: Learning activities programs generate learning through exercises and developing skills and are controlled by the system.

Information-gathering programs can currently be divided into three types: hypermedia/hypertext, multimedia books, and multimedia databases.

- *Hypermedia/hypertext* programs use highlighted text or terms the user selects to receive more information, such as a definition, graphic, or animation about that term or to link to another area or topic. The World Wide Web is a hypermedia/hypertext system.

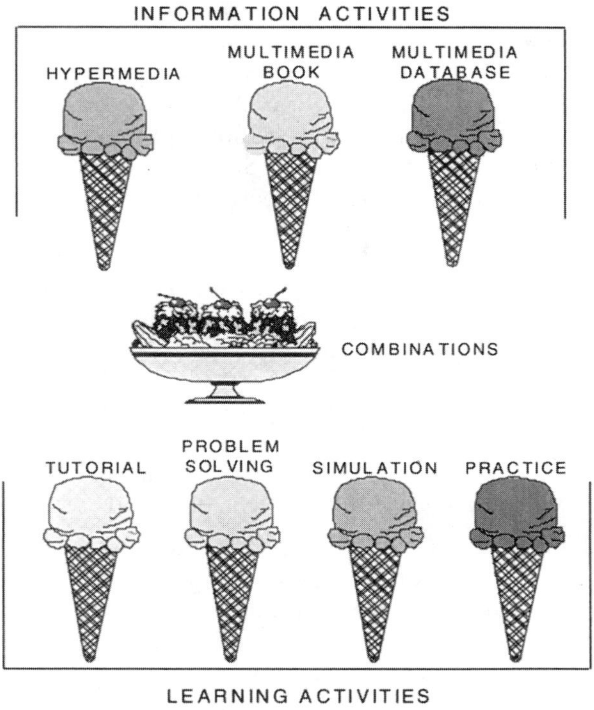

FIGURE 10.2. The many "flavors" of multimedia.

- *Multimedia books* are electronic versions of conventional textbooks. In addition to text and images, they contain video and audio clips and allow the reader to interact dynamically with the content.
- *Multimedia databases* are set up as records and fields such as the conventional text-based databases with which readers are already familiar. The difference lies in the fact that there is user-controlled access to all the "pieces" that comprise multimedia, such as graphics and video.

Learning activities programs fall into four basic categories: tutorials, simulation, practice, and problem-solving.

- *Tutorial* is the category in which one would place classic computer-assisted instruction (CAI). Historically, the user was presented with some information followed by an activity such as a question, with appropriate feedback for a wrong response. CAI has evolved so much over the years that some use this term to mean multimedia or refer to it as multimedia CAI. However, because of the negative connotation associated with the term CAI, meaning merely drill and practice format, which was all early computers were capable of doing, the term has fallen into disfavor. A modern multimedia tutorial attempts to mimic a live lecture that takes the user through

a series of objectives but allows the user to undertake the operation at their own pace and still provide the option of interactivity with the "teacher." The main difference is an emphasis on thinking and motivation rather than a simple stimulus response. Several national nursing organizations, including the Canadian Nurses Association and the National Council of State Boards of Nursing in the United States, have developed computerized testing programs to measure competence as a component of licensure or specialty certification examinations.
- *Simulations*, in the health sciences, are usually of patients. The patient simulation attempts to provide the user with the same type of experience with patients they would encounter in a clinical environment. Health-related examples are programs such as "Ethical Dilemmas in Nursing" by the *American Journal of Nursing.*
- *Practice programs* allow the user to develop skills by using repetition. They somewhat overlap simulation programs.
- *Problem-solving* programs present the user with a problem, provide a number of resources to solve the problem, and let the user come up with the correct answer on their own.

Several resources discuss the process of authoring and delivery of multimedia material (Hannah, 1998; Jerram and Gosney, 1996; Kristof and Satran, 1995; Locatis, 1992; Lopuck, 1996). It should be noted that many available programs are so varied in content and presentation that they use combinations of these categories. An excellent example is the program "Learning and Using ICNP" (http://www.omv.la.se/icnp).

What Is Worldware

Definition

Worldware can be defined as software that isn't specifically developed for instruction but can be educationally valuable. Word processors, e-mail, and the Internet are all examples of Worldware. A practical example of integrating these applications would be Web-based on-line courses using discussion boards and e-mail. Worldware packages are valuable for a variety of reasons. They are in instructional demand because students know they need to learn to use them and to think with them. Instructors are already familiar with them as a result of their daily academic activities, and vendors have a large enough market to make it financially feasible to provide continual upgrades and enhancements. New versions of worldware are usually compatible with their older counterparts, which eases the burden on instructors when it comes to updating and modifying their courses, year after year, without last year's material becoming obsolete (and thus unusable) because of the software format.

Learning and Using ICNP

The software package called Learning and Using ICNP is a prototype of a web-based environment for learning to navigate within the International Classification for Nursing Practice (ICNP). It is also an interactive tool for nurses in practice or research and nursing students around the world to share their experience of nursing; it contributes to the continuing development of a unifying classification. Nurses can participate and contribute to this ongoing process of development to make sure that the ICNP continues to be developed as an international, practice-based instrument for nurses. (This paragraph was provided by Gunilla Nilsson and Lars Rundgren Lund University, Lund, Sweden.)

This application is designed to acquaint the user with the ICNP. Interactive procedures according to learning needs and requirements are built into the application to facilitate learning and training within the classification of nursing phenomena. There are opportunities in each module to make comments, statements, and suggestions and to submit them to a database for retrieval. There are also opportunities to create various exercises and assignments for use in learning environments.

Nursing Education Settings Using Computers

Whether used for information gathering or learning, the computers are being used in all facets of nursing education. Their use in basic nursing education at both the diploma and baccalaureate and graduate levels is widely reported. In addition, their use in continuing education programs and in-service education is growing at a logarithmic rate. Most educational institutions and many hospitals and clinics now provide Internet access. An excellent source of information on the Internet can be found in *The Internet for Nurses and Allied Health Professionals* (Edwards, 2002).

One of the largest growth areas during the last few years is distance learning, on-line learning, or e-learning. It is generally agreed that these terms are basically synonymous in that they represent any learning that takes place with the instructor and student physically separated from each other. This process can occur by mail, video, interactive or cable television, satellite broadcast, e-mail, or the World Wide Web (or any combination of these technologies). It appears that the health sciences sector has preferentially chosen the term e-learning over any other. In its broadest sense, e-learning can be defined as any type of learning that utilizes a network for delivery, with student–instructor interaction (e-learners, 2005).

There are many software packages used to deliver e-learning in nursing, but two predominate, WebCT and BlackBoard with WebCT being the most popular in nursing circles. There is little discernible difference between the two, and the choice of one or the other is largely based on personal preference (Anthony, 2002).

Whether attempting to establish an e-learning component to a curriculum or initiating just one course, several key factors must be addressed (Adams, 2004; Longman and Gabriel, 2004).

1. A commitment by the instructor and the administration to make the program successful by believing that for the right subject e-learning can achieve the same results as the conventional classroom
2. To provide relevant, high-quality, learner-centered course material
3. Financial support to provide continuous evaluation of the program

In summary, traditional paper-based distance education courses and e-learning courses have many similar pros and cons when compared to classroom teaching. However, e-learning when compared to paper-based courses, excels in interactivity and access to information.

Effectiveness of Multimedia Technology

Many studies of learner achievement using classic computer-assisted instruction (CAI) have been conducted in undergraduate nursing education. These studies consistently conclude that classic CAI is at least as effective as other teaching strategies in effecting behavioral changes in students (Nyamathi et al., 1989). Substantial reductions in the time spent learning subject matter have been shown in studies of classic CAI (Chang, 1986). Similarly, when classic CAI was compared with traditional strategies, significant cost benefit in favor of CAI was shown. These findings, regarding the effectiveness of nursing CAI with respect to learner achievement, time savings, and cost benefit, are consistent with findings in the health professions collectively and with findings in general education. The consensus among findings from a variety of disciplines, however, lends support to the generalization that classic CAI is at least as effective as other means of teaching (Belfry and Winne, 1988; Gaston, 1988).

The development of multimedia computers and software and the resulting enhanced capabilities have led to yet another round of comparison studies. The time has come finally to accept that computers are now as effective as any other traditional teaching tool—no better, no worse. Several factors are involved with determining the effectiveness of computer instruction, including the quality of the programs, environment of use (location and accessibility of computers), and characteristics of the learner (e.g., anxiety, level of computer knowledge) (Khoiny, 1996). Future research should be aimed at developing tools for evaluating new programs and determining how students learn with computers so existing programs and new programs can be improved rather than continual comparison with other teaching methods.

Limitations of Multimedia Technology

Limitations that emerge from detailed study of computer usage in nursing education include the following.

- *Cost factors*: The initial time investment in developing good programs is extensive. For example, to author 1 hour of effective, terminal-tested tutorials requires 120 to 150 hours of work. Once instructors become more adept at design strategies, the time required is reduced. However, extensive analyses of cost benefit and detailed studies of cost figures for the development and operation of nursing CAI programs are unavailable. Although the cost of the hardware may be dropping consistently, software development costs are not. Hopefully, in the future institutions will enter into joint development projects to control costs. One such enterprise is called MERLOT, an acronym for Multimedia Educational Resource for Learning and On-line Teaching; it is a consortium of U.S. and Canadian universities that maintains an on-line peer reviewed catalog of learning materials that are easily incorporated into faculty-designed courses. Although all university disciplines are represented, nursing is extremely active in the submission and peer review process of the organization, resulting in large number of learning materials encompassing all aspects of nursing (MERLOT, 2005).
- *Content control*: Unless more nurse educators become knowledgeable in the area of multimedia, there could be a tendency to abdicate the preparation of computer programs for nursing to educational computer software firms. Decisions about nursing and nursing education could slip out of nursing hands. Nursing educators must monitor their own learning programs to ensure that decisions related to nursing remain in the hands of nursing content experts. Conversely, without a firm foundation, a sophisticated computerized nursing curriculum, instead, become a patchwork coverage of course material.
- *Altered professorial roles*: Teachers who have felt secure in their role as dispensers of information may feel uncomfortable as they find their role changing to that of facilitators, moderators, and coordinators. In addition, active involvement by faculty members in computerized instruction requires that a reward structure exists that places value on published instructional design efforts to the same extent that it values research and other publication activities.
- *Technology*: The dominance of the Windows and Macintosh personal computer operating systems, along with Internet access, has greatly facilitated the sharing of programs within and among institutions. However, many programs are still locked into a single proprietary computer language and hardware system. Translating an existing program from one computer operating system and language to another may require more programming

time than was required to produce the original. This is an impediment to wider dissemination of nursing material. For this reason, there is probably a redundancy of lessons among nursing users.

- *Large central (or mainframe) computer systems or centrally controlled servers*: These systems place the nurse user at the whim of the individual or group controlling the system. The autonomy and control provided by personal computers has removed this limitation. Nursing multimedia is now dominated by the personal computer world. However, with the number of programs available on the Internet increasing at a dramatic rate [at the time of writing, the MERLOT catalog housed 129 groups of nursing lessons (MERLOT, 2005)] and with the huge potential of distance education via the Internet soon to be realized, nursing institutions must consider developing a balance between personal computers and large computer systems.
- *Lack of formal communication among users*: In North America most information about multimedia in nursing education is communicated among nursing educators who meet at annual conferences, such as the American Medical Informatics Association (AMIA) annual fall conference, or MERLOT, the American Nurses' Association Council on Continuing Education. International exchanges, such as Medinfo and the International Symposium on Nursing Informatics, also permit formal and extensive exchange of information about the quality and quantity of available nursing programs.

Summary

The objective of this chapter has been to provide a macroscopic perspective and conceptual framework concerning the place of computers in nursing education. The "third wave" requirements of education are here. The deficits in the existing system and the capability of using the computer to resolve those deficits must be acknowledged. Taking advantage of these capabilities means changes for educators, learners, and healthcare professionals, as well as changes in work processes and the educational system. The potential of multimedia technology offers education and healthcare professionals the opportunity to move out of the reactive positions into which they have been forced. Success will be achieved when these professionals contribute their efforts to these phases.

1. Adapt the technology to the needs of the professions
2. Provide users with quality, professionally validated educational resources
3. Develop, update, and monitor multimedia resources
4. Support the utilization of multimedia technology by healthcare professionals

Commitment to these efforts will lead to innovation and transformation in learning. Although education will surely continue in the classroom, it will also expand beyond it and into every area of professional life. Indeed, far from making traditional approaches obsolete, multimedia technology can become a source of revenue for institutions now hard pressed to make ends meet. The demand for effective learning resources is great.

Computer technology is an exciting addition to the repertoire of teaching strategies available for use by nurse educators. Its use must be based on substantive content expertise, however, and its success will be dictated by the imagination and creativity of nurse educators who author multimedia materials.

References

Adams, A.M. (2004). Pedagogical underpinnings of computer-based learning. *Journal of Advanced Nursing 46*(1):5–12.

Anthony, D. (2002). Online courses in the therapies survey. *Information Technology in Nursing 14*(4):13–25.

Belfry, M.J., & Winne, P. (1988). A review of the effectiveness of computer-assisted instruction in nursing education. *Computers in Nursing 6*(2):77–85.

Bitzer, M.D., & Bitzer, D.L. (1973). Teaching nursing by computer: an evaluative study. *Computers in Biology and Medicine 3*:187–204.

Chang, B. (1986). Computer-aided instruction in nursing education. In: Werely, H.H., J. Fitzpatrick, & R. Traunton, (eds.) *Annual Review of Nursing Research,* vol. 4. New York: Springer, pp. 217–233.

Edwards, M.J.A. (2002). *The Internet for Nurses and Allied Health Professionals, 3rd ed*. New York: Springer.

e-learners.com Inc. (2005). *What Is e-Learning?* http://www.elearners.com/-resources/elearning-faq1.asp (accessed February 21, 2005).

Gaston, S. (1988). Knowledge, retention and attitude effects of computer-assisted instruction. *Journal of Nursing Education 27*(1):30–34.

Hannah, R.S. (1998). *Designing Multimedia for Health Education*. Unpublished.

Harless, W.G., Drennan, G.G., Marxer, J.J., Root, W.G., & Miller, G.E. (1971). CASE: a computer-aided simulation of the clinical encounter. *Journal of Medical Education* 47:443–448.

Jenkins, T.M., Ball, M.J., & Bruns, B.M. (1983). The state of the art in technology assisted learning. In: *AAMSI Proceedings*.

Jerram, P., & Gosney, M. (1996). *Multimedia Power Tools*. New York: Random House.

Khoiny, F.E. (1996). Factors that contribute to computer-assisted instruction effectiveness. *Computers in Nursing 13*(4):165–168.

Kristof, R., & Satran, A. (1995). *Interactivity by Design,* Mountain View, CA: Adobe Press.

Locatis, C. (1992). Authoring Systems. Bethesda, MD: US Department of Health and Human Services, Public Health Service, National Institutes of Health, National Library of Medicine.

Longman, S., & Gabriel, M. (2004). Staff perceptions of E-learning. *Canadian Nurse 100*(1):23–27.

Lopuck, L. (1996). *Designing Multimedia: A Visual Guide to Multimedia and Online Graphic Design.* Berkeley, CA: Peachpit Press.

MERLOT. (2005). MERLOT Tasting Room. *http://taste.merlot.org* (accessed February 21, 2005).

Nyamathi, A., Chang, B., Sherman, B., & Grech, M. (1989). Computer use and nursing research: CAI versus traditional learning. *Western Journal of Nursing Research* *11*(4):498–501.

11
Research Applications

WITH CONTRIBUTIONS BY ANN CASEBEER

> For many nurse researchers, computer-mediated communication has become as essential as the telephone.
>
> —(Norris, 1999, p. 197)

Computer applications are an integral part of most research. Computing hardware and software comprise useful timesaving tools and information-gathering sources that are used regularly by researchers of all kinds (Parker, 2003). Whereas the basic principles and approaches to the conduct of nursing research have remained relatively constant, great strides continue to be made in the ways researchers can access evidence and manage and transfer data and findings (Cotton, 2003b). This chapter focuses on some of the ways in which nursing research can be enhanced by computer applications and the research information and analytical tools to which they provide access.

Nursing, as a profession, must continue to develop a research-based body of nursing practice knowledge as a central means to continuous improvement of patient care. Nursing research also has an expanding role in contributing to broader interdisciplinary health research focused on identifying and implementing better healthcare practice. Therefore the focus in this chapter is on clinical nursing practice research rather than on research related to nursing education or nursing administration, although many of the principles and approaches discussed apply equally well to these areas. It is not our purpose to provide a comprehensive discussion of clinical nursing research [see Gillis and Jackson (2002) and Polit and Beck (2004) for an extensive description of the principles and methods of nursing research]. Rather, the purpose of this chapter is to provide an overview of the use of computer technology and the web-based information to which it allows access in support of clinical nursing research. Clinical nursing researchers must exploit all available tools to aid the development of empirically based nursing practice.

The beginnings of clinical nursing research can be traced to Florence Nightingale. In *Notes on Nursing,* Nightingale stated her firm belief in applied nursing research: "Averages again seduce us away from minute observation. . . . We know, say, that from 22 to 24 per 1000 will die in London next year. But minute enquiries enable us to know that in such a district, nay, in such a street—or even on one side of the street, in a particular house, will be the excess of mortality, that is, the person will die who ought not to have died before old age" (Nightingale, 1860/1969, p. 124). Unfortunately, much of nursing practice has been founded on intuition-based apprentice training programs. Much of that intuition was experiential, either the nurse's or the nursing teachers', and was passed on to new learners using practitioner authority as validation. The nursing profession is making a concerted effort in its quest for empirical knowledge that will develop a scientific structure for the practice of nursing. To know the true effectiveness of nursing actions, practice-oriented research grounded in sound theoretical concepts is essential (Polit and Beck, 2004). Nursing must continue to challenge and examine its traditions, experiences, and intuitive actions by actively engaging in nursing research.

Searching the Literature

Nursing research is predicated in part on the ability of the nurse researcher to carry out a comprehensive review of the relevant literature and, in turn, to appraise this literature critically (Brettle and Gambling, 2003; Griffin-Sobel, 2003). This task used to be conducted manually by spending untold hours in the library thumbing through the cumulative indexes and journals. This time-consuming task may or may not allow the researcher to locate relevant material and most certainly would not result in a comprehensive collection of all pertinent evidence. Computer-assisted systematic reviews yield much more complete and valid compilations of the most relevant and up-to-date information related to research and practice questions (Egger et al., 2003; Helmer et al., 2001).

The advent of computerized databases of literature during the 1960s allowed researchers, initially with the help of librarians, to search rapidly and retrieve abstracts of literature immediately. University and college libraries as well as the libraries of many large teaching hospitals continue to provide this mediated literature searching to their staff, faculty, and students. Many databases that were available only from online vendors have been mounted locally by hospitals, colleges, and universities through a subscription process enabling end-users to search these databases themselves via the Internet. Many less commonly used databases are still available only through on-line vendors, requiring password access from an organization or subscription. Databases of primary interest to nurses conducting literature searches include CINAHL and MEDLINE. A description of these and other relevant databases is found in Appendix G.

Even with easier, more rapid direct access to databases, effective literature searching remains a skilled process that must be acquired either through training or through the assistance of someone with the expertise required.

Literature searches of certain types are more problematic than others. For example, finding relevant "gray" (unpublished) literature may be important to the clinical research of interest but difficult to locate and evaluate (Conn et al., 2003). Additionally, searching for qualitative evidence often pertinent to nursing research poses unique problems. Barroso and colleagues (2003) discuss the challenges of searching for qualitative research and made recommendations for improving the quality of such searches.

In mediated literature searching, a professional librarian works with the researcher to identify appropriate keywords and subject headings to generate a printout of citations and abstracts related to the topic. With the abstracts, the researcher can determine the relevance of a particular article to the research question before attempting to locate the article in a database, local library or ordering it through an interlibrary loan system. Researchers who choose to conduct their own searches should both acquire training and seek the advice and assistance of a professional librarian. Library staff can provide guidance in the selection of keywords and subject headings, as well as the correct search protocol for a given database, saving the user hours of frustration. The capacity of a researcher to personally search the literature provides the opportunity for browsing and the serendipitous discovery of information, which might appear unrelated to another researcher or librarian but is important to the particular research question or problem being pursued. Another innovation that helped researchers was the development of on-line full-text information services. For example, Ovid Technologies Inc. provides enhanced electronic full text to more than 1500 leading scientific, academic, and medical journals and books (http//www.ovid.com). Ovid is available through libraries and also as an individual subscription.

Once the researcher has searched appropriate literature databases, identified potentially useful citations, located and read the articles, and determined which are relevant to the research question, there is the matter of indexing and filing the information that has been so laboriously gathered. While it is still possible to use a manual system involving index cards or photocopied pages covered with highlighter pen, general-purpose database software packages are available for both office and personal computers. Bibliographic packages have undergone many changes and improvements in the past several years. These packages allow the researcher to set up a personal database of bibliographic references. Further, most of these packages allow reformatting of entries automatically with only one command. If, for example, the researcher has entered all the references in a personal bibliographic file in APA format but the journal to which a paper is being submitted requires Terabian format, the researcher selects the appropriate references, issues a command, the computer automatically reformats the selected references, and they are ready to be printed out. Commonly used programs in biomedical/nursing research are Reference Manager, ProCite, and EndNote (Nicoll, 2003).

Preparation of Research Documents

The bane of every researcher's existence is the paperwork. Grant proposals, correspondence with funding agencies, consent forms, data-gathering forms and instruments, ethics applications, consent forms, progress reports, grant renewals, manuscripts for publication, all require multiple copies of essentially the same information with minor modifications or slight revisions. The advent of electronic text editing facilities and word processing equipment has been a boon to all researchers when preparing research documents. The speed and ease of computer use is well established—assisting in the preparation, revision, and formatting of research documents and reducing the time spent on the paperwork associated with research. Today's research environment demands a high level of computer literacy from all researchers who intend to compete for grant funding and who wish to collaborate effectively with other colleagues in obtaining existing evidence or creating new knowledge for future improvement in clinical practice.

Text editing facilities today are a regular component of all word processing software available for computers. Standard software packages (such as Microsoft Word or Word Perfect) have become increasingly sophisticated and easy to use. Centers of nursing research and learning resource centers now include computers with appropriate word processing and other software packages as required equipment for their researchers. Journal manuscripts are typeset directly from the word-processing file prepared by the nurse researcher. Additionally, many journals are now available only electronically, not in a print version. For these journals, the author's article file is reformatted for online presentation. Similarly, book publishers, including this book's publisher, Springer, are typesetting books directly from authors' electronic files sent via the Internet. Web-based publishing is creating expanded opportunities to publish and access research. It is also raising issues around ownership and production costs for both online and off-line journals and literature generally (Graczynski and Moses, 2004).

The benefits of computerized methods of producing research documents include reduced costs and fewer errors resulting from repeated retyping of the manuscript, increased control of the document by the author, faster production of the finished work, and greater ease of revision. In other words, speed, accuracy, flexibility, and control are the result. The costs incurred are the investment of the researcher's time in acquiring keyboarding skills, locating appropriate software, and learning to use the available software tools. Additional costs are purchase, lease, or rental of appropriate equipment and software. All these are one-time costs that provide long-term benefits. Access to and ability to use computerized word-processing packages has become essential. As practitioners and researchers, we live in a computerized world, and basic computer and word-processing skills and technology access are essential areas of professional competence.

Data Gathering

There has been an explosion in the range and scope of accessible data of potential value to nursing researchers. Researchers use technology to manage the data gathering process. Facts (or data) originate with the patient. Nurse researchers who seek to gather reliable and accurate facts should ensure that the data capture occurs as closely as possible to its source, i.e., the subject/patient. Technology can be helpful to the systematic collection, management and transfer of accurate data. Nurse researchers are increasingly using a variety of input devices including digital photography, biometric probes and bar code generators and readers as well as hand held computers and personal digital assistants (PDAs) for source data capture in nursing research studies. (See Chapter 7 for more information on source data capture.) The archiving and transfer of digital and live images is a reality in practice and accessible to researchers (Blackmore et al., 2003; Moloney et al., 2003).

The conduct of web-based research is becoming an acceptable method of data collection, adding to the possibilities for direct input of research findings prior to management and interpretation (Birnbaum, 2004). Research on and through the Web is clearly a breakthrough in terms of reaching some research participant populations; at the same time issues of data accuracy and security are heightened and have created significant ethical issues and debates (Cotton, 2003a; Ellett et al., 2004).

Increasingly, data are automatically and directly entered into a database on a personal computer for analysis. There are far fewer opportunities for coding or transcription errors with this method of data capture and transfer. This is now an easily accessible option, as is direct input from patients or clients themselves as well as practitioner input and access to relevant data at the desk or bedside.

Principles of source data capture can also be applied to computer-assisted interviewing methods. Computer-assisted interviewing methods allow the researcher to capture the data immediately in the computer in a usable format. Using these methods eliminates the step of data entry and has the potential to improve data quality, as errors are commonly found in the transcription from code sheet to computer. Computer-assisted interviewing can be accomplished either with the subject being physically present in the computer-base interviewing room or through the use of Internet-based tools subjects can use in the location of their choice (Read, 2004; Rew et al., 2004). There are three types of computer-assisted interviewing.

- Computer-assisted self-interviewing (CASI): Research subjects answer on-screen questions by selecting their response with a keyboard, light pen, or touch screen. This method has been used in areas such as lifestyle risk assessment, nutritional surveys, and health behavior studies.

- Computer-assisted telephone interviewing (CATI): When using CATI, a telephone interviewer reads each question from a computer screen. The answer to the question is entered through the keyboard. The answer is immediately placed in the correct preprogrammed row/column position. The captured data are then already in the final form necessary for analysis.
- Computer-assisted personal interviewing (CAPI): Laptop computers allow the researcher to use the CATI process in a face-to-face setting. Questions are posed on the screen. Answers are entered immediately in a form ready for analysis. Both open-ended and closed-ended questions can be posed with these systems.

Advantages of Computer-Assisted Interviewing

- Automatic branching can be programmed, thereby decreasing errors that result from incorrectly followed skip patterns.
- Text can be inserted into later questions. For example, if a current nursing diagnosis or patient problem has been previously entered, a subsequent question would replace "patient problem/nursing diagnosis" with the answer given. This personalizes the interview.
- Question order and response categories can be automatically randomized. When long lists of choices are given, particularly during telephone interviews, respondents tend to select from those at the end of the list. Random reordering of the responses is one way to address this problem.
- On-line editing and consistency checking allow the interviewer to check data captured while still interviewing. Many programs do not allow out-of-scope answers to be recorded. This also increases the precision of the data gathered.
- Typing is faster than writing when capturing answers to open-ended questions. Software resident spellcheck programs can then clean the captured data. Content analysis of captured data is facilitated because the information does not have to be entered from written notes.

Considerations When Using Computer-Assisted Interviewing

- Each question is restricted to the size of the computer screen. If a question scrolls to a second page, the speed of screen redisplay is important. Each new screen must be immediately useful.
- Provision must be made for nonstandard movement through the questionnaire. The interviewer or respondent must be able to go back to a previous question and check or change an answer.
- A major consideration is the up-front cost in both time and money to acquire the hardware initially and develop the software and questionnaires.

Use of Clinical Databases

Much clinical nursing research requires descriptive studies (i.e., initial gathering of a database from which inferences and conclusions are drawn). With the introduction of computerized information systems in healthcare institutions, nurses' opportunity to access large databases of nursing practice documentation has become a reality in many such institutions. Health and hospital information system databases provide unique possibilities for retrospective studies generating nursing research questions and descriptive nursing research. However, not all systems are equally suitable for the storage or manipulation of data relevant to nursing research, nor do all systems retain on-line information for extended periods of time. From a nursing research perspective, there are several considerations and problems associated with the data currently being accumulated in many computerized hospital information systems. Too often such data are formatted and retrievable merely as patient record data rather than with any view to retrieval for research purposes. The introduction of relational database management systems has been most supportive of achieving the goal of simultaneously gathering clinical documentation for the purposes of both legal records and nursing research.

Data Mining

With the advent of widespread use of source data capture and the electronic health record, healthcare clinical databases have grown exponentially in both size and complexity. It has become increasingly difficult and now nearly impossible for the researcher to manually analyze the massive amounts of clinical data available from these large institutional or governmental databases. Data mining, a step in the knowledge discovery in databases (KDD) process, offers an approach to extracting useable and useful information from large data sets. Data mining has been defined as "the semiautomatic exploration and analysis of large quantities of data in order to discover meaningful patterns and rules" (Berry and Linhoff, 1997, p. 5). As the definition infers, data mining is generally focused on discovery, looking for patterns in the vast amount of data available related to a particular question. For example, researchers Goodwin and Iannacchione (2002), looking for factors that predict which women are at risk for preterm birth, used data mining techniques to examine the relationship between gestational age at delivery and more than 4000 perinatal data variables. Manual analysis could not accommodate such a large number of possible relationships, but data mining identified seven key variables that could then be tested further for their ability to predict the risk of preterm birth (Goodwin and Iannachione, 2002).

There are challenges to using data mining techniques. The largest challenge arises from the lack of standardized data measurement and labeling.

Clinical data require considerable preprocessing to standardize labels, remove redundant data, and complete necessary data transformations. For example, "myocardial infarction" and "MI" refer to the same diagnosis, so rules must be applied to account for multiple labels representing the same category (Berger and Berger, 2004). Goodwin and Iannachione (2002) note that data mining makes sense when there are large stores of data to be searched, where the computing power is available to process the massive analysis, and when the people exist to prepare and analyze both data and output. Although computer systems complete the processing of the data sets, knowledgeable domain experts, such as nurse researchers are required to transform the resulting information into useful and understandable knowledge to guide nursing practice (Berger and Berger, 2004).

Technology is now available to allow interfacing among computers within a single institution as well as between computers in different institutions or facilities. For example, it is possible to use the computer in one site via a modem and telephone lines or cable or wireless connection to merge existing data with data entered on, and processed by, a computer at another location. This technology of intercomputer communication, or networking, allows creation of larger, more diverse databases. Random sampling, large samples, and control groups may be easier to delineate using the database linkage provided by computer networking.

Furthermore, networking makes collaboration with colleagues in widely separated geographic locations possible through the use of electronic mail and other Internet-based collaboration tools. Researchers now have the means at their disposal to collaborate with colleagues having similar research interests and expertise, regardless of the fact that they may live and work in locations that are widely separated geographically.

Using electronic means of communication, dialogue and exchange of ideas, refinements in protocols, and interpretation of data occur in a timely fashion. Previously, these interactions among investigators had not been possible unless the investigators lived and worked in close geographic proximity to each other. The regular interactions and contact vital to the outcome of any research study are fully available to all investigators working on a project, independent of location. Thus, both data gathering and data analysis are enhanced by the use of computer networking and telecommunications.

There are also concerns along with the benefits of technologically enhanced access including the potential for an overloading of communication and information—an explosion of data that can lead to paralysis of sorts (Mathieson, 2003; Radner, 2004). As well, the emergence of viruses that infect databases and e-mail transfers can corrupt the quality of accessible and reliable information for research and practice alike (Reid, 2002). It is essential to establish effective communication and information-sharing protocols as well as to employ sophisticated virus protection software.

Data Analysis

A critical part of any research process involves analyzing data. Research data can include numerical information of a quantitative or statistical nature or take the form of narrative text providing qualitative information. Computerized software packages can assist both types of data manipulation. As nurse researchers work with others in increasingly multidisciplinary research and practice teams, their own scope of research interest and analytical competencies grow.

Most experienced nurse researchers are familiar to a greater or lesser degree with the use of computers in statistical analysis. There are hundreds of software packages for use in carrying out statistical analysis on computers. The best known and most widely used include BMDP (Biomedical Data Processing), EPINFO (Epidemiological Information), SAS (Statistical Analysis Software), and SPSS (Statistical Packages for the Social Sciences). Institutions in which research is being conducted have these packages available through their main computing facility or network. These particular software packages are widely available internationally and on the Internet; they have demonstrated consistency and stability, provide a wide variety of statistical treatments, and are fairly easy to learn and use. They are also powerful enough to handle large volumes of data.

Statistical software packages are increasingly designed for use on personal computers. Some packages, such as EPINFO, are available free of charge on the Internet (www.cdc.gov/epiinfo/). Five fundamental criteria originally identified by Francis (1981) have long been regarded as guidelines for novices to use when evaluating the utility and quality of statistical programs: capabilities, portability, ease of learning and use, reliability, and cost. Although they are not as powerful as the statistical packages available on larger computer systems or those linked from dedicated servers, researchers may, for a variety of reasons, wish to carry out data analysis on a personal computer (Anthony, 2004). If so, in addition to the criteria just mentioned, researchers must consider the compatibility of their hardware and operating system with what the software package requires, the quality of the documentation provided by the software distributor regarding how to use the system, and the availability of technical support online or via telephone. Other important considerations are limitations in the volume of data that can be manipulated and stored as well as constraints regarding the number of statistical functions that can be performed, although these capacity limitations are rapidly being addressed in powerful microcomputers.

One of the more innovative applications of computers in data analysis is the use of text editing programs in qualitative research (Wietzman, 2002). Any researcher who has conducted qualitative studies is well aware that the volume of field notes and interviews to be transcribed is enormous, costly, and frequently overwhelming. Qualitative data analysis packages, such as

Atlas/ti, Ethnograph, and NUDIST, provide a way to enter these data into computer files. These programs then use computer technology to search the text for occurrences of particular words or phrases indicative of data related to a specific category or cluster (Morse and Richards, 2002). Using these programs for qualitative research permits illustrative blocks of text to be copied and moved easily into another file for use when composing the final report.

Graphics

Remember the well-known phrase, "A picture is worth a thousand words"? Before the advent of computer graphics, researchers were confronted with mounds of paper containing the outcome of statistical processing of their data. As they attempted to aggregate and interpret this mound of paper, researchers often sketched graphs and charts of the results. These rough sketches were useful when summarizing data and reducing it to a manageable scale. Eventually, these sketches were refined and given to an artist, who produced the formal published versions that were used in research reports to illustrate the findings. Computers have the capacity to produce, rapidly and inexpensively, a wide variety of graphs, scattergrams, histograms, and charts simultaneously with the numerical data analysis. People can retain only a limited number of figures in their heads at one time. These pictorial representations greatly assist the investigator's progress in interpreting the data. At the same time, the use of computer graphics to prepare illustrations to accompany research publications also is accelerating the rate and reducing the cost at which findings can be prepared for publication.

Summary

The advantages of computers to researchers are speed, accuracy, and flexibility. In common with most researchers today, nurse researchers must know how to use automated information systems to their advantage to provide them with better information at all phases of the data gathering, data analysis, and communication of research findings. These computer applications must be combined with well developed critical appraisal and research methods skills. This allows increased creativity and aids the development of the body of scientific knowledge on which nursing theory, practice, and education are based and through which nurses make important contributions to wider health systems research. Nurse researchers and practicing nurses alike must become proficient in the application and uses of computer technology to forward the development and use of an empirical base for nursing practice. Nursing research plays a critical role in enhancing nursing practice and contributing to the wider body of clinical research necessary to patient care and population health protection and improvement.

References

Anthony, D. (2004). Using a computer to perform statistical analysis. *Nurse Researcher 11*(3):7–27.

Barroso, J., Gollop, C.J., & Sandelowski, M., et al. (2003). The challenges of searching for and retrieving qualitative studies. *Western Journal of Nursing Research 25*(2):153–78.

Berger, A.M., & Berger, C.R. (2004). Data mining as a tool for research and knowledge development in nursing. *CIN: Computers, Informatics, Nursing 22*(3):123–131.

Berry, M.J.A., & Linhoff, G. (1997). *Data Mining Techniques for Marketing, Sales and Customer Support.* New York: Wiley.

Birnbaum, M.H. (2004). Human research and data collection via the internet. *Annual Review of Psychology 55*:803–832.

Blackmore, C.C., Richardson, M.L., & Linnau, K.F., et al. (2003). Web-based image review and data acquisition for multiinstitutional research. *American Journal of Roentgenology 180*(5):1243–1246.

Brettle, A., & Gambling, T. (2003). Needle in a haystack? Effective literature searching for research. *Radiography 9*(3):229–236.

Conn, V.S., Valentine, J.C., Cooper, H.M., & Rantz, M.J. (2003). Grey literature in meta-analyses. *Nursing Research 52*(4):256–261.

Cotton, A.H. (2003a). Ensnaring webs and nets: ethical issues in Internet-based research. *Contemporary Nursing 16*(1–2):114–123.

Cotton, A.H. (2003b). The discursive field of Web-based health research: Implications for nursing research in cyberspace. *Advances in Nursing Science 26*(4):307–319.

Egger, M., Juni, P., Bartlett, C., Holenstein, F., & Sterne, J. (2003). How important are comprehensive literature searches and the assessment of trial quality in systematic reviews? Empirical study. *Health Technology Assessment 7*(1):1–76.

Ellett, M.L., Lane, L., & Keffer, J. (2004). Ethical and legal issues of conducting nursing research via the Internet. *Journal of Professional Nursing 20*(1):68–74.

Francis, I. (1981). *Statistical Software: A Comparative Review.* Amsterdam: North-Holland Elsevier.

Gillis, A., & Jackson, W. (2002). *Research for Nurses: Methods and Interpretation.* Philadelphia: Davis.

Goodwin, L.K., & Iannachione, M.A. (2002). Data mining methods for improving birth outcomes prediction. *Outcomes Management 6*(2):80–85.

Graczynski, M.R., & Moses, L. (2004). Open access publishing—panacea or Trojan horse? *Medical Science Monitor 10*(1):ED1–ED3.

Griffin-Sobel, J.P. (2003). Research in practice: the literature review. *Gastroenterology Nursing 26*(1):47–48.

Helmer, D., Savoie, I., Green, C., & Kazanjian, A. (2001). Evidence-based practice: Extending the search to find material for the systematic review. *Bulletin of the Medical Library Association 89*(4):346–352.

Mathieson, S. (2003). E-novation. spam with everything. *Health Service Journal 8* (suppl 4):113.

Moloney, M.F., Dietrich, A.S., Strickland, O., & Myerburg, S. (2003). Using Internet discussion boards as virtual focus groups. *Advances in Nursing Science 26*(4):274–286.

Morse, J., & Richards, L. (2002). *Readme First for a User's Guide to Qualitative Methods.* Thousands Oaks, CA: Sage.

Nicoll, L.H. (2003). A practical way to create a library in a bibliographic database manager: Using electronic sources to make it easy. *CIN: Computers, Informatics, Nursing 21*(1):48–54.

Nightingale, F. (1969). *Notes on Nursing.* New York: Dover Publications Inc. (original work published 1860).

Norris, J.R. (1999). The Internet: Extending our capacity for scholarly inquiry in nursing. *Nursing Science Quarterly 12*(3):197–201.

Parker, M.E. (2003). The Internet . . . as a research tool: Finding the balance. *Registered Dental Hygienist 23*(9):78–81.

Polit, D.F., & Beck, C.T. (2004). *Nursing Research: Principles and Methods*. Philadelphia: Lippincott Williams & Wilkins.

Radner, G. (2004). Editorial: Web-based technology—a lifeline for managing information overload. *Journal of Asset Management 4*(6):364.

Read, C.Y. (2004). Conducting a client-focused survey using email. *CIN: Computers, Informatics, Nursing 22*(2):83–89.

Reid, G. (2002). Protecting yourself against cyberterrorism. *Tech Directions 61*(6): 9.

Rew, L., Horner, S.D., Riesch, L., & Cauvin, R. (2004). Computer-assisted survey interviewing of school-age children. *Advances in Nursing Science 27*(2):129–138.

Weitzman, E. (2000). Software and qualitative research. In: Denzin, N.K., Lincoln, Y.S. (eds.) *Handbook of Qualitative Research,* 2nd ed. Thousand Oaks, CA: Sage.

Additional Resources

Brink, P.J., & Wood, M.J. (2001). Basic Steps in Planning Nursing Research. Boston: Jones & Bartlett.

Crombie, I.K. (1996). *The Pocket Guide to Critical Appraisal.* London: BMJ Publishing Group.

Egger, M., Davery Smith, G., & Altman, D. (Eds.) (2001). *Systematic Reviews in Healthcare*, 2nd ed. London: BMJ Books.

Garrand, J. (1999). *Health Sciences Literature Review Made Easy*. Gaithersburg, MD: Aspen.

Gift, A.G. (1997). *Clarifying Concepts in Nursing Research*. New York: Springer.

Hulley, S.B., Cummings, S.R., & Browner, W.S., et al. (2001). *Designing Clinical Research*. Philadelphia: Lippincott Williams & Wilkins.

Lakeman, R. (1997). Using the Internet for data collection in nursing. *Computers in Nursing 15*(5):269–275.

Milley, A. (2000). Healthcare and data mining. *Health Management Technology 21*(8):44–46.

Peckham, M., & Smith, R. (Eds.) (1996). *Scientific Basis of Health Services.* London: BMJ Publishing Group.

Websites of Internet

CINAHLdirect: http//www.cinahl.com
International Healthcare Research Guide: http//www.health.ucalgary.ca/
National Institute of Nursing Research (NINR): http//www.nih.gov/ninr
National Institutes of Health: Scientific Resources: http://www.nih.gov/science
Research Institutes: http//pie.org/E21224T3783
SVR Nursing Connections Links to Nursing E-Journals: http//homel.inet.tele.dk/box4280/nursedk/journ.htm
Newsgroups: Usenet newsgroup:sci.research

Part IV
Infrastructure Elements of the Informatics Environment

12
Nursing Data Standards

Nursing Values Related to Health Information

The initial systems for gathering minimum uniform health data can be traced back to systems devised by Florence Nightingale over a century ago (Verney 1970). Nightingale (1859) asserted the need for nurses to use their powers of memory and nonsubjective observation to track the condition of those in their care. Subsequently (Nightingale 1863), she provided forms and definitions for the collection of uniform hospital statistics. In conclusion, she wrote (Nightingale 1863):

> I am fain to sum up with an urgent appeal for adopting this or some *uniform* system of publishing the statistical records of hospitals. There is a growing conviction that in all hospitals, even in those which are best conducted, there is a great and unnecessary waste of life;... It is imperative that this impression should be either dissipated or confirmed.
>
> In attempting to arrive at the truth, I have applied everywhere for information, but in scarcely an instance have I been able to obtain hospital records fit for any purpose of comparison... if wisely used, these improved statistics would tell us more of the relative value of particular operations and modes of treatment than we have any means of obtaining at present. They would enable us, besides, to ascertain the influence of the hospital... upon the general course of operations and diseases passing through its wards; and the truth thus ascertained would enable us to save life and suffering, and to improve the treatment and management of the sick and maimed poor.

The needs have not changed. Nurses must be able to manage and process nursing data, information, and knowledge to support patient care delivery in diverse care delivery settings (Graves and Corcoran, 1989). Ozbolt, (1999) maintained that:

> Standard terms and codes are needed to record as structured data the problems and issues that nurses and other caregivers address; the actions they take to prevent,

ameliorate, or resolve the problems; and the results of their care. Such data could be used to increase the effectiveness of care and control costs.

There is an essential linkage among access to information, client outcomes and patient safety. "As Lang has succinctly and aptly described the present situation: If we cannot name it, we cannot control it, finance it, teach it, research it or put it into public policy" (Clark and Lang, 1992). Access to information about their practice arms nurses with evidence to support the contribution of nursing to patient outcomes. Outcomes research is an essential foundation for evidence-based nursing practice. Evidence-based practice is a means of promoting and enhancing patient safety.

Evolution of Nursing Information and Nursing Data Elements

There are a variety of concepts that interlink when considering the capture of nursing practice data. Figure 12.1 illustrates the derivation, from nursing practice, of nursing classification, nursing terminology, minimum data sets, reference terminology models, and the resulting feedback loop.

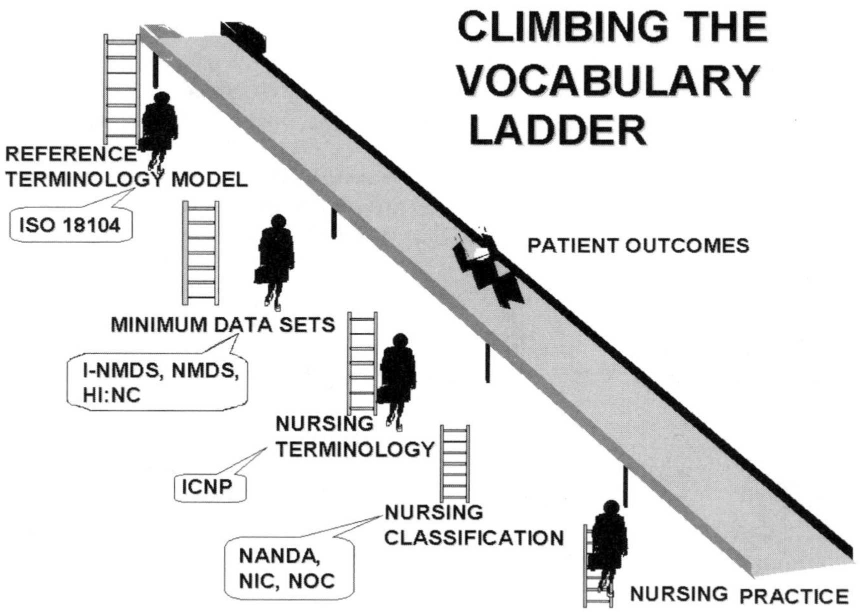

FIGURE 12.1. Relationships between nursing practice and classification, terminology, minimum data sets, and reference terminology model.

United States

Uniform Hospital Discharge Data Set

In the United States, the Uniform Hospital Discharge Data Set (UHDDS) was developed over a 5-year period during the early 1970s. It identified the minimum basic set of data elements to be collected from all hospital records at the point of patient discharge from hospitals. In 1974, the UHDDS was adopted and mandated by the Secretary of the Department of Health and Human Services for collection by the U.S. National Committee on Vital and Health Statistics (Abdellah, 1988; Pearce, 1988). The UHDDS provided the model for the hospital discharge abstract that was subsequently developed in Canada and ultimately evolved into the Discharge Abstract Database (DAD), now maintained by the Canadian Institute for Health Information (CIHI).

The care items included in the UHDDS focused on physician-derived clinical data (specifically, medical diagnosis and procedures based on medical treatments). There were absolutely *no* nursing clinical data included in this data set. Patient care is not exclusively physician-directed; therefore, a data set of this nature falls short of providing a complete, accurate representation of information related to the operation of hospitals.

Nursing Minimum Data Set

In response to recognition of the information gap created by the exclusion of nursing data elements from the Uniform Hospital Discharge Data Set, Werley and colleagues developed the Nursing Minimum Data Set (NMDS) through a consensus conference at the University of WisconsinMilwaukee School of Nursing in 1985 (Werley and Lang 1988). The NMDS was defined as "a minimum set of items of information with uniform definitions and categories concerning the specific dimension of professional nursing, which meets the information needs of multiple data users in the healthcare system" (Werley and Lang 1988). There were five purposes of the NMDS.

- Establish comparability of nursing data across practice settings and geographic boundaries
- Capture descriptors reflecting the nursing care of clients and their families in a variety of settings
- Project trends in nursing care needs and resource use according to health problems
- Provide a database for nursing research
- Provide data about nursing care for consideration by individuals involved in health policy decision-making

The NMDS consisted of nursing care elements, patient demographic elements, and service elements. The nursing care elements of nursing diagnosis, nursing intervention, nursing outcome, and intensity of nursing care drew on the nursing process used by nurses to plan and provide patient care in any setting. The patient demographic and service elements, except health record number and the unique number of the nurse provider, are data elements contained in the UHDDS and could be accessed through linkage with this data set (Werley and Lang, 1988). Once the NMDS was agreed upon, uniform definitions for each of the data elements and standard classification systems were necessary for collection of uniform, accurate data to be feasible.

Classification Systems for NMDS Data Elements

The North American Nursing Diagnosis Association (NANDA) initiated the development of labels for the clinical phenomena for which nurses provide care (i.e. nursing diagnosis) in 1973. NANDA has defined nursing diagnosis as "a clinical judgment about individual, family, or community responses to actual and potential health problems and life processes. Nursing diagnoses provide the basis for selection of nursing interventions to achieve outcomes of which the nurse is accountable" (Carpenito, 1989).

The Visiting Nurses Association (VNA) of Omaha developed the problem classification scheme, intervention scheme, and problem rating scale for outcomes related to community health client problems and nursing problems used for documenting community health nursing services. The Omaha classification system defined a problem as "a clinical judgment about environmental, psychosocial, physiologic and health related behavior data that is [*sic*] of interest or concern to the client" (Martin, 1988; Martin and Scheet 1992).

The Home Healthcare Classification (HHCC) was developed at the Georgetown University School of Nursing from 1988 to 1991 to assess and classify home health Medicare clients for predicting their need for nursing and other home care services as well as for measuring outcomes and data on the resources employed (Saba, 1992). Nursing interventions were defined in the HHCC: Nursing Interventions as a nursing service, with significant treatment, intervention, or activity identified to carry out the medical or nursing order (Saba, 1992). Nursing interventions were considered critical measures of the resources used.

The Nursing Interventions Classification (NIC) and Nursing Outcomes Classification System (NOC) were developed by a large research team (the Iowa Intervention Project) led by McCloskey and Bulechek at the University of Iowa. This team defined nursing interventions as "any treatment, based upon clinical judgment and knowledge, that a nurse performs to enhance patient/client outcomes. Nursing interventions include both direct and indirect care; both nurse-initiated, physician-initiated and other-provider-initiated treatments"(McCloskey and Bulechek, 1996). NIC was coded to be consistent with the Current Procedural Terminology, American Medical Association, and the Healthcare Financing Administration's Common Procedure Coding System and was included in the Library of Medicine's *Metathesaurus for a Unified Medical Language.* Additionally, it has been endorsed by the

American Nurses Association (ANA) for inclusion in the proposed Unified Nursing Language System (McCloskey and Bulechek, 1996; McCormick et al., 1994). NIC provides a standardized language that can be used across settings and across healthcare disciplines (McCloskey and Bulechek, 1996). Independent and collaborative interventions as well as basic and complex interventions were included. A nursing outcomes classification (NOC) system has also been developed in conjunction with the NIC through the Iowa Intervention Project Johnson et al., 2000).

The Unified Medical Language System (UMLS) includes NANDA, the Omaha System, the HHCC, and the NIC. The UMLS is a long-term research project developed by the U.S. National Library of Medicine to integrate clinical vocabularies from various sources so data from each can be cross-referenced when needed. In addition all four of these classifications have been incorporated into the International Classification for Nursing Practice (ICNP).

International Classification for Nursing Practice (ICNP)®

The International Council of Nurses (ICN), as a component of its commitment to advance nursing thought the world, initiated a long-term project to develop an international classification for nursing practice (ICNP) in 1990. The motivation was to support the processes of nursing practice and to advance the knowledge necessary for cost-effective delivery of quality nursing care (Ehnfors, 1999; Nielsen and Mortensen, 1999). The intent was to establish a common language about nursing practice that was capable of describing nursing care, permitting comparison of nursing data, demonstrating or projecting tendencies, and stimulating nursing research (International Council of Nurses, 1993, 1996, 1999). In 1993, a draft of the classification was proposed that included virtually all of the nursing classification schemes that had been developed internationally. The aim was to provide worldwide input into the construction of a comprehensive classification scheme that could eventually be used by nurses around the world. The Alpha Version was released for comment and critique in 1996, followed in 1999 by a Beta Version. The Beta 2 version was published in 2002 (International Council of Nurses, 2002b)® and Version 1 was released at the ICN Congress in 2005 (ICN 2005).

The ICNP® is a classification of nursing phenomena, actions, and outcomes. It provides a terminology for nursing practice that serves as a unifying framework into which existing nursing vocabularies and classifications can be cross-mapped to enable comparison of nursing data (International Council of Nurses, 2002b).

The initial objectives of the ICNP® were reviewed by the ICNP Evaluation Committee in 2000. The objectives were revised to direct the aims of the ICNP® program.

- Establish a common language for describing nursing practice to improve communication among nurses and between nurses and others

- Represent concepts used in local practice across languages and specialty areas
- Describe the nursing care of people (individuals, families, communities) worldwide
- Enable comparison of nursing data across client populations, settings, geographic areas, and time
- Stimulate nursing research through links to data available in nursing and health information systems
- Provide data about nursing practice to influence nursing education and health policy
- Project trends in patient needs, provision of nursing treatments, resource utilization, and outcomes of nursing care

Europe

Telenurse

European nurses also recognized that their health systems need to include nursing data elements that are significant in the nursing decision-making process. A research initiative entitled "A Concerted Action on European Classification for Nursing Practice with Special Regard to Patient Problems/Nursing Diagnosis, Nursing Intervention, and Outcomes" (TELENURSING) was launched in 1991. The objectives of TELENURSING were to create a network of nurses interested in the classification of patient problems/nursing diagnosis, nursing interventions, nursing outcomes; minimum data sets and healthcare informatics; raising the awareness among nurses of standardization efforts in healthcare informatics; and linking the technical approach of national groups and the professional approach of international groups with regard to the development of classifications of healthcare. The TELENURSING group established evidence of an interest in developing data standards and a nursing minimum data set. The next step was to promote standardization of definitions, classification, and coding of data as initial work that may contribute to the development of internationally comparable nursing minimum data sets (Mortensen et al., 1994). The second phase of the project was TELENURSE, which stood for telematic applications for nurses. TELENURSE was a dedicated effort to the following goals (Mortensen, 1997).

- Disseminate and promote the ICNP in Europe in collaboration with the ICN and the national member organization in Europe
- Build consensus among European nurses
- Demonstrate how comparative telematics-based nursing data could be used in nursing modules of electronic patient records

The final phase, TELENENURSE ID, was the development, testing, and evaluation of software products using the ICNP® in electronic health records.

This phase also included translation of the alpha version of ICNP® into 14 European languages and collaboration with the ICN in the preparation of the beta version of ICNP® (Mortensen, 1999).

European Standardization Committee

The European Standardization Committee (Comite European de Normalisatrion) Technical Committee 251 on Medical Informatics (CEN TC 251) brought together the efforts of the ICNP program (Coenen et al., 2001; Hardiker and Rector, 1998; Hardiker et al., 2000; Mortensen, 1997, 1999; Nielsen and Mortensen, 1996; Ozbolt, 2000b), Telenurse ID (Mortensen, 1999; Nielsen and Mortensen, 1996), and other European efforts such as nursing activities in the Galen projects (Hardiker and Rector 1998; Hardiker et al., 2000) into a Prestandard—CEN prENV 14032 (Ozbolt, 2000b). The CEN Prestandard broadly addresses categorical structures for nursing diagnoses and nursing actions (ISO, 2002, 2003).

Canada

Nurses in Canada who were monitoring development of the NMDS in the United States urged Canadian nurses to initiate similar activity. The Canadian Nurses Association responded to a resolution calling for a national consensus conference "to develop in Canada a standardized format (NMDS) for purposes of ensuring entry, accessibility, and retrievability of nursing data" (Canadian Nurses Association 1990). The NMDS conference was held in Edmonton, Canada in 1992. The overall objective of this working conference was to develop an NMDS in Canada to ensure the availability and accessibility of standardized nursing data. Because of recognition of the paucity of dialogue that had taken place on the topic among Canadian nurses and the inappropriateness of attempting to achieve consensus on the topic at such an early stage, the invitational conference brought together those individuals best able to formulate a plan for initiating the development of an NMDS in Canada. The Canadian NMDS conference culminated in the identification of five elements.

- *Client status* is broadly defined as a label for the set of indicators that reflect the phenomena for which nurses provide care relative to the health status of clients (McGee, 1993). Although client status is similar to nursing diagnosis, the term client status was preferred because it represents a broader spectrum of health and illness. The common label "client status" is inclusive of input from all disciplines. The summative statements referring to the phenomena for which nurses provide care (i.e., nursing diagnosis) are merely one aspect of client status at a point in time, in the same way as medical diagnosis.
- *Nursing interventions* refer to purposeful and deliberate health affecting interventions (direct and indirect), based on assessment of client status,

that are designed to bring about results that benefit clients (Alberta Association of Registered Nurses, 1994).

- *Client outcome* is defined as a "clients' status at a defined point(s) following healthcare [affecting] intervention" (Marek and Lang, 1993). It is influenced to varying degrees by the interventions of all care providers.
- *Nursing intensity* "refers to the amount and type of nursing resource used to [provide] care" (O'Brien-Pallas and Giovannetti, 1993)
- *Primary nurse identifier* is a single unique lifetime identification number for each individual nurse. This identifier is independent of geographic location (province or territory), practice sector (e.g., acute care, community care, public health), or employer.

Group deliberations on each of the data elements are summarized elsewhere (Canadian Nurses Association, 1993a). These nursing data elements were proposed for addition to existing national data sets as a next step toward a cross sectoral, multidisciplinary, longitudinal national health database in Canada (Canadian Nurses Association, 1993a). However, some individuals and national organizations in Canada perceived the Canadian use of the term "nursing minimum data set" to portray a stand-alone nursing data set such as that in the United States. In Canada, this was not the intent. It is essential in Canada that the nursing data elements constitute one component of fully integrated health information data, such as the Canadian Institute for Health Information (CIHI) discharge abstract data set (Canadian Institute for Health Information, 2002) or an electronic health record (EHR) such as that being developed under the leadership of Infoway. Therefore, the five nursing data elements were identified collectively as the Nursing Components of Health Information (Health Information: Nursing Components, HI:NC) (Canadian Nurses Association, 1993b).

Following the Conference in 1992, CNA's Working Group on the Nursing Components of Health Information (HI:NC Working Group) continued to build on the work that had been started. In 1997 a national consensus was reached on three clinical nursing care data elements: client status, nursing intervention, and client outcome as well as nursing resource intensity and nurse identifier (Canadian Nurses Association, 2001a).

Identifying data elements that represent the most important aspects of nursing care is only the first step. In Canada, nurses face an immediate challenge to determine the most effective and efficient means to collect and code data elements that reflect nursing practice. To collect the data reflecting nursing contributions within the larger health information system, there is a need for consistent data collection using standardized languages to aggregate and compare data (Canadian Nurses Association, 1998).

In October 1999, a meeting was held at the CIHI in Toronto. Representatives of CIHI and CNA, as well as nurse researchers and nursing informatics specialists, from across the country discussed the gaps and opportunities for nursing data in the national health databases held by CIHI. A number of nursing informatics leaders representing CNA supported ICNP in principle as the most universal, generic, comprehensive foundational classification system for nursing at the time. CIHI representatives committed to exploring inclusion of the five data elements comprising the Nursing Components of Health Information in their national databases. Regrettably, CIHI's investigation of the version of ICNP available at the time (early beta version) revealed that the lack of a coding structure was a significant barrier to implementation at that time. This barrier has now been eliminated in Version 1. Another barrier was the apparent lack of awareness and consensus among nurses about the need for and importance of capturing nursing data nationally. As discussed in the following paragraph, the second barrier has been substantially reduced during the intervening 4 years since the CIHI analysis of ICNP.

In March 2000, CNA completed a discussion paper (Canadian Nurses Association, 2000) proposing that registered nurses in Canada support ICNP in principle as the foundational classification system for nursing practice in Canada. Responses and feedback received from the consultation related to this discussion paper indicated strong support from CNA's member jurisdictions for investigating how ICNP might be adapted for use in Canada (Canadian Nurses Association, 2001a). The result was a CNA position statement (Canadian Nurses Association, 2001b).

In Canada, nurses have come to recognize the need to incorporate the Nursing Components of Health Information into the national health information infostructure (national data bases and EHRs) as federal and provincial health information systems are being restructured. To ensure that nursing data are incorporated into the national health infostructure, nurses must participate in the design, standards development, and pilot studies to ensure capture of data that are essential to reflect the contribution of nursing to healthcare in Canada.

Current State of Nursing Information in Clinical Nursing Practice

Internationally

International Classification for Nursing Practice (ICNP)®

Nursing information and specifically nursing data elements with their associated definitions and classification systems evolved simultaneously in disparate parts of the world. Efforts at consensus and convergence among these classification systems led to the development of the ICNP® by the ICN. The beta 2 version of the ICNP® was released in 2002. The differences between the beta and the beta 2 versions of the ICNP® are mainly editorial corrections. The ICNP® Beta 2 provided a version for ongoing testing and evaluation. Continuing development, revision, and updating based on research and experience with *ICNP®* resulted in the production and release of ICNP® Version 1 at the ICN Congress in Taiwan in 2005. ICNP® Version 1 is a mature product with a level of stability that can provide vendors confidence to encourage incorporation into software products. In addition to maintenance and release of updated versions of the *ICNP*®, the ICNP® program established formal evaluation and review processes to advance the ongoing maintenance and advancement of the ICNP® (International Council of Nurses, 2002c).

As shown in Table 12.1 the International Council of Nurses (2002a) has identified work under way on developing and refining the ICNP® in one

Table 12.1. ICNP® Projects registered with the ICN (International Council of Nurses, 2005)

Country	Project
Austria	ICNP® German Browser
	Using ICNP® in Hospital Information Systems
Botswana	ICNP® in Botswana (W.K. Kellogg/ICN)
Brazil	A linguistic analysis of the ICNP® Beta Version
	Social violence: A case for classification as a sub-phenomenon of community in the ICNP®
	ICNP Project in Brazil (W.K. Kellogg/ICN)
Canada	Authenticating the Voice of Nursing Through the Use of ICNP in Capturing Nursing Data from Multiple Practice Settings
	Collecting Data to Reflect Nursing Impact
	The Use of the International Classification for Nursing Practice for Capturing Community Health Nursing
Chile	ICNP® Project in Chile (W.K. Kellogg/ICN)
Colombia	ICNP® Project in Colombia (W.K. Kellogg/ICN)
Czech Republic	ICNP® User Group
Denmark	Classificatory Review of the ICNP
	ICNP® Going Live in Nursing Homes
Estonia	Implementation of the ICNP into nursing practice
European Union	Telenurse ID
Germany	Conceptual System Design and Implementation of a web-based Classification-Browser for Documentation of Nursing Practice with PHP and XML
	Using the ICNP® in Continuity of Care in the Osnabrück Region
	Introduction and evaluation of nursing documentation systems
	Nursing Classification system-practical use and integration in a clinical information system (CIS) on the example of the ICNP® Beta Version
Italy	Testing of the International Classification for Nursing Practice to define nursing diagnosis and procedures: usage in the electronic nursing record and in the implementation of pressure ulcers prevention plan
	Translation and Testing ICNP® in Italy
International	ISO—Integration of a Reference Terminology Model for Nursing
Japan	Evaluation at Nine Months after the Establishment of Nursing Care Support System with Reference to ICNP
	Fundamental research on development of community nursing assessment and evaluation for elderly people
	Development of the Standardized Nursing Language System in Japan
	Validation study of select ICNP® terms
	Nursing practice in transurethral ureterolithotripsy treatment
Korea	Development of electronic nursing record model through application and evaluation of ICNP® in Nursing

Table 12.1. (*Continued*)

Country	Project
Mexico	ICNP® in Mexico (W.K. Kellogg/ICN)
Netherlands	Cross-mapping ICNP® and ICF
New Zealand	An International Classification for Nursing Practice: Terms used by Community-based Mental Health Nurses to Describe their Practice
Norway	Evaluating the beta-version of the International Classification for Nursing Practice (ICNP®)
Pakistan	Nursing Care Plan in Pakistan
Poland	ICNP® in Poland
Portugal	Nursing Information Systems: Support, Structure and content-an action research approach
	Study about the cultural adequacy of ICNP concepts and definitions on an hospital obstetric unit and content-an action research approach
	Clinical evaluation of ICNP® in a Portuguese perioperative nursing setting
	Study about the relevance of nursing documentation for the continuity of care along nursing shifts on a hospital unit
	Study of the benefits for citizens, related with the implementation of an automated articulation between hospitals and health centers by means of nursing information systems
	Study about the intensity of nursing care in primary health care
	The ICNP Beta and the terms used by the Nurses of Madeira Autonomous Region
Slovenia	ICNP Browser in Slovenia
	Translation and dissemination of the ICNP® in Slovenia
South Africa	ICNP and the electronic record
	ICNP® Project in South Africa (W.K. Kellogg/ICN)
Swaziland	ICNP® in Swaziland (W.K. Kellogg/ICN)
Sweden	Learning and Using the ICNP® on the Web
	Swedish Nursing Terminology Workgroup
Switzerland	Deriving Nursing Workload Data from the Electronic Health Record NURSING Data
	German Speaking ICNP® Development and Evaluation Project
Taiwan	ICNP® Validation Project in Taiwan
	Development of Integrated Multi-modal Interface for Recording Nursing Care Activities
Thailand	A Study of Nursing Minimum Data Set in Inpatients Departments of Queen Sawangwattana Memorial Hospital at Sriracha
	Nursing Diagnosis Used in Nursing Practice among Professional Nurses at Nan Hospital
	RTG/WHO: Nursing Minimum Data Set and Preliminary Nursing Classification
UK	Testing Reference Terminology
USA	A content coverage study: Coded terminologies and post acute care data sets
	Evaluation of the ICNP®
	Multinational Validation Study of Dignified Dying
	The International Study of Certified Nurses: Implications for the ICNP
	International Nursing Minimum/Essential Data Set (i-NMDS)
	Use of terminology tools to ease use of ICNP® in selected American graduate nursing schools
Zimbabwe	ICNP® in Zimbabwe (W.K. Kellogg/ICN)

international project and 64 other projects in 30 countries. There does not seem to be any country where the ICNP is being used nationwide in clinical nursing practice.

International Standards Organization Technical Committee on Health Informatics (ISO TC 215)

Nursing terminologies, in either paper-based or computer-based form, have been designed as enumerated classifications and implemented as interface terminologies at the point of care and as administrative terminologies to examine nursing data across settings. As discussed in the previous sections, many standardized terminologies exist and no single standardized terminology is complete for the domain of nursing in terms of breadth or granularity. The most comprehensive of the classifications systems is the ICNP.

Experts in the field of concept representation (Bakken and Mead, 1997; Campbell et al., 1997; Ingenerf, 1995; Ozbolt, 2002) widely recognize that classifications are useful to people as a means of communicating and understanding. However, classifications are not sufficiently granular or specific for use in electronic information systems (Bakken and Mead, 1997; ISO, 2002, 2003). Such systems require a formal terminology that Ingenerf (1995) defined as

> based on concepts or units of thought, rather than on lexical expressions or terms. Formal terminologies also have explicit rules for combining simple concepts into sensible complex concepts. Finally, formal terminologies have a knowledge representation scheme, or formalism, for depicting the relationships among the concepts.

The International Standards Organization Technical Committee 215 on Health Informatics Standards (ISO TC 215) has facilitated an international convergence and consensus-building process to develop a formal terminological model for nursing. Currently the only concept-oriented terminology that integrates the domain concepts of nursing in a manner suitable for computer processing is the ISO's International Standard 18104—"Integration of a Reference Terminology Model for Nursing." This international standard was accepted by the ISO member nations on December 15, 2003 (ISO, 2003). The Reference Terminology Model for Nursing (RTMN) is being reviewed and evaluated by each member nation for national adoption and use in electronic information systems as the standard for linking nursing classification systems. It was approved as a national standard of Canada in March 2005.

The ISO's International Standard 18104 (ISO, 2003) focuses specifically on the conceptual structures that are represented in a reference terminology model rather than in other types of information models. Moreover, toward the goal of integration with other healthcare models, the reference terminology models for nursing diagnoses and nursing actions in the ISO international standard reflect harmonization with evolving terminology and information model standards outside the domain of nursing (ISO, 2003).

The stated purpose of International Standard 18104 (International Standards Organization, 2003) is to establish a nursing reference terminology model consistent with the goals and objectives of other specific health terminology models in order to provide a more unified reference health model. The International Standard 18104 (ISO, 2003) includes the development of reference terminology models for nursing diagnoses and nursing actions and relevant terminology and definitions for its implementation. The anticipated uses (ISO, 2003) for the reference terminology model are the following.

- Support the intentional definition of nursing diagnosis and nursing action concepts
- Facilitate the representation of nursing diagnosis and nursing action concepts and their relationships in a manner suitable for computer processing
- Provide a framework for the generation of compositional expressions from atomic concepts within a reference terminology
- Facilitate the construction of nursing terminologies in a regular form that makes mapping among them easier
- Facilitate the mapping among nursing diagnosis and nursing action concepts from various terminologies including those developed as interface terminologies and statistical classifications
- Enable the systematic evaluation of terminologies and associated terminology models for purposes of harmonization
- Provide a language to describe the structure of nursing diagnosis and nursing action concepts to enable appropriate integration with information models (e.g., Health Level 7 Reference Information Model).

The ISO 18104 Reference Terminology Model for Nursing (ISO, 2003) is already guiding the efforts of the team modeling nursing concepts and relationships for SNOMED-CT. SNOMED-CT will contain the first realization of a formal reference terminology for nursing. Because SNOMED-CT will encompass virtually all of healthcare, nursing's formal terminology will be integrated de facto into a broad healthcare terminology (Bakken et al., 2001). HL7 is beginning to register nursing vocabularies that satisfy that organization's standards for sending messages containing healthcare information (Ozbolt, 2002). In addition, LOINC (Logical Observations, Identifiers, Names, and Codes) has adapted its standards to accept nursing information and has added terms for nursing assessment data (Bakken et al., 2000).

United States

The Nursing Terminology Summit began in 1999 and has been held annually at Vanderbilt University (Ozbolt, 2000a, 2000b, 2000c). These summits bring together the developers of nursing vocabularies with leaders of professional associations and standards developing organizations, developers and vendors of healthcare information systems, and representatives of government agencies concerned with healthcare terminology standards. Efforts of this group have focused on contributing to the development of a formal, concept-based terminology model for nursing to which the preceding classifications as well as other sets of nursing terms could be mapped. The intent is to resolve ambiguities among representations of nursing concepts and relationships between evolving standards being produced by standards bodies such as the International Standards Organization Technical Committe on Health Informatics (ISO TC 215), Health Level 7 (HL7), and Logical Observations, Identifiers, Names, and Codes (LOINC) and incorporation of the formal terminology into information systems. Over four years, the major accomplishments of the Terminology Summit are:

- Identified the need for a formal, concept-based terminology for nursing to which classifications and other sets of nursing terms could be mapped.
- Determined that the first step in developing a formal concept-based terminology was to depict the model of nursing concepts and relationships that would subsequently be populated by terms providing specific instances of the concepts.
- Facilitated collaboration among participants toward developing a nursing concept model.
- Reviewed, analyzed, and critiqued the European CEN TC 215 "Categorical System for Nursing," a model with characteristics approximating a nomenclature.
- Supported a proposal to ISO TC 215 to create a formal reference terminology model for nursing and to integrate it with other standards for healthcare data. This proposal integrated previous efforts by the terminology summit, European CEN TC 215, ICN, and the Nursing Informatics Group of the International Medical Informatics Association (IMIA).
- Resolved ambiguities between the representation of nursing concepts and relationships in the evolving ISO reference terminology model and their representation in the reference information model (RIM) of the standards organization called HL7. As a result of summit collaboration, HL7 has begun to register nursing vocabularies that satisfy that organization's standards for sending messages containing healthcare information. Similarly, the standards organization called LOINC has adapted its standards to accept nursing information and has added terms for nursing assessment data.
- Supported use of ISO's Reference Terminology Model for Nursing to guide the efforts of the team modeling nursing concepts and relationships for SNOMED-CT. SNOMED-CT likely will contain the first realization of a formal reference terminology for nursing. Because SNOMED-CT will encompass virtually all of healthcare, nursing's formal terminology will perforce be integrated into a broad healthcare terminology.
- Initiated exploration of ways to incorporate the formal terminology into information systems.

Canada

The clinical data elements comprising the Nursing Components of Health Information (i.e., client status, nursing interventions, client outcomes) are not formally captured in a standardized terminology in any national database or EHR. There is a paucity of Canadian research related to the clinical data elements of the Nursing Components of Health Information. Only one completed Canadian study (Loewen, 1999) and two studies in progress (Kennedy, 2002; Pringle and White, 2002) were identified. The Nursing and Health Outcomes Project (Ontario) aims to identify nursing-sensitive patient outcomes and their attendant inputs and processes that could be entered on, and abstracted from, patients' charts or provided in other formats (Canadian Institute for Health Information, 2002).

Summary

Much remains to be accomplished in research to continue to develop a formalized clinical nursing vocabulary common among nurses. Nurse educators must become more aware of the importance of nursing data standards and become familiar with the content and substance of standardized clinical nursing vocabulary so they incorporate this knowledge throughout nursing education curricula. Similarly, practicing nurses need to understand the importance of nursing data standards for use in documenting clinical practice in a fashion that enables data analysis of the nursing impact on patient outcomes. Nurse managers need to become familiar with nursing data standards and their role in providing evidence to substantiate the value of the nursing contribution to patient care.

References

Abdellah, F.G. (1988). Future directions: Refining, implementing, testing, and evaluating the nursing minimum data set. In: Werley, H.H., & Lang, N.M. (eds.) *Identification of the Nursing Minimum Data Set.* New York: Springer, pp. 416–426.

Alberta Association of Registered Nurses (AARN) (1994). *Client status, nursing intervention and client outcome taxonomies: a background paper.* Edmonton: AARN.

Bakken, H.S. & Mead, C.N. (1997). Nursing classification systems: necessary but not sufficient for representing "what nurses do" for inclusion in computer-based patient record systems. *Journal of the American Medical Informatics Association 4*(3):222–232.

Bakken, S. et al. (2000). Evaluation of the clinical LOINC specification as a terminology model for standardized assessments. *Journal of the American Medical Informatics Association* 7(6):529–538.

Bakken, S., J. et al. (2001). An evaluation of the utility of the CEN categorical structure for nursing diagnoses as a terminology model for integrating nursing diagnosis concepts into SNOMED. Proceedings of *Medinfo 10*(Pt):151–155.

Campbell, J.R., Carpenter, P., Sneiderman, C., et al. (1997). Phase II evaluation of clinical coding schemes: Completeness, taxonomy, mapping, definitions, and clarity; CPRI Work Group on Codes and Structures. *Journal of the American Medical Informatics Association 4*(5):238–251.

Canadian Institute for Health Information. (2002). http://www.cihi.ca/.

Canadian Nurses Association. (1990). *Report of the resolutions committee*. Ottawa, Unpublished report.

Canadian Nurses Association. (1993a). *Papers from the Nursing Minimum Data Set Conference,* Ottawa.

Canadian Nurses Association. (1993b). *Policy statement on health information: Nursing components (HI:NC)*, Ottawa.

Canadian Nurses Association. (1998). *Policy statement: Evidence-based decision-making and nursing practice,* Ottawa.

Canadian Nurses Association. (2000). *Collecting data to reflect nursing impact: A discussion paper*, Ottawa.

Canadian Nurses Association. (2001a). *Making nursing evident: Nursing informatics strategy session*. Ottawa, unpublished report.

Canadian Nurses Association. (2001b). *Position statement: Collecting data to reflect the impact of nursing practice*, Ottawa.

Carpenito, L.J. (1989). Nursing diagnosis. In: *Classification Systems for Describing Nursing Practice. Working Papers*. Kansas City: American Nurses' Association, pp. 13–19.

Clark, J. & Lang N. (1992). Nursing's next advance: An international classification for nursing practice. *International Journal of Nursing 39*(4):102–112, 128.

Coenen, A., Marin, H.F., Park, H.-A., & Bakken, S. (2001). Collaborative efforts for representing nursing concepts in computer-based systems: international perspectives. *Journal of the American Medical Informatics Association 8*(3):202–211.

Ehnfors, M. (1999). Testing the ICNP in Sweden and other Nordic countries. In: Mortensen, R.A. (ed.) *ICNP and Telematic Applications for Nurses in Europe: The Telenurse Experience.* Amsterdam: IOS Press, pp. 221–229.

Graves, J.R. & Corcoran, S. (1989). The study of nursing informatics. *Image: Journal of Nursing Scholarship 21*(4):227–231.

Hardiker, N.R., Hoy, D., & Casey, A. (2000). Standards for nursing terminology. *Journal of the American Medical Informatics Association* 7(6):523–528.

Hardiker, N.R. & Rector, A.L. (1998). Modeling nursing terminology using the GRAIL representation language. *Journal of the American Medical Informatics Association, 5*(1):120–128.

Ingenerf, J. (1995). *Taxonomic Vocabularies in Medicine: The Intention of Usage Determines Different Established Structures*. MedInfo 95. Vancouver, British Columbia: Healthcare Computing and Communications.

International Council of Nurses. (1993). *Nursing's next advance: An international classification for nursing practice (ICNP)—a working paper*, Geneva: ICN.

International Council of Nurses. (1996). *International Classification for Nursing Practice (ICNP)—alpha version*, Geneva: ICN.

International Council of Nurses. (1999). *ICNP: International Classification for Nursing Practice, beta version.* Geneva: ICN.

International Council of Nurses. (2002a). ICNP® research and development projects. http://www.icn.ch/database1.htm **(accessed December 27, 2002)**.

International Council of Nurses. (2002b). ICNP® International Classification for Nursing Practice, beta 2. Geneva: ICN.

International Council of Nurse. (2002c). ICNP introduction. http://www.icn.ch/icnpupdate.htm#Intro (**accessed December 27, 2002**).

International Council of Nurses. (2005). ICNP® Research and Development Projects. http://www.icn.ch/database1.htm (**accessed February 8, 2005**).

International Council of Nurses. (2005). ICNP® International Classification for Nursing Practice, Version 1. Geneva: ICN.

International Standards Organization. (ISO) (2002). *Integration of a reference terminology model for nursing. working document* TC 215/WG 3.

International Standards Organization. (ISO) (2003). *Integration of a reference terminology model for nursing.* TC 215/WG 3. Geneva: ISO.

Johnson, M., Maas, M., & Moorhead, S., Eds. (2000). *Nursing Outcomes Classification (NOC)*. St. Louis: Mosby.

Kennedy, M.A. (2002). *Authenticating the voice of nursing through the use of ICNP in capturing nursing data from multiple practice settings.* Unpublished doctoral research proposal, University of South Australia.

Loewen, E.M. (1999). *The Use of the International Classification of Nursing Practice for Capturing Community-Based Nursing Practice*. Winnipeg: Faculty of Nursing, University of Manitoba.

Marek, K. & Lang, N. (1993). Nursing sensitive outcomes. In: *Papers from the Nursing Minimum Data Set Conference.* Ottawa: Canadian Nurses Association, pp. 100–120.

Martin, K.S. (1988). Nursing minimum data set requirements for the community setting. In: Werley, H.H., & Lang, N.M. (eds.) *Identification of the Nursing Minimum Data Set* New York: Springer, pp. xxii, 474.

Martin, K.S. & Scheet, N.J. (1992). *The Omaha System: Applications for Community Health Nursing.* Philadelphia: Saunders.

McCloskey, J.C. & Bulechek, G.M. (1996). *Nursing Interventions Classification (NIC)*. St. Louis: Mosby.

McCormick, K.A., Lang, N., Zielstorff, R., et al. (1994). Toward standard classification schemes for nursing language: recommendations of the American Nurses Association Steering Committee on Databases to Support Clinical Nursing Practice. *Journal of the American Medical Informatics Association 1*(6):421–427.

McGee, M. (1993). Response to V. Saba's paper on nursing diagnostic schemes. In: *Papers from the Nursing Minimum Data Set Conference*. Ottawa: Canadian Nurses Association, pp. 64–67.

Mortensen, R.A. (1997). *ICNP in Europe: TELENURSE*. Amsterdam: ISO Press.

Mortensen, R.A., Ed. (1999). *ICNP and Telematic Applications for Nurses in Europe: The Telenurse Experience* (Vol 61: Studies in Health Technology and Informatics). Amsterdam: IOS Press.

Mortensen, R.A., Mantas, J., Manuela, M., et al. (1994). Telematics for healthcare in the European Union. In: Grobe, S.J., & Pluyter-Wenting, E. (eds.) *Nursing Informatics: An International Overview for Nursing in a Technological Era.* Amsterdam: Elsevier, pp. 750–752.

Nielsen, G.H. &. Mortensen, R.A. (1996). The architecture for an international classification of nursing practice (ICNP). *International Nursing Review 43*(6):175–182.

Nielsen, G.H. & Mortensen, R.A. (1999). ICNP time for outcomes: Continuous quality development. In: Mortensen, R.A. (ed.). *ICNP and Telematic Applications for Nurses in Europe: The Telenurse Experience.* Amsterdam: IOS Press, pp. 79–102.

Nightingale, F. (1859). *Notes on Nursing: What It Is, and What It Is Not.* London: Harrison.

Nightingale, F. (1863). *Notes on Hospitals.* London: Longman, Green, Longman, Roberts, and Green.

O'Brien-Pallas, L. & Giovannetti, P. (1993). Nursing intensity. In: *Papers from the Nursing Minimum Data Set Conference*. Ottawa: Canadian Nurses Association, pp. 68–76.

Ozbolt, J. (1999). Testimony to the hearings on medical terminology and code development. Washington, DC: *National Committee on Vital and Health Statistics (NCVHS).*

Ozbolt, J. (2000). Towards a reference terminology model for nursing: the 1999 nursing vocabulary summit conference. In: *Proceedings of Nursing Informatics 2000.* Auckland, NZ, p. 267.

Ozbolt, J. (2000 a). Terminology standards for nursing: collaboration at the summit. *Journal of the American Medical Informatics Association* 7(6):517–522.

Ozbolt, J. (2000 b). Focus on the nursing vocabulary summit. *Journal of the American Medical Informatics Association* 7(6):517–549.

Ozbolt, J. (2002). *International standards for nursing terminology: effects on nursing diagnosis.* Presented to the Japanese Nursing Diagnosis Association. Unpublished.

Pearce, N.D. (1988). Uniform minimum health data sets: Concept, development, testing, recognition for federal health use, and current status. In: Werley, H.H., & Lang, N.M. (eds.) *Identification of the Nursing Minimum Data Set.* New York: Springer, pp. 260–279.

Pringle, D. & White, P. (In progress). The nursing and health outcomes project (Ontario). http://www.gov.on.ca/health/english/program/nursing/nursing_mn.html (**accessed December 16, 2002**).

Saba, V.K. (1992). Diagnosis and interventions. *Caring 11*(3):50–57.

Verney, H. (1970). *Florence Nightingale at Harley Street*. London: Dent & Sons.

Werley, H.H. & Lang, N.M.(Eds.). (1988). *Identification of the Nursing Minimum Data Set*. New York: Springer.

13
Defining Information Management Requirements

JANE CURRY

The mantra of informatics is "getting the right information to the right people at the right time." The requirements definition phase is determining (and making sure everyone agrees with) what is the right information, who are the right people, and when is the right time. The most important decisions require that everyone involved agree on the anticipated benefits and the expected scope of information system use.

The use of computers has changed over the last 50-plus years. At first, computers were used as fast calculating machines (hence the name). Later, manual processes that involve moving pieces of paper from one person to another were automated so the paper was replaced by electronic data storage and screens, or printers were used to retrieve the information. Still later, as computers and networks became more readily available and affordable, information systems were used to enable communication between people located across time and space. The newest use of computers is to manage complexity—there are simply too many interdependent elements in the health system for people to be able keep track of all of them and their changes with sufficient reliability.

Introducing any kind of automated information system involves changing the way people get their work done. Simply replacing paper with information systems without understanding how the change affects the minute-to-minute activities of the people involved cannot produce the benefits anticipated. Rather than saving time and improving information quality and availability, introducing information systems may increase people's frustration and decrease the quality of information. This is especially true when adding yet an other information system into an environment in which information systems are already in use. Getting information systems to work effectively together is an additional activity that usually takes more time and effort than anticipated. Making information systems truly useful requires that many activities be done well. None of the technical activities can be effective without first having a shared understanding of what the collection of information systems is supposed to do to help people get their work done.

Stages in System Development/Acquisition

Information systems are not introduced in a vacuum. What activities are undertaken depends on what information systems already exist and how the information systems are managed. The most successful organizations manage information systems as assets of the organization as a whole, with each new information system or major change to an existing information system being managed as an individual project. Managing all the information systems together is often called "information systems architecture management" and involves planning for change, setting standards, and keeping track of all the information systems and the interdependence of their components.

Each information system project goes through a process that roughly falls into the following stages.[1]

- *Initiation*: getting approval for the project, organizing the people affected, clarifying the expected benefits, planning, and assembling a team to do the project
- *Elaboration*: one or more iterations (or mini-phases), each verifying requirements, identifying interdependencies among components, aligning with industry and organizational standards, testing major technical assumptions, analyzing and specifying component design details, and building core components
- *Construction*: refining information systems requirements, refining information system design details, building and testing interdependent information system components, piloting the resulting information system with a small group
- *Transition*: introduce a new information system across all environments, train people to use and support the information system, manage data archiving and conversion, integrate with other information systems
- *Production*: support the information system, including ongoing training and help support
- *Retirement*: ensuring information system is appropriately withdrawn from the environment, archive and convert historical information

In general, the broader the expected scope of information system use, the more attention that is needed during the earliest phases. Many information systems being acquired or developed in healthcare organizations today cross boundaries and are expected to be used by multiple disciplines, across multiple organizational units, and spread across multiple sites and even between multiple organizations operating in different jurisdictions. Such projects require careful planning and coordination to be successful.

---

[1] Although many information system development methodologies exist, emerging industry best practices are being based on a methodology called "unified process." One proprietary source that supports a unified process within an enterprise management approach is found at http://www.enterpriseunifiedprocess.info/.

The details of what the information systems are expected to do must be determined within a set of activities that includes providing ongoing communication to everyone affected and coordinating change to align activities, roles, policies, and procedures to accompany the introduction of the information system.

Requirements Definition

Requirements definition is the process of ensuring a common understanding of just what an information system is supposed to do and how it fits into the daily lives of the people expected to use it. The process is essentially the same whether an information system project is expecting to acquire a commercial information system, modify an existing information system, develop an information system from scratch, or integrate many information systems to work together.

People communicate with each other in a dialogue fashion, allowing each individual to clarify meaning and intent and make sure the information provided is suitable to the purpose. This form of person-to-person communication is highly effective so long as all parties understand the same "language." Language is not just a matter of being able to speak and understand or to read and write in a common human language such as English or French, it also refers to the use of terms and a shared context. People use short cuts in communicating all the time. Acronyms and jargon abound in healthcare, and often clear understanding is local to a work setting among people in a common discipline. People from different disciplines, or teams, must work out a common language whether the form of communication is person to person or person to paper to person.

People excel at clarifying ambiguity in language and can often understand terms within a context without resorting to formal definitions. Computers do not tolerate ambiguity. Information systems rely on extremely specific instructions to do anything. The goal of the requirements definition is to make sure enough details are known and accepted about what information is required by whom at which point in time to accomplish the purpose of allowing a computer to carry out the tasks necessary to make the information system useful in the expected environment. Most information systems allow at least some customization to accommodate the differences in the way people work in different settings. The most challenging part of the requirements definition is gaining agreement among groups of people who need to cooperate to be able to accomplish a common goal. The more an information system is expected to do to make work more effective, the more important it is to make sure the details are explicit and accepted by everyone who needs to use the information system. Because it is not possible to ask every person's opinion in advance, it is especially important that the people who are chosen for the requirements definition team of the information systems project can adequately delineate the interests of the group of people they represent.

The suite of information systems supporting healthcare in a particular setting are becoming increasingly complex. There are many combinations of hardware and software components that exchange information to accomplish a stated purpose, and these combinations are changing all the time as new information is required or old systems are retired. Keeping track of these complex environments is a task that requires information system support. Information system architecture management uses information system tools to help make sure the suite of information systems supporting the healthcare organization is as effective as possible with the least cost.

Information system management tools are also being used to make sure the details captured during the requirements definition are sufficiently specific and consistent. One of the most effective techniques in managing anything highly complex with interdependent components is to show the components and their relationship in a visual diagram. The analogy of a blueprint used to build a building is often used to talk about what an information system is supposed to do. The blueprint is made up of a series of related diagrams each specifying details supporting a different discipline, such as structural or mechanical engineering or carpentering. The advantage of using diagrams is that attention can be focused on one topic at a time until it is sufficiently understood, with the information system management tool keeping track of the details so no gaps or overlaps occur. Different views of the blueprint are used to inform different audiences at different levels of detail. Everyone has a different perspective and considers a complex topic with a focus point representing what they care about. The center of the diagram typically has many details about components and their relationships. The edges of a diagram tend to be less detailed and relationships to components exist but are not shown. Diagrams are supported by text to add further clarity for people to read, as well as highly structured data that allow the information system tool to manage the interdependence among views and components.

The types of diagrams have evolved over time but are beginning to converge around an information technology industry standard called the unified modeling language.[2] The following discussion of diagram types helps clarify which diagram is used to capture the details of the *information* needed by *which people* at *the time* to accomplish *what purpose*.

The purposes for information systems vary widely but must be explicitly understood and accepted. This is particularly important when information recorded for one purpose is made available to someone else to avoid their

[2] Unified modeling language (UML) is an information technology standard managed by the Object Management Group. More information can be found at http://www.uml.org/.

redundantly collecting information or to reuse information collected for one purpose for a different purpose. Information quality, in terms of precision of measure, timeliness, accuracy, and relevance, must be considered in the context of both the circumstances under which it was initially recorded and when it is subsequently used. Information sharing can improve the coordination of care and reduce the cost of maintaining information—but only when the information's quality is preserved. Examples of information recording purposes include the following.

- Recording reminders to self
- Recording activities performed to demonstrate accountability for actions
- Recording requests for someone else to do something
- Recording direct observations or measures to monitor the condition of a subject of interest
- Record the outcome of activities that affect the availability of resources, such as money in an account, time spent by a specific human resource, amount of time a specific piece of equipment was used
- Record the authorization to do something or acknowledge a decision
- Calculate new measures or summaries from information already available

Using diagrams during the requirements definition phase and recording the resulting pictures in information system tools that support requirements definition helps to maintain a clear linking of requirements to delivered information systems over time. As information systems are added and changed, the impact on other information systems or related activities can be predicted. Integration of the specific diagrams and the accompanying detailed information into requirements definition tools ensures that each perspective is adequately represented and that all the details are recorded that make up the accurate specification of just what an information system is supposed to do and how it is integrated into daily activities. Figure 13.1 represents how people with different viewpoints would view a complex information system. If each circle represents the scope of interest of a different perspective, it is easy to see that complete understanding is impossible by considering only a single perspective. Effective information systems need to be built from specifications that integrate the multiple perspectives into a congruent whole. The ability to view different aspects individually, however, ensures that each perspective is accommodated and allows the appropriate people to validate that their needs have been met. The requirement definition tools also help identify how the activities of people and the corresponding roles and responsibilities along with the organizational policies and procedures must be adjusted to make the whole work environment more effective as new information systems are implemented.

The following diagrams are often used during the requirements definition phase. There are 13 types of diagram available in UML, each of which adds clarity to some aspect of the requirements definition or component analysis, design, and deployment management.

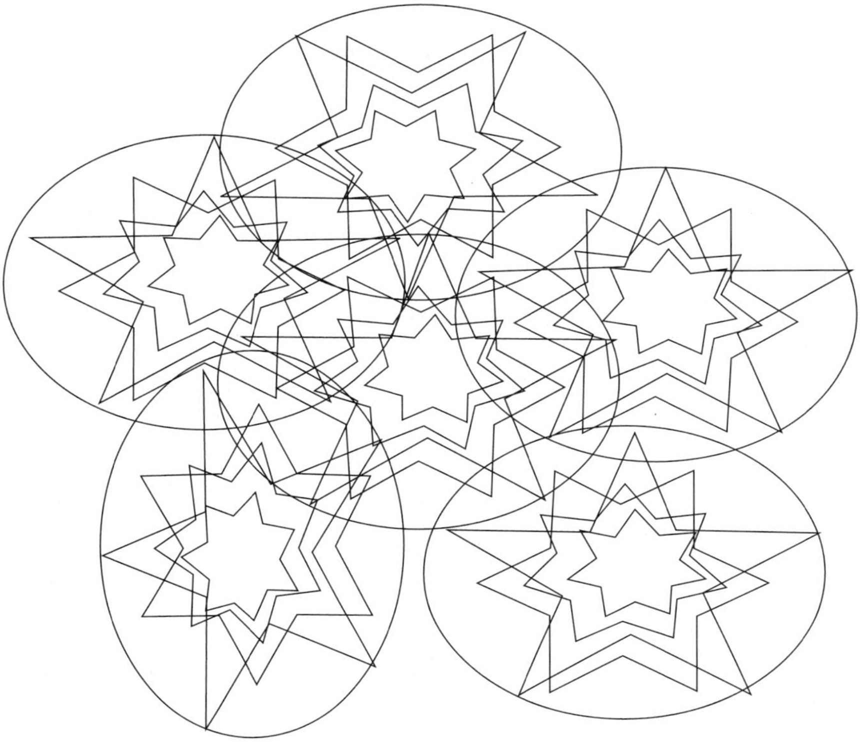

FIGURE 13.1. Scope of interest of different perspectives.

Use Case Diagram

A use case diagram specifies which people use an information system to accomplish what purposes. It shows the set of roles involved in using an information system to achieve a purpose. People are represented by a stick figure called an actor. The name of the actor is a specific role that has a defined set of responsibilities and permissions to use an information system to accomplish specific tasks, or use Cases. Use cases are represented by ovals inside a box that represents the information system boundary. The use cases can be specified at different levels of detail and may be related to each other. This is a useful convention because exception processes can be understood without distracting attention from the "mainline" processes typically used to achieve the purpose. Figure 13.2 is an example of a simple use case diagram. It shows that although both physicians and nurses have access to a clinical information system, it is the nurse who is expected to record vital signs and the physician who is expected to record medication prescriptions. Both are expected to verify patient demographics.

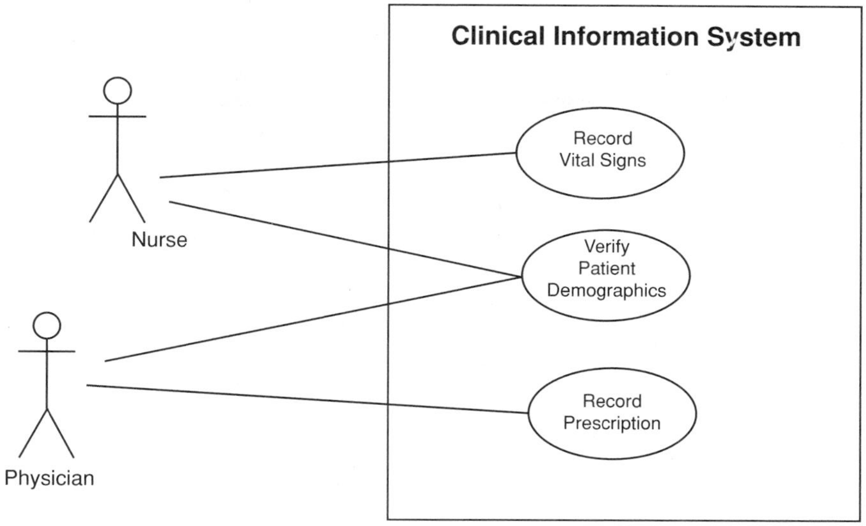

Figure 13.2. Use case diagram.

Activity Diagram

An activity diagram specifies the responsibility for processes, the sequence in which they are performed, and any decision points. These diagrams are useful for clarifying how information systems are used across organizations, disciplines, or systems. Sometimes called a "swim lane" diagram because the processes are organized to show which actors (which may be information systems) are responsible for what processes. This diagram is especially useful for clarifying the "hand-off" of responsibility and can serve to focus attention on aligning policies, responsibilities, and information definitions associated with the performing cooperating processes. A simple example is depicted in Figure 13.3.

In this example, a discharge planner is interacting with a placement system to determine if a patient should be discharged home or to a long-term care residence or if alternative arrangements are needed while the patient is on a waitlist for transfer. The use case starts when the patient needs are assessed. The placement system calculates a resource requirement and, based on the outcome, arranges for patient transfer with the long-term care coordinator if the patient needs that level of care and a place is available. Otherwise, the patient is placed on a waitlist, or the discharge planner is notified that long-term care is not suitable. The discharge planner arranges for discharge home, transfer to long-term care or alternative arrangements, depending on the outcome of decisions made. Note that this activity diagram would be used to explore the responsibilities associated with each role, the rules required to

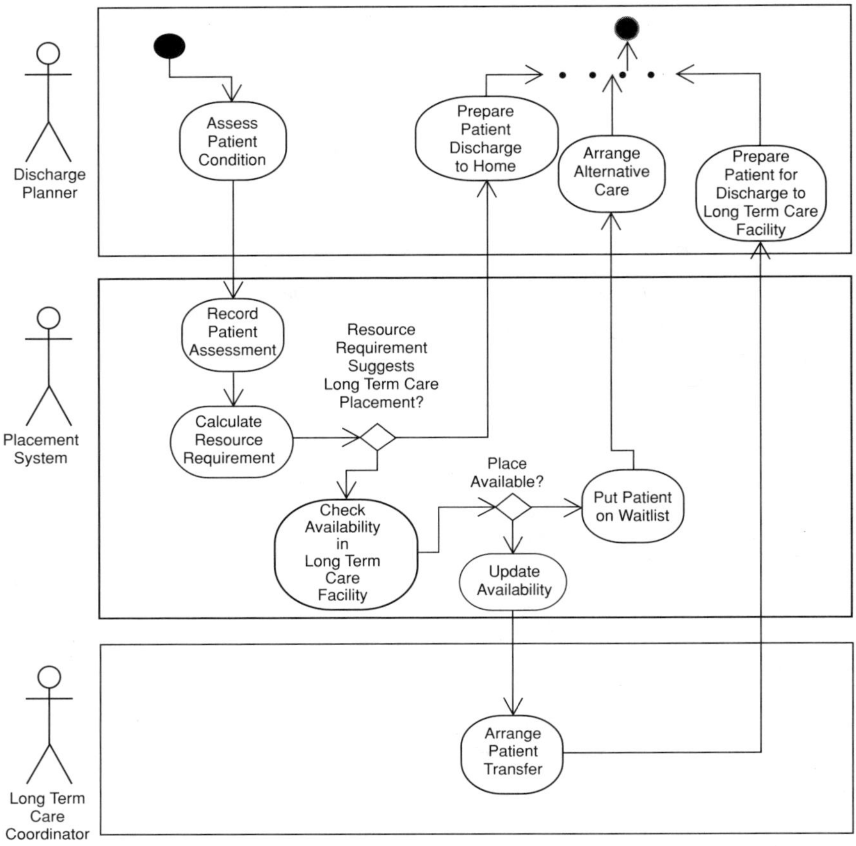

Figure 13.3. Swim lane diagram.

determine placement, and any other policy or procedure alignment among the organizations.

Information Model Diagram

Information is understood only in a specific context. However any information has certain core subjects that correspond to real-world factors that must be tracked over time. Information models are diagrams that depict items and information about them that are required to support an organization and all its information systems. Diagrams that visually display items and the relationships among them have evolved over time but have always been intended to help the user clearly understand what people, places, factors, rules, and events are important to keep track of over time and the meaning of their important characteristics and relationships.

Diagrams of these "information classes" help specify the "right information" that must be maintained by information systems. Information modeling has often been represented as entity/relationship diagrams, although more recently class diagrams have become more accepted. Understanding information as descriptions of things whose characteristics change over time and as they are affected by particular events, helps not only to design information systems that are adaptable as circumstances change but also to help organizations take on appropriate accountability for the quality of information used to support many purposes. Not all information about classes can be shown on a diagram. Accompanying definitions for each element in the model are also required. For example, it is important to understand how each characteristic can be expressed so an information system can process it correctly and what would be considered valid content for each characteristic. It is also important to determine how each class might change over time, either through changes as processes effect a class or as part of a normal life cycle. Additional considerations involve determining sensitive information that must be protected with additional security and access permission. Such additional details may be expressed in related diagrams or as narrative text in a related glossary.

Figure 13.4 depicts a simple class diagram that helps clarify that it is important to understand a person as a unique individual and what the role of patient really means in the context of a specific healthcare encounter. A box represents a named class, with characteristics of interest appearing below the line. The lines between the boxes represent key relationships and may be named with notation on the ends indicating whether the relation is optional and whether more than one relation of that type can exist between the classes. The diagram in Figure 13.4 can be interpreted to mean that a person can play the role of either a patient or a healthcare practitioner. A patient is a person with a relation with a healthcare organization. A person in the role of a patient participates as a subject during an encounter, whereas a person

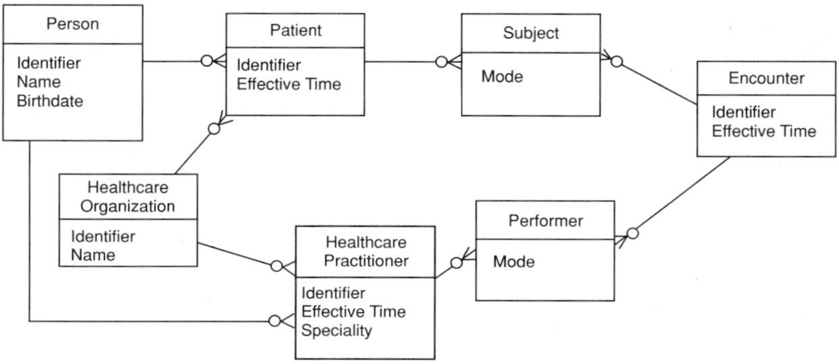

FIGURE 13.4. Class diagram.

in the role of a healthcare practitioner participates as a performer during the encounter. An encounter can be with more than one patient and involve more than one healthcare practitioner who may be participating is different modes: physically present or remotely.

This model is drawn from a health information standards development organization, Health Level 7 (HL7),[3] which has produced a reference information model that is now being used across the world to help information systems share information with the same meaning. Other standards development organizations are working on developing common terminology to be used by information systems. Having these health information standards available during requirements definition helps people recognize that their unique information needs can be met using a "common language" that is sufficiently precise that computers can process it and expressive enough that detailed requirements can still be met.

Summary

Participating in the requirements development phase of an information systems project is challenging but rewarding. It is an opportunity to help an organization acquire the best possible information systems that support the daily activities of the people who use them and help coordinate care over time and across disciplines and organizations. Most of the effort is spent working with other people to reach a consensus of just what the information system is to do and making sure there is a common understanding of the specific activities and the information captured and used to achieve the stated purposes. One way to gain understanding is to tell specific stories of just what the future would look like when the information system is in place. Use the diagrams and accompanying detailed information as the "bones" of the story, but flesh out the story and dress it up by using real-world examples in reasonable detail. These stories carry over into the next phases of information systems projects and can become test cases that help make sure that the information systems do what they are supposed to do—before they are implemented.

---

[3] Health Level Seven has many activities focused on supporting information sharing with the same meaning across information systems. More information is available at http://www.hl7.org/.

14
Selection of Software and Hardware

With contributions by Eleanor Callahan Hunt, Sara Breckenridge Sproat, and Rebecca Rutherford Kitzmiller

Selection Process and the Role of Nursing

The installation of a clinical information system does not just happen, nor is it a mysterious process. The process starts with identifying a need, conducting a feasibility analysis, creating a selection team who gathers information and develops vision and goals, promoting executive buy-in and funding commitments. After a clear vision and goals are identified, a request for proposal (RFP) is sent out to the vendor field. Vendor responses are evaluated, site visits and on-site vendor fairs are arranged, and the system selection decision is made. While the contract is being negotiated, funding is confirmed and an implementation team is formed. The implementation team configures the system, deploys it to users, and evaluates and maintains the system. This entire process from initial idea to deployment is summarized in Figure 14.1.

A clinical system implementation provides nursing the opportunity to help clinical staff optimize their workflow and improve patient care by harnessing technology and using it to advantage. A system implementation project marks its beginning from its earliest conception, perhaps a clinician with an idea inspired to find a better way to solve workflow issues, reduce errors, or improve patient outcomes. As the idea develops, buy-in from senior leadership and the executive level formalizes the project. Although the selection process may appear lengthy, it serves multiple purposes, such as engaging all potential users, promoting buy-in and ensuring that all embrace the same shared vision (Hunt et al., 2004). Depending on the experience level and knowledge of the staff working on a particular implementation, this process can be abbreviated for smaller projects (Hunt et al., 2004). Through thoughtful, deliberate information gathering, analysis, and decision making, a system that enhances clinician decision making, optimizes staff work, and improves patient care will be selected and implemented. It is imperative that

The contents of this chapter are opinions of the authors only and do not reflect those of the US Army Medical Department or the US Army.

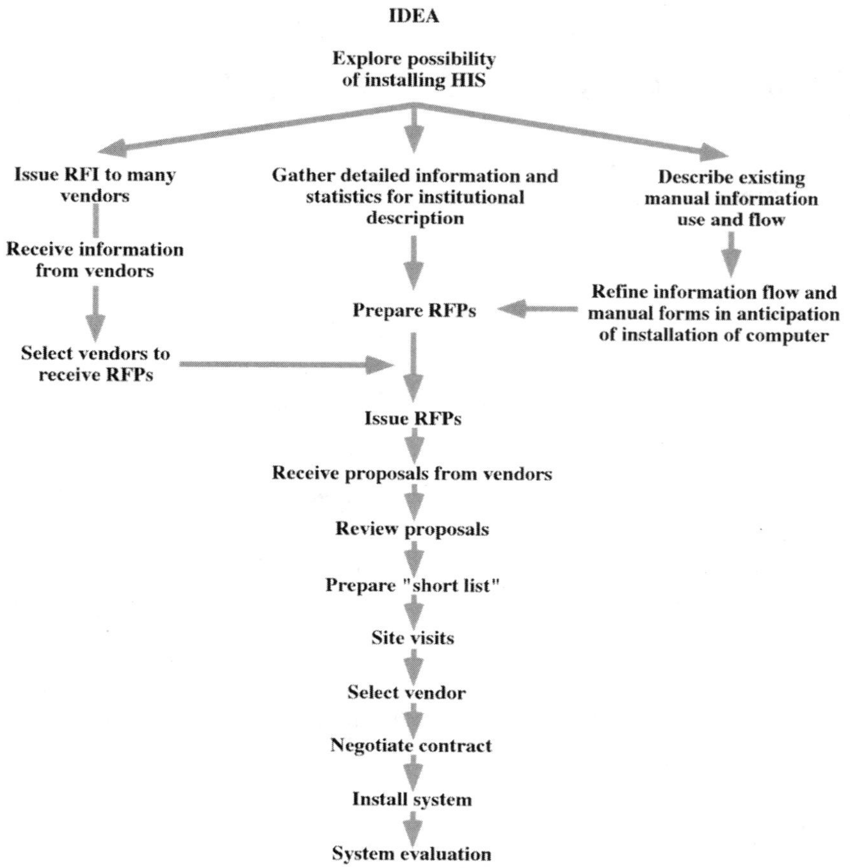

FIGURE 14.1. Hardware and software selection process. HIS, health information system; RFI, request for information; RFPs, request for proposal.

nursing be actively involved at every stage of the process from beginning to end (Hunt et al., 2004; Manning and McConnell, 1997; Mills, 1995).

Once the need for a system has been identified, the initial step is to form a selection team to choose the solution. The formation of the selection team committee depends on how the organization typically handles projects and committees. This committee is usually composed of various department heads or designates (including nursing) in the organization, but it can and should include other disciplines as needed. It is important to identify all of the organizational departments that will be affected by the system installation and ensure that their interests are adequately represented. Membership can include both permanent and ad hoc representation of the core group of users (Hunt et al., 2004). Communication mechanisms must be made more formal as the size of the group grows to ensure effective meetings and to keep the process moving along. Large groups require documented meeting agendas, meeting minutes, assigned responsibilities, and subcommittees reporting progress. Small groups could accomplish similar tasks with handwritten agendas, round-table discussion, and documentation only as decisions are made.

One of the first tasks addressed by the selection committee is to gather detailed information and statistics about the organization. This baseline description includes information about the type of healthcare organization, daily patient census and workload, number of staff, number of prescriptions dispensed, specialty units, level of patient acuity, organizational design, administrative structure, and geographic area served. Other tasks at this stage are to complete a needs analysis; develop the vision, mission, and goals of the project; determine how the system selection decision is to be made; identify a budget range for system installation and maintenance; and create a broad timeline. Information gathered is used for many purposes throughout the life cycle; for the RFP it is used to compare and evaluate vendor proposals, implement the chosen system, and evaluate system effectiveness after installation. The process of gathering information and arriving at common goals provides the opportunity to gain buy-in of the user base and to cultivate appropriate user expectations. Obviously, during this phase the nursing department has a great deal of information to provide as end-users of many of the clinical systems installed in an organization.

It is wise to capture existing information flow, document additional data needs, and examine data usage while gathering descriptive information about the organization. Often, existing systems are cumbersome, inefficient, and error-ridden, which is why the team is seeking a replacement. There is no point in continuing such processes. Self-evaluation reveals areas and processes needing minor improvements, modifications, or even major revisions. Often immediate time and cost savings can be realized by simply refining current information-handling procedures in preparation for installation of a computerized information system. This self-evaluation and documentation may be conducted by the selection committee, the information computer services department, or a hired systems analysis consultant. Documenting initial information handling provides a means by which one can evaluate the final product of a computerized information system. In addition, this self-evaluation phase facilitates early identification of gaps or inequities in the existing information management methods. Such knowledge permits initiation of remedial action. For example, when patient care plans are to be included in the computerized information system, the information analysis may reveal that there is no standard format for patient care plans in the organization or that there is a standard format but it is not used consistently by all patient units. Consolidating or making practice consistent prior to the start of an implementation makes deployment of the system easier. Implementing a familiar documentation method in a new clinical system is easier than implementing a new documentation method in a new clinical system, and it will meet less resistance (Hunt et al., 2004).

The Request for Information (RFI)

Members of the selection team or the manager of information services distributes a request for information (RFI) to as many vendors as possible. An RFI provides demographic information about the organization, such as size and mission, and requests a general response from vendors regarding the types of products they manufacture and market. The RFI addresses the basic system description, desired capabilities, and scope of the intended project. It is usually the first contact with a vendor and is used to obtain vital information about the products and services offered by the company. An RFI announces to vendors that the organization is in the preliminary phase of considering installation of a system and provides the organization with a quick, albeit superficial, educational overview of what is commercially available. The RFI also narrows down options and eliminates vendors that cannot meet basic requirements. Once the vendor field has been whittled down, vendors are asked to respond to the more detailed RFP.

An alternative to sending out an RFI is attending a clinical conference that has a large clinical system vendor presence. Conferences are valuable for the sessions on implementing clinical systems as well as providing opportunities to see and touch the systems, network with colleagues evaluating similar systems, and selecting pertinent literature to share with the rest of the selection team.

The Request for Proposal (RFP)

The RFP is the way the selection team gets detailed information from vendors. An RFP is prepared from the information received from evaluating RFI materials returned by vendors, as well as organizational summaries of the site, technology infrastructure, existing and desired information use, and flow (see Chapter 13). An RFP is sent to selected vendors, inviting them to submit a detailed response or proposal describing how they would meet the needs of the organization. Be aware that it is expensive for a vendor to prepare a thorough RFP, and it is costly to evaluate RFPs returned. It is important to narrow the list of vendors sent RFPs to those that are likely to meet an organization's needs.

The RFP may be assembled by the chief executive officer, a project officer, the information systems department, a nurse informaticist, or an independent consultant. It reflects decisions and specifications provided by the selection committee. Each member of the committee reviews the final document before it is issued, further reinforcing the team's effort and input. The format for an RFP varies depending on the organization and the author(s). Appendix I contains a detailed example of an RFP for an inpatient clinical system. The RFP should give vendors enough detailed information to respond to the questions asked in the RFP. The format of the RFP may vary from one organization to another and in the level of detail provided.

If written well and unambiguously, the RFP elicits accurate responses from vendors. Vendors do not mistakenly indicate that their system can meet the requirement when it does not, nor do they misinform the system selection committee. RFP questions must be phrased so the vendor can answer most questions with one of four answers: yes; yes, with customization; yes, available in the future; or No. An area should be left for comments if explanation is needed (Hunt et al., 2004). Clearly, the nursing perspective at this point in the process is crucial. "It is the nurse who must integrate and collate all the information into a logical format and develop a comprehensive plan of care for the individual patient. Information the nurse collates is captured by registration, medical records, physicians, laboratory, pharmacy, radiology, physical therapy, dietary, and many other departments" (Jenkins, 2000).

Although it is helpful to start with an example, vendors naturally have a strong self-interest in this process, and therefore organizations should not accept any vendor's offer of assistance with the preparation of an RFP, no matter how apparently innocent and well intentioned the offer. (It is likely that the RFP would request system features the vendor's system would be able to provide.) The high cost of preparing an RFP rests in the cost of gathering and compiling information. Care should also be taken to ensure that if an outside consultant prepares the RFP there is also no bias toward a particular vendor in final selection.

Vendors interested in competing for the opportunity to sell their product to the organization then submit proposals and costs estimates in response to the RFP. These documents specify the vendor's proposed means of meeting the specifications outlined in the RFP. Details include hardware and software descriptions, including number, type, location, and specifications; installation information, including location, wiring, delivery times; staff training requirements; and a multiplicity of other specifications, including travel expenses (Hunt et al., 2004).

When all the proposals have been received from the vendors, the organization must select vendors whose proposals they wish to pursue. The proposals from the competing vendors are reviewed and evaluated by the selection committee. It is imperative that nursing representatives on the committee are knowledgeable about nursing's processes and issues and are empowered to make decisions. Some (among many) criteria considered during the evaluation process are as follows.

- Timeliness of response. Did the proposal meet the deadline for submission? If not, what is the assurance that the vendor will meet other deadlines and internal milestones?
- Degree to which the proposed solutions for each area meet the evaluation criteria stipulated in the RFP. Are there many "No" or "Available in the future" answers?
- Compliance with system specifications stated in the RFP.
- Soundness of the vendor's technical approach.

- Past and current experience of the vendor with similar installations. Ask for references and visit or call those sites that are organizationally similar in size and mission.
- Qualifications of proposed implementation staff and consultants to be provided by the vendor.
- Financial stability or business health of the vendor.
- Cost-benefit ratio to include total system costs over the expected system lifetime.

Incorporating the established criteria into a grading tool can greatly assist the selection team when documenting their evaluation. The tool also serves as a reminder of the agreed-upon decision-making process at the beginning of the process when determining the overarching goal(s) of the project. Existing tools can be found in the literature on total quality management (TQM) and continuous quality improvement (CQI) and are easily adapted to technology projects (Hunt et al., 2004).

The effectiveness of an information system depends on nursing input and use along with satisfaction with the system from patient care, clinical, and administrative perspectives. Input during the RFP evaluations is crucial. The outcome of the evaluation process is a consensus on rank ordering of all proposals based on comparisons across all the evaluation criteria. This rank ordering identifies the two to four vendors whose solutions seem most acceptable on paper. They are often comprise the "short list" of vendors competing for the business.

Vendor Demos and Site Visits

While the list of vendors is being whittled down and top choices become apparent, arrange vendor fairs and site visits to locations where computer systems similar to the one being proposed by the vendor are installed and operational. The purpose of site visits is to see systems under consideration in operation and being used by clinicians. The importance of nursing's representation on these site visit teams cannot be understated. Each member of the site-visiting team is visiting with a different perspective, with interview questions developed before departure and after input from the total selection committee. Manning and McDonnell (1997) and Hunt et al., (2004) have provided lists of questions and guidelines about need, safety and security, effectiveness, efficiency, and the economic and social impact. The purposes of these site visits are to see the system, clarify understanding of the system, and verify vendor claims. The site-visiting team is optimally small, composed of four to six members chosen from among senior administrators and end-users who are also members of the selection committee. Site-visit locations are suggested by the vendor, but contacts and scheduling of visits are usually arranged directly between the prospective purchaser and the organization to be visited. Site visits should conform to a predetermined structure so each system function or lack of function is exposed and allowed fair evaluation across vendors (Staggers and Repko, 1996). In addition to looking for specific functional criteria, the team should try to gain a general opinion of the system.

In addition to arranging site visits where the systems are functioning, many consider inviting vendors to set up a training environment in their organization to demonstrate their product to the selection team and larger groups of users if appropriate. The vendor should use a functional system with 'live' data, with a "script" developed by the selection team to demonstrate the functionality described in the RFP. It is most important to structure these vendor visits and utilize the same criteria for all vendors (Staggers and Repko, 1996). If the team does not control demonstration sessions, each vendor may discuss different aspects of a system and few comparisons can be made between vendors, making evaluation difficult. Each representative should be encouraged to point out unique features of his or her product, but the overall format should be similar (Hunt et al., 2004).

There is always a trade-off between the number of companies under consideration and the depth to which each product can be investigated. A large number of vendor companies involved at the beginning preclude a detailed investigation of each. As the field is narrowed and decisions must be made on an increasingly detailed level; in-depth demonstrations of selected systems can provide greater detail and assist with prioritizing the short list.

Here are some things to watch for or do during site visits.

- Observe the general state of cleanliness and order around the terminals: a smooth running system tends not to have dozens of little "helpful hints" notes stuck to the walls or terminal.
- Observe the response time of the system, particularly when it is busy.
- Observe whether all staff use the system or just selected staff (e.g., clerks).
- Ask the staff if they would prefer to go back to a "traditional" method.
- What aspects of care has the system improved? What is the best feature?
- Attempt to speak to staff other than the ones the vendor has arranged for you to see.
- Ask the staff what they do when the system "goes down" or stops working. What you want to hear is "the system rarely goes down."
- Ask "who fixes the system when it stops working." This can illuminate how many people really support the system.
- This is also the time to ask about training. How long did it take the staff to learn the system and who trained them?
- How responsive is the vendor? How easily and quickly are customizations made?

The final selection of the vendor is based on information presented in the proposal and on the site visit. A contract is negotiated between the vendor and the organization; the system is installed and evaluated.

Developing a Short List of Vendors

Below is a suggested phased approach aimed at minimizing the time required to evaluate lengthy RFPs and providing a structured means for all participants to contribute.

- *Phase I: narrowing process*. Eliminate vendor proposals that fail to meet all mandatory requirements or that arrive late (unless contacted prior to deadline). Distribute the remaining responses to the RFP to all committee members. Each member should review the responses and decide whether the proposal addresses essential requirements. Utilize a tracking tool to keep members focused and to organize responses. The idea is to reduce the number of proposals to a workable number, such as three to five. Then correlate the team's findings. Discuss the areas of the proposal where members held different views.
- *Phase II: telephone survey and site visits*. A telephone survey can help determine what sites might be visited. Call those suggested by the vendor as well as organizations that may not be suggested by the vendor to gain a better overall, unbiased picture of the system. Ask each location specific questions about the system: Does it meet their needs, why did they choose a particular vendor, what type of computer hardware and software is required to use the system, would they be willing to have a visit? Site visits help minimize the risk of a wrong choice of vendor or system and allow valuable observations of the system in use. Use them wisely but also be aware that some organizations charge for such visits.
- *Phase III: vendor demonstrations*. Bring the top vendors in for a demonstration. Provide the vendor with a scripted demo of typical scenarios in advance. (Note: these scenarios are also useful during the system testing phase.) Consider inviting a broader group of users and have them fill out evaluation surveys. Collect and evaluate the data submitted on these surveys to see if the selection committee is representing the user base appropriately.
- *Phase IV: decision making*. Using the decision-making criteria determined at the start of the selection process, choose the factors that are important to the success of the system in your organization. Assign a weight, or "score," to each vendor's response for their system (Hunt et al., 2004). For example, response and stability may be more important to your organization than a flashy graphical user interface (GUI) front end that your users may desire. Being able to rank certain areas of the RFP with more "points" provides more accurate scoring of the RFPs.
- *Phase V: technical analysis*. An organization's information services department needs to evaluate vendor offerings to ensure that the proposed system integrates easily in the existing technical infrastructure and can be supported after installation. If additional infrastructure must be purchased or incorporated into planning to allow the purchased system to be

installed, the cost must be incorporated into the financial analysis of the final vendors.

- *Phase VI: financial analysis*. Remember to consider all the financial costs. There can be front-end costs: installation, conversions from old systems, interfaces to existing systems, renovations to facilities, hardware and software, training. Operating costs include hardware and software maintenance, insurance, supplies, ongoing training, and staffing. The goal is to try to compare the proposals objectively and consistently. Bring together the entire package of price versus performance combined with financial information. Identify the vendor or system that gives the most results for the least investment. However, keep in mind that price should not be the overriding consideration: It just happens to be one that is foremost in everyone's mind.

Contract Negotiations

The definitive legal document that defines the relationship with a consultant or the purchase of hospital information systems or stand-alone computer systems in the nursing department, laboratory, or pharmacy is a contract. A successful contract represents a "win-win" solution and leaves both parties feeling positive (Marreel and McLellan, 1999). The contract is the legal umbrella that defines a mutually acceptable set of understandings and commitments between a vendor and an organization. Generally, the contract outlines the products purchased, required data gathering for planning, the implementation plan and timeline, and evaluation criteria. Given the importance of this document and potential consequences, it follows that the contract must be precise, comprehensive, and reviewed by legal advisors and contract experts because it serves both user and vendor for the duration of their relationship (Hunt et al., 2004).

The points discussed here are broad in nature and are meant only to kindle awareness in the reader regarding the importance and consequent implications of a computer contract. The objective of this section is to point out the need for an effective legal document and importance of accurate advice before contract signing. The following is a list of items to help the first-time purchaser of computerized healthcare systems. These tips are offered to avoid major problems that have been encountered.

- Involve an attorney at the beginning of the contract negotiation—not just any lawyer but a lawyer who understands healthcare and technology.
- Ensure that you have the authority to sign a contract and obligate your organization. Often this power or ability resides in certain individuals in the organization who tend to be experts in contracts and should be consulted early in the contracting process (Hunt et al., 2004).

- Be a firm negotiator but not unreasonable. Be demanding of special items your organization has defined as essential while you negotiate the contract with the vendor.
- "It is not so much that the buyer beware but that the buyer should always be aware."
- Avoid signing a vendor's standard contract. It is their contract and is primarily protecting the vendor's interest, not that of the organization.
- Make sure everything is in writing; do not accept verbal promises.
- Read the fine print.

Several key steps can be taken before entering into a contractual relationship.

- Prepare the RFP as clearly as possible, paying specific attention to the fact that those requirements stated in the RFP will become part of the final contract.
- Request that vendors include any additional contractual requirements to their response to the RFP.
- When comparing systems and while doing the final systems evaluations, keep in mind that decisions about modifications to the existing system must be a major part of the final contract.
- A reference check on vendor performance and a check on the financial stability of the vendor(s) being considered is crucial.

The user or purchaser must have some notion of how to negotiate a contract. Certainly, the overall purpose of a contract is to have a comprehensive document that provides the decision-makers with the flexibility to monitor the performance of the vendor. It is extremely important to remember that the final contract must be signed before the actual purchase of the system. If the hardware or software is installed before contract signing, additional problems are introduced.

It is to the buyer's disadvantage if only one vendor is being considered during the final negotiation period. At least two vendors should be considered until the contract is signed. The contract is also much more effective if top-level management from both organizations are present in the final phases of contract negotiations. By this time, the hospital, including the nursing department, should have clearly defined its needs and be able to document its requirements in the contract.

Ask your legal counsel to define the element of profit for the vendor. What will the effect be on the vendor of having you as a user? Consider the time and other resources invested in the proposal preparation, site visits, and demonstrations by the vendor. Is the vendor strictly a provider of the healthcare computer services you need, or is it a larger company marketing many healthcare or even general computer services? This information gives you some idea as to how the vendor values your business.

All these points can help develop a strong negotiation strategy. A few more logistical points are of interest.

- It is advantageous for the buyer to maintain control over what is being negotiated and how it is being negotiated.
- The buyer should have an agenda and set the times and locations of negotiation.
- The buyer should decide the chronological order of items to be negotiated.
- A healthy two-way negotiation of give and take should be established to reach desired goals.
- The buyers should always have a set of alternatives, but it is essential that a position statement be developed from which no compromise is possible (the bottom line).
- To draw an analogy, when bidding at an auction, the buyer has a set price on each item over which he or she will not bid. Working with a contract is similar. There must always be limits, or the game is lost before you start.

The ultimate purpose of contract negotiation, however, is to produce a workable arrangement that satisfies the buyer and can be carried out by the vendor. Compromise is almost essential even on key issues of importance to the buyer. The buyer must remember that if the contract becomes too restrictive or burdensome for the vendor, the relationship can end up in legal friction to the point of nonperformance. Negotiation is an art; in a good contract, both parties believe they have won.

A sensible contract differs according to the objectives of the purchaser. One basic similarity remains: A contract is the written document of mutual consent made between the buyer and seller or vendor. The contract stands as the written testament of the legal obligations of both parties. It should be written to anticipate problems and should establish an ordered mechanism as to how these problems will be remedied. In addition, the contract should deal with the following (Hunt et al., 2004).

- Specific hardware and software being purchased and when (if spread over several fiscal years)
- Financing or a payment plan if tied to vendor deliverables or systems acceptance
- Implementation schedules and major milestones
- Configuration, software modifications, upgrades
- Acceptance criteria
- Ownership of software source code
- Warranties and liabilities
- Detailed set of descriptions of responsibility for both parties, including software, maintenance, and support functions
- Remedies for nonperformance and default of warranties; technical and legal standards to measure success or failure of the implementation
- Vendor presence during deployment

Using a Consultant

All nursing directors or administrators during the course of their administrative responsibilities must at times make the decision to consider various forms of assistance. Although system implementation is relatively new in comparison to the history of nursing in general, there are still lessons learned and captured in current literature that can be used as tools. The intent of this textbook is to provide nurses with a means for learning about computers and information systems and to provide further references for information. However, not all nurses need to be computer experts. Those nurses in decision-making positions may choose to seek advice from a nursing informatics or healthcare informatics consultant.

When choosing a nursing informatics or healthcare informatics consultant, a nursing director or administrator should be aware of the available options. One option is an internal consultant who is a member of the organization and who is most knowledgeable in a certain aspect of the organization (e.g., patient care, nursing education, information services). The second option is to tap into the expertise of a similar healthcare system or an informatics expert in academia. The third option is an independent professional consultant.

In many cases, an internal consultant can serve as a liaison with a consultant brought in from the outside, as internal consultants are more intimately involved and knowledgeable about the organization. There is no doubt that there is a place for each of the three types of consultants, but it is up to each nursing director or administrator to choose from the various alternatives on the basis of need, expertise offered, and financial resources.

When Is a Healthcare Computer Consultant Needed?

Employing a competent healthcare information systems consultant should be considered when computerized patient information systems are under consideration. The organization greatly benefits from one or two people who have experience facilitating successful use of information systems. For what amounts to a minimal financial commitment, the organization thus engages someone with an unbiased, broad perspective that specifically addresses its defined needs. However, as with any type of advice, administrators must use the advice of healthcare information systems consultants with discretion; after all, consultants do not have to live with their proposed solutions. Consultants' advice must always be tempered by the administrator's common sense, intimate knowledge of the organization, and a deep and abiding faith in personal knowledge of the nursing discipline. There are a number of specific reasons for bringing in additional assistance in the form of consultants.

- Need advice and support of an outside consultant to justify or modify the current operation of a department.

- Need advice on a specific management or technical problem requiring an expert opinion of a specialized nature.
- Offer an outside, unbiased opinion on major equipment decisions, reorganizations, and financial commitments and assist in decision-making.
- Provide an overview of the current healthcare, hospital, or clinic situation with a view toward developing a long-range strategic plan for the organization.
- To provide a state-of-the-art evaluation of the current information systems. This can often focus and/or reduce the time it takes an organization to develop an RFP.
- To analyze current operations with the intent of providing recommendations for improvement.
- To perform a rescue operation, usually at the request of the board of trustees, in the areas of management replacement or cost reductions. This reason is applicable when drastic action is required.

It is important to note that an effective consultant seldom makes definitive decisions but, rather, develops and presents a set of viable alternatives for the client. The role of the consultant can be viewed in the broad context, not only as a specialist who might be called on for specific advice but also as a generalist to whom the nursing department can turn to at regular intervals for the purpose of addressing unanticipated problems.

What Is a Qualified Healthcare Informatics Consultant?

One of the most difficult tasks for the nursing administrator or director is defining what a qualified healthcare informatics consultant is. Often the best person for this position is a nurse informaticist who meets the following criteria (Welebob, 2000).

- Relevant professional preparation
- Significant experience with more than one type of information system
- Recognition in the field
- Recommendations tailored to needs of the client
- Reports delivered on time and within budget
- Ability to accomplish change
- Effective communication skills

Where Can a Healthcare Informatics Consultant Be Found?

One of the best ways to ensure competent consulting assistance is to check with colleagues who have already worked with a consultant and can make a recommendation. Second, the prospective employer should check the credentials of computer healthcare consulting firms. Another avenue is to work through various national professional organizations, which are often willing to suggest several private consultants who might be in business for themselves or who are affiliated with major universities. It is important to identify whether a consultant or their agency has arrangements with a particular vendor(s). Having an affiliation with a particular vendor may be acceptable after a system has been chosen but having an affiliation during system selection may lead to a conflict of interest, with the risk of having a system chosen that may or may not meet an organization's needs.

At this time, it is relevant to point out that it is up to the individual who is hiring the consultant to define precisely the parameters of the consultant contract. It is often most valuable to have a preliminary meeting with the consultant in question. At that time, financial compensation and the duration of the consultant's employment should be discussed. In addition, a written agreement about expected outcomes is mandatory. In the overall consideration, employers should be aware of what can and cannot be expected from a consultant. A competent healthcare informatics consultant is able to review the present information system and anticipate future needs; usually suggests alternative solutions for various organizational, technical, and system problems; offers advice about how the system can be integrated with other information systems in the organization; and assists with contract negotiations.

One might think that a consultant can solve all the problems encountered in the organization. However, a consultant cannot, or at least should not, make basic decisions for the administrator. A healthcare informatics consultant cannot assist in fighting private, internal political battles or be expected to solve fundamental management or organization problems. This is a job for a management consultant.

Linking Nursing and Healthcare Information Systems

The object of this section is to impart an understanding and recognition of the importance of nurses being educated about computer systems as a way of ensuring the success of such information systems. One of the essential aspects of a successful information system projectlies is establishing effective communication between and among the various professionals, technicians, consultants, and administrators in a healthcare organization. This section emphasizes a few basic rules that have been effective in closing the communication gap between nurses and the information technology (IT) department. In other chapters, basic computer concepts and details of information systems have been expanded upon, but the emphasis here is to make the reader aware of the importance of establishing a basic conceptual understanding between these two professional groups.

Hostility toward technology produces definite obstacles in the course of system implementation. It is therefore vital that nursing management be fully committed to the changeover, thereby making the transition smooth and sustaining the morale of the nursing staff. Given the fullest commitment by all parties, it is still difficult to implement technology solutions. One of the most glaring problems encountered is the gap in communication between the nurses and the IT professionals. Most tasks in the healthcare computing field require the expertise of both disciplines. An effective working relationship is a prerequisite for the accomplishment of these complex tasks.

The basic characteristics of the average IT professional are that he or she is energetic, is anxious to help the user, wants to be creative, is convinced that the computer can help solve problems, and is totally unaware of the user's real problem. The willingness and technical capabilities of these individuals must not be underestimated. How, then, can the health professional best utilize these highly motivated, specially trained individuals who are eager to lend their talents to improving the delivery of healthcare?

To work effectively with clinical information systems, it is essential to recognize the principles and methods of modern information processing. One should look forward to this learning opportunity. Nurses can learn or gain command of basic concepts, such as design of computer-compatible records and transformation of plain English statements into logical computer-compatible systems, and recognize the benefits and risks of electronic storage of medical information. On the other hand, to achieve a mutually beneficial working relationship, the computer professional must learn the terminology and practice of modern nursing. The following suggestions are helpful for integrating computer systems into the various areas of nursing practice.

1. Have the workflow or operation of the department well defined. One must know what is happening in the department before undertaking the task of implementing a system that computerizes it. All activities of the operation must be documented, and the sources and recipient of all transactions must be identified (see Chapter 13). The smallest detail must be explainable. If you do not know what is going on, there is no way to make the computer help you. If anything, you would then have a more serious problem on your hands. You must precisely define the input to the new system to begin the task of developing a useful tool.
2. Know what you want to do. One must know what is desired as output—the end result must be well defined. If you want nurses' notes in a certain format, be able to articulate to the IT professional why you want it that way. Do not worry at the design stage about how the data are manipulated by the computer; be more concerned with what you want to get out of the system. Draw a detailed picture of your desired report's data elements. Realize that appearances can be changed so it is the content that needs to be captured accurately and communicated (Hunt et al., 2004).
3. Be aware of all the exception conditions. An exception condition is any statement where the user says, "this is true except when...." For

example, temperature is expressed in Fahrenheit degrees except on the pediatrics unit, where it is expressed as Celsius degrees. This is the most difficult part of designing, configuring, and implementing any system. Discovering and satisfying all the exceptions that can arise during the implementation of a new system eliminates most of the traumatic situations that might occur. The more precise the identification of exception conditions during the design/configuration phase of the project, the smoother and more well accepted is the final system.

4. Ask questions. No one enjoys talking about his or her work more than a dedicated IT professional. Get explanations about the purpose of each device your application is using. "Oh, you wouldn't understand" is a response that should not be accepted; convince the IT professional to be your teacher. Build a relationship and learn what you can about their field, as they learn about yours. Unless you understand what facilities the computer has available and what their functions are, the mystique of *Do not fold, spindle, or mutilate* will inhibit you from taking full advantage of the computer's capabilities. It is wise to remember that a little knowledge is dangerous. Make sure you understand the answers to your questions.
5. Obtain explanations of the computer solution. The computer user must understand how the computer is maintaining the data for the system. Nurses must be able to compare the computer workflow with the workflow that occurs in the current system. The IT professional typically thinks logically, and many of the techniques implemented in a computer system could also be valuable if adapted to the manual system. It has been said that the best method of developing a good manual system is to plan for a computerized one. Develop a complete computer system and design a manual backup system that emulates the computer system; then install the manual backup system. This may be a bit extreme, but it emphasizes the fact that much can be learned by comprehending the computer solution to your problem. This can be done prior to actual implementation, and it is especially recommended if the workflow is going to change dramatically.
6. If you are not getting what you need, speak up. Once the computer system is installed and running, keep the data processing or IT support personnel informed about what they need to do to make the system better fit the requirements. If all you do is complain to your coworkers about how bad the computer is, it will never work satisfactorily. You have to tell the people who can do something about it. A good system is never quite complete and must be evaluated and enhanced to stay up to date with current clinical practice.
7. Make constructive suggestions. Do not limit your criticism of the computer system to "that dumb computer does not work." Tell the computer programmer or analyst, specify the problem, and participate in problem-solving. A successful well received computer system is a partnership between the end-users and the data-processing people who implement the

system (Clough, 1997). Effective communication between these groups is essential for the realization of a successful system.

8. Do not be overly impatient. It took a long time for your system to evolve to the point at which it was decided to use a computer. Computer systems are not created in a day. Extensive work must be done in system design, programming, and interfacing to have a current operational system. Ask the IT staff for time estimates to implement the enhancements and respect these estimates. Add in extra time because configurations often take longer than estimated—but never shorten the estimates. If you force a "quick and dirty implementation," the system will not be what you want and will require a great deal of your time to correct or work around. Instead, consider phased approaches if something is absolutely time-boxed for a particular date.
9. Be considerate of the IT professional's problems. Computer professionals are humans too and therefore have all the emotional conflicts, problems, and stresses to which any other person is subject. A family member may get sick or other priorities arise, all of which can affect implementation schedules. They endure similar frustrations of everyday workdays. Treat the IT staff as you would any other valued clinician, and the world will be more pleasant for everyone involved.
10. Understand the system's limitations. After you have a functioning system, it is easy to escalate your desire to the unattainable. One must understand restrictions well enough to not make impossible requests. There are many reasons a computer cannot fulfill all workflow requests or scenarios. Talk to the IT systems people about this aspect; perhaps there is an intermediate solution. Try to keep your dreams realistic and stay within reasonable demands. On the other hand, do not settle for inconvenient workaround steps because the IT staff is too busy. Ask for time estimates, options for phasing in components you want and can use, and hold the IT staff accountable for the dates provided.

The entire organization can derive significant benefits by the early establishment of several IT and user committees. These committees should represent every department of the healthcare organization and focus on particular priorities. For example, an IT steering committee may look into the future for IT planning versus only one project or solution. Find out what committees your organization has and who the nursing members are on those committees.

Summary

There are incredible opportunities when selecting a clinical system. Of utmost importance is that it helps clinicians provide quality patient care. This chapter has considered various aspects of the preparation required when selecting computer applications for patient care settings. The focus has been on selections that meet the needs of clinical applications, but the same principles apply for administrative, educational, or research applications. System selection is also the time to start encouraging change, getting end users excited about the new system, and establishing appropriate user expectations, thereby improving eventual system implementation success.

The following "common sense" guidelines might be of help during the selection process.

- Understand the process.
- Write down what is not clear.
- If you do not understand something, say so.
- Keep documents simple, write for clarity, and be concise. Do not try to "snow" others.
- Realize you cannot know it all.
- Assign responsibility for tasks.
- If someone else drops the ball, pick it up.
- Be proactive and head off trouble before it occurs.
- Two heads are sometimes better than one.
- Avoid distractions.
- Isolate tasks; do things one step at a time; use a time line.
- Be patient; involved problems take time to solve.
- Be willing to follow up.
- Do not be afraid to fail; we all learn from our mistakes.
- Do not hesitate to ask questions.
- Do not hesitate to ask for outside opinions.
- Know that what you do will make a difference.

To prepare nurses for the widespread use of information systems in healthcare, there is a strong need for continuing education, in-service education, and undergraduate education programs that provide nurses with general knowledge about information systems. Informatics nurses obtain more advanced education about information systems to enable them to maintain their nursing focus and serve as interpreters between information systems people and nurse users of information systems. This preparation makes the nurse knowledgeable about both nursing and information system science. When asked, all nurses are responsible for full participation and representation of nursing in the selection, development, implementation, or evaluation of clinical information systems.

References

Clough, G.C. (1997). Getting the right system: The CHIPS experience. In: Gerdin, U., M. Tallberg, & P. Wainwright (eds.) *Nursing Informatics: The Impact of Nursing Knowledge on Healthcare Informatics.* Amsterdam: IOS Press, p. 569.

Hunt, E., Breckenridge-Sproat, S., & Kitzmiller R. (2004). *The Nursing Informatics Implementation Guide*. New York: Springer-Verlag.

Jenkins, S. (2000). Nurses' responsibilities in the implementation of information systems. In: Ball, M.J., Hannah, K.J., Newbold, S.K., & Douglas, J.V. (eds.) *Nursing Informatics: Where Caring and Technology Meet*, 3rd ed. New York: Springer-Verlag, p. 211.

Manning, J., & McConnell, E.A. (1997). Technology assessment: A framework for generating questions useful in evaluating nursing information systems. *Computers in Nursing 15*(3):141–146.

Marreel, R.D., & McLellan, J.M. (1999). *Information Management in Healthcare*. Albany, NY: Delmar Publishers, Inc.

Mills, M.E. (1995). Nursing participation in the selection of HIS. In: Ball, M.J., K.J. Hannah, S.K. Newbold, & J.V. Douglas (eds.) *Nursing Informatics: Where Caring and Technology Meet*, 2nd ed. New York: Springer, pp. 233–240.

Staggers, N., & Repko, K.B. (1996). Strategies for successful clinical information system selection. *Computers in Nursing 14*(3):146–147, 155.

Welebob, E.M. (2000). Nursing informatics consultancy: how to select a nursing informatics consultant. In: Ball, M.J., K.J. Hannah, S.K. Newbold, & J.V. Douglas (eds.) *Nursing Informatics: Where Caring and Technology Meet*, 2nd ed. New York: Springer, pp. 179–180.

15
Data Protection

The issue of privacy is difficult. The individual has the inherent right to control personal information. However, to provide the best possible care and service to the individual, the public, and private organizations must know some of that information. The issue is further complicated because "privacy" has not been defined in a way that is widely and generally accepted. Actions such as collecting and storing unnecessary personal data, disclosing data to individuals or organizations that do not have a genuine need for it, or using private information for something other than the original purpose could be considered intrusive.

Since the 1960s, the widespread use of computers has led to concern about the large mass of data collected through sophisticated data linkage capabilities. The following sociolegal concerns are widespread among the public.

- How and what information is collected
- How the collected information will be used; who will have access to it
- How the collected information can be reviewed and, if necessary, corrected

Within the nursing community, concern over data protection has always been present. The power provided by technologies such as computers and the Internet has heightened the concern of nurses for these reasons.

- More data and information are available.
- More possibilities exist for errors in the data.
- Organizations rely on information systems for essential functions.
- More data are shared between disciplines and organizations/institutions/facilities.
- Public concern over possible abuse of information and privacy is strong.

Until recently, terminology in the area of data protection has not been uniform. However, a standard is emerging, based on the headings used by Working Group 4 of the International Medical Informatics Association (IMIA) (Hoy, 1997). In the area of data protection, then, data security is the overarching concept, with three subareas.

- Usage integrity, more commonly called confidentiality
- Data or program integrity
- Availability

This chapter provides a foundational understanding of the concepts contained in usage integrity (confidentiality), data or program integrity, and availability. The major focus has been on addressing usage integrity (confidentiality). As approaches to data usage integrity have been identified and implemented, more attention has been focused on data/program integrity and availability.

Usage Integrity (Confidentiality)

Exchange of information is a cornerstone of the provision of healthcare. Nurses are continually asking patients to share information relating to their health, including work, home, and social life. When a patient shares something with the expectation that the information is for a limited audience only, it is called confidentiality. The formal definition for *confidentiality* is respect for the privacy of information being disclosed and ethical usage of that information only for the original purpose. *Privacy* is the right of individuals and organizations to decide for themselves when, how, and to what extent information about them is transmitted to others.

Some degree of anonymity in the environment is necessary for mental and physical well-being. On the other hand, the needs of society often supersede the individual's right to privacy. As computer databanks proliferate, the public's concern rises. In a 1994 survey, 52% of respondents thought that computer records were more secure than written records. Surprisingly, when the same survey was conducted in 1995, only 42% thought this (McKenzie, 1996). The increased use of automated personal data systems creates a serious potential for abuse and for "invasion of privacy." Today, systems abstract a uniform data set from medical records at the hospital level and forward it to local, state, and federal organizations. The exchange of medical records information between hospitals and third parties has been made easier by computers. This exchange will increase in the future.

To date, these exchanges usually have the personal identifying data removed. The main problem with automated medical records is the *potential* for breach of privacy. Many health professionals, citizen groups, and other individuals directly affected by such systems consider them to threaten the basic rights of the individual. Underlying these attitudes is a deep concern for confidentiality.

Data collection did not originate with the use of computers. In 1918, physicians began, as a matter of practice, to record information in a medical record. Today, the record is the vehicle for communicating information among healthcare professionals. A health team administering comprehensive care to the patient develops and uses the patient record. Healthcare professionals assume that patients fully disclose all information related to their condition so proper care and treatment can be given. For an effective relationship to exist between the healthcare professional and the patient, the patient must believe that all information provided will be treated confidentially. Unless patients feel assured that the highly sensitive personal information they share with healthcare professionals will remain confidential, they may withhold information critical to their treatment. This need for assurance existed before computerized records. However, the introduction of computerized healthcare records has brought the issue of confidentiality and security to the forefront.

The capabilities of modern technology have created a public awareness regarding the loss of confidentiality inherent in the systems being developed and installed. People other than the direct caregivers have become responsible for the storage and safekeeping of records. Other uses of individual information—for accounting, administrative decision making, and biomedical and healthcare research—are being explored now because the information is easy to retrieve. The flowchart in Figure 15.1 suggests the multitude of possible uses for healthcare data. The ability of computers to match data from diverse sources, to handle large quantities of data, and to maintain records over time has resulted in an unprecedented risk to personal privacy. Record keeping and record protection (i.e., data security) are only parts of the problem. It is access to records for "secondary" purposes that poses the major risk to maintaining confidentiality.

Demands for computerized patient data in the healthcare setting, other than for the actual administration and delivery of an individual's medical care, include the following.

- Utilization of facilities and standards reviews
- Epidemiological studies
- Program evaluation
- Biomedical, behavioral, and health services research
- Financial/billing purposes

Putting private and personal information to "secondary" uses poses a major threat to patient privacy and creates complex social and ethical dilemmas in healthcare. Examples of misuse of confidential information—from old medical files left in the trash to identification left on computerized health databases—are readily found in the newspapers. This sort of abuse does little to reassure the public. Possible linking of various databases and fast retrieval and distribution capabilities have increased concern over how private this information might truly be. The need of users (i.e., physicians, nurses, police, insurers) to have easy access to medical information systems must be balanced with the need of the individual for privacy.

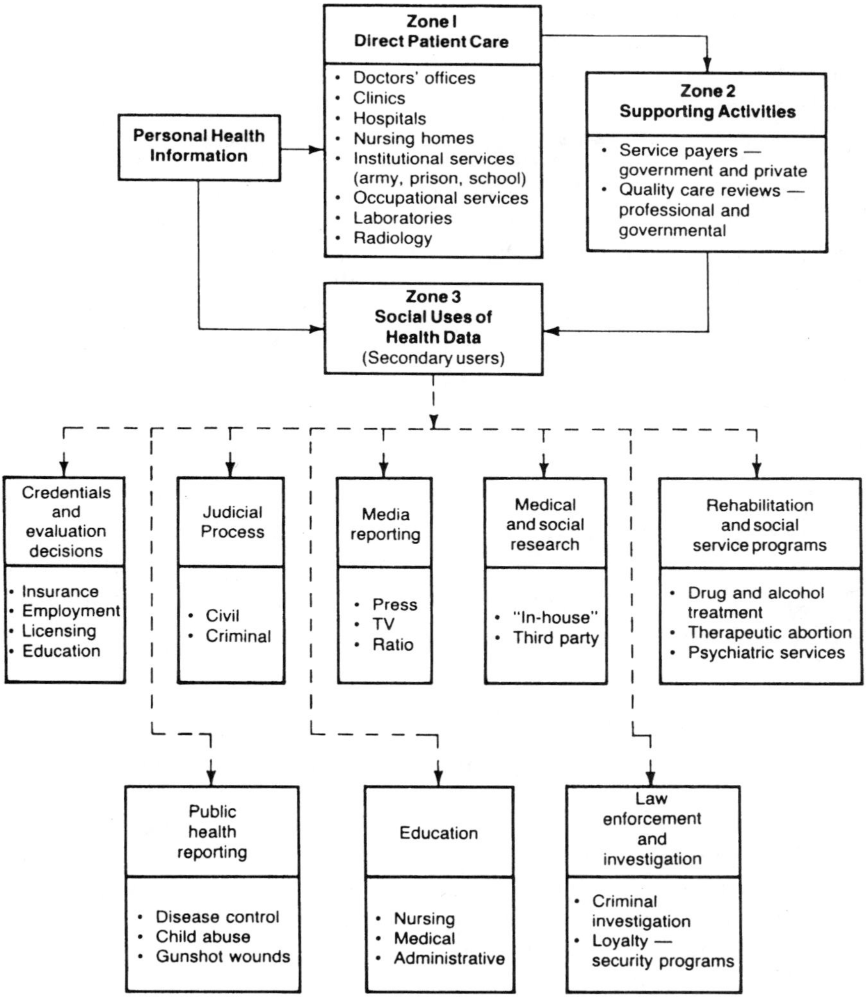

FIGURE 15.1. Possible uses of healthcare data.

Data Security Breaches

There are many outcomes that can occur as a result of breaches in data security (Barber, 1977, p. 62).

- Public embarrassment or loss of public confidence
- Question of personal safety
- Infringement of personal privacy

- Failure to meet legal obligations
- Question of commercial confidentiality
- Financial loss
- Disrupted activities

Damage to patients is of vital concern; however, other types of damage are also important. Legal cases, financial loss, and loss of public confidence can cause great damage to organizations. To address these concerns before problems occur, it is essential that nurses be involved in formulating specific, documented policies related to data security. When such policies are in place, nurses are not left in the dangerous situation of having to make judgments about use of data without any regulations to assist them. The three areas identified here must be considered when defining data protection policies. Data protection policies will contribute to an overall organizational disaster plan, as discussed in Chapter 17.

Protecting Data Usage Integrity

Three approaches to protecting data usage integrity are suggested: hardware, software, and organizational.

Hardware Approach

Hardware security is concerned with the protective features that are part of the architectural characteristics of the data-processing equipment. It also includes the support and control procedures necessary to maintain operational integrity of those features. Hardware security features include hardware identification, isolation features, access control, surveillance, and integrity. Specific protection could include physical barriers such as special doors, locks on individual machines, and control over the use of communication links to the system.

Software Approach

Software security requires the operating system to provide the same features as the hardware security system. It must be able to identify and authenticate, to isolate, to control access, and to have surveillance and integrity features. Security mechanisms designed to protect patient confidentiality generally rely on some combination of authentication, authorization, and auditing (Bowen et al., 1997).

Authentication refers to the methods by which a system verifies the identity of a user, usually based on passwords or physical tokens. Passwords, although a useful approach, have many inherent problems. Users exchange passwords,

passwords are left written down by the computer, common words are used, and passwords are not changed on a regular basis.

Authorization denotes access controls or other means used to provide specific information to a given user. Systems that implement authorization procedures generally attempt to determine whether a given user has a need to know the requested information. Some of the dimensions considered when formulating mechanisms for making such decisions include user roles, types of database interaction, and the purpose for which the information will be used. Commercial programs exist to aid this process.

Auditing is used to record and review a user's interaction with the system. These user records create an audit trail. Depending on the system, auditing may be unapparent to the user. Audit records can then be used to identify unauthorized attempts at access and patterns of access. The threat of sanctions is often sufficient to deter abuse of information access. However, such systems depend on users being aware of and sensitive to the consequences of abuse. Another problem associated with the use of auditing as a security approach is that it is retrospective (Bowen et al., 1997). Depending on the design of the processes to review auditing records, much time can pass, with the result of having continued information security breaches before the unauthorized usage is detected and confronted.

Organizational Approach

The procedural considerations that bring together computing equipment, software, and data in an operational electronic data-processing environment are collectively called *operations security*. These procedures must provide for secure processing during data input, processing, storage, and output. The administrative and organizational component of privacy protection involves the development and dissemination of policies, procedures, and practices related to privacy of patient information. Administrative policies and procedures must be put in place to protect the privacy and confidentiality of patient information. Such measures include disciplinary action for violation. An initial concern is the question of which individuals or categories of workers should have access to what information in a hospital information system. These are difficult decisions. Each user's or department's needs must be considered, along with those of the patient. The committee who makes these decisions and the information systems staff most likely know how best to access the entire patient record. Yet even then there is potential for violation of confidentiality. For example, some institutions employ data entry clerks to enter previously written data. These employees have access to the entire patient chart while the data are being entered but are not bound by a "code of ethics" as are other healthcare personnel. This could be a strong argument against using these employees to enter data. It might be better to have all professionals enter and retrieve their own data. Other considerations include where terminals, printers, and data storage are located. Portable computers and bedside terminals are liable to theft and may allow the patient or visitors unauthorized access to the system. The organizational decisions about ways in which physical items are sited influence the hardware and software approaches to security that must be taken.

Data/Program Integrity

Data must be collected, stored, and transmitted in a manner that preserves the integrity of the data. Accurate collection of data along with mechanisms for reviewing and correcting specific information are essential for preserving data integrity. The use of source data capture technologies enhances the probability of collecting accurate data (see Chapter 6). A key concern of consumers is the ability to view personal data and correct it as required. Accuracy is the foundation for data integrity. Arduously protecting the storage and transmission of that which is fundamentally flawed is a strong possibility if attention is not paid to all three aspects of data integrity.

There has always been concern about protecting the storage of data. In times past, the primary threat was from natural disasters such as fires, floods, tornadoes, or earthquakes. Electronically stored data are also open to these threats. However, the more common threats to data and storage integrity come from system malfunctions, either accidental or malicious. Computer viruses that corrupt individual data or entire system are a major threat to the security and integrity of data storage. The viruses are commonly introduced into an organization's information system by users transferring infected files between their personal computers and the organization's computers. Another threat to the secure storage of data is the ability of users to copy data files onto personal computers to work at home. Confidential patient information may be left on a CD-ROM that is then partially copied over and given to someone else, with identifiable data remaining accessible. As part of an overall data security plan, organizations must develop and enforce policies related to the transfer of information between the organization's information system and an individual user's personal computer.

The transmission of electronic data within an organization and with outside agencies provides another significant opportunity for exposure to security threats. Many organizations have developed policies to deal with the security of data transmitted within the organization (e.g., between departments). However, the exponential growth of the use of the Internet for secure data transmission requires a fresh look at transmission policies. The level of concern about Internet security depends on how an organization is using the Internet. Even organizations that have not connected their networks to the Internet are at risk as staff members use the organization's systems and networks to connect to the Internet using their personal subscriptions. Organizational use of the Internet can be roughly divided into three categories, each with specific data transmission security concerns (Miller, 1996).

1. Using the Internet as an information resource or on-line library includes searching the CINALHDirect database or other on-line databases for articles and downloading articles from a website. The risk here is not from inappropriate transmission of secure data but of downloading a virus along with the article. The installation and maintenance of antivirus software should protect data from corruption from an Internet connection.
2. Using the Internet as a communication vehicle. Sending and receiving e-mail, participating in mailing lists or discussion groups, and making information available to the public through a website are examples of the Internet's use as a communication tool. As a communications tool, the Internet should not be considered secure. Messages may be read by many other persons in addition to the intended recipient. The message may be stored on a variety of computers before delivery, or the recipient may make copies or forward the message to any number of people. Transmitting electronic patient data to other healthcare professionals via e-mail, for either consultation or research, must also be regulated for the reasons stated above. Communicating with patients via e-mail may pose risks to the patient's privacy and data security, especially if the e-mail is directed to the patient's employment e-mail address. Policies must be developed to govern communication using the Internet so as to preserve data transmission integrity.
3. Use of the Internet as an extension of the organization's network, including linking your computer systems to another organization's computer systems (e.g., to participate in a joint research project) or providing remote access for staff members or transfer of files to other organizations. File transfers should be used with caution. When files are transferred into an organization, there is a risk of downloading software in violation of copyright or infecting the organization's computers with viruses. Transferring files outside the organization runs the risk of disclosing confidential patient or proprietary information either in the file transfer itself or as a result of the way in which the information is handled in the receiving organization. Research and policy discussions about the secure transmission of electronic patient information are accelerating as the electronic health record becomes a reality in many jurisdictions.

System Availability

A system must be available in the right place at the right time. Overloading may slow down a system's response, and other, more serious problems may shut it down altogether. All computer users live in fear of their system becoming unusable because of failure of the machine or its power supply. Solutions may involve uninterruptible power supplies and backup hardware on standby and certainly should include backup of patient data on a regular basis to ensure that no information is lost if a system problem occurs.

Buildings that house computer equipment require precautions against natural and manmade hazards. Chapter 17 contains detailed information related to disaster recovery planning.

Legislation and Standards

As healthcare institutions use computerized medical records in more ways and as demands for personal data increase, public concern will continue to rise unless fears regarding potential abuse of information are addressed. In an effort to strike a balance between institutional objectives and public concerns, legislators have proposed or enacted policies to control and regulate the creation and use of large databases. However, many of these proposals have created legal conundrums because of their conflict with existing laws or through the resulting division of power between the various levels of government. Because of these problems, there has been greater emphasis on the voluntary establishment of standards and codes of ethics within the data processing and medical record management communities. Internationally, the Organization for Economic Cooperation and Development (OECD) (1981) held that

> although national laws and policies may differ, member countries have a common interest in protecting privacy and individual liberties, and in reconciling fundamental but competing values such as privacy and the free flow of information.

This belief led to the adoption by member countries of a set of guidelines that should be minimum standards for handling personal data relating to an identifiable individual. The Guidelines on the Protection of Privacy and Transborder Flows of Personal Data, adopted in 1980, continue to represent the international consensus on general guidance concerning the collection and management of personal information: http://www.oecd.org/document/20/0,2340,en_2649_201185_15589524_1_1_1_1,00.html (OECD, 1980). The eight guidelines are as follows.

1. *Collection Limitation Principle.* Collection of personal data should be limited. It must be done through lawful and fair means and, whenever possible, with the knowledge and consent of the subject.
2. *Data Quality Principle.* Data should be relevant to the proposed usage, accurate, and complete; and it should be kept up to date.
3. *Purpose Specification Principle.* The intended use of data should be stated at the time of collection, and subsequent usage should be limited to that purpose or such other that is not materially different from the stated intended purpose.
4. *Use Limitation Principle.* Data should not be disclosed, made available, or used for purposes other than those specified without the consent of the subject or unless authorized by law.

5. *Security Safeguards Principle.* Personal data should be protected by reasonable security safeguards against such risks as loss or unauthorized access, destruction, use, modification, or disclosure of data.
6. *Openness Principle.* A general policy of openness should exist about developments, practices, and policies with respect to personal data. Means should be readily available for establishing the existence and nature of collected personal data and the main purpose of their use, as well as the identity of the collector of the data.
7. *Individual Participation Principle.* An individual should have the following rights.
   - Be able to obtain confirmation as to whether data relating to himself or herself exists
   - Be able to have data relating to him or her made available within a reasonable time, at a reasonable cost, in a reasonable manner, and in a form that is readily intelligible
   - Be given reasons for refusal of a request made under the first two rights
   - Be able to challenge data relating to him or her and, if successful, to have the data erased, rectified, completed, or amended
8. *Accountability Principle.* A data controller should be accountable for complying with measures that give effect to these principles as just stated.

The principles embodied in the OECD guidelines are evident in many privacy-related laws passed in member countries and in principles and guidelines adopted by national professional organizations.

In the United States, the Health Insurance Portability and Accountability Act (HIPAA) of 1996 was enacted to allow employees and their families to transfer insurance benefits from one employer to another or to extend coverage if the employee was terminated or left the job (portability) and to protect the way electronic health information is stored and exchanged (accountability) (Follansbee, 2002; Trossman, 2003). Although there are nursing implications related to portability, the major implications of HIPAA in the area of accountability are addressed here. The Administration Simplification addresses accountability through "The Privacy Rule" and "The Security Rule."

> In response to the HIPAA mandate, HHS published a final regulation in the form of the Privacy Rule in December 2000, which became effective on April 14, 2001. This Rule set national standards for the protection of health information, as applied to the three types of covered entities: health plans, healthcare clearinghouses, and healthcare providers who conduct certain healthcare transactions electronically. By the compliance date of April 14, 2003 (April 14, 2004, for small health plans), covered entities must implement standards to protect and guard against the misuse of individually identifiable health information. Failure to timely implement these standards may, under certain circumstances, trigger the imposition of civil or criminal penalties. [http://www.hhs.gov/ocr/hipaa/guidelines/overview.pdf]

Under the Privacy Rule, health plans, healthcare clearinghouses, and certain healthcare providers must guard against misuse of individuals' identifiable health information and limit the sharing of such information, and consumers are afforded significant new rights to enable them to understand and control how their health information is used and disclosed. [http://www.cms.hhs.gov/hipaa/hipaa2/regulations/privacy/finalrule/privrulepd.pdf]

HIPAA places comprehensive restriction on the use and disclosure of individual health information in any form including computer diskette or CD-ROM, storage on a computer server, e-mail, voice recordings, and other similar media as well as anything derived from these sources (Follansbee, 2002). "Covered entities" include health insurance plans, healthcare clearing houses, and healthcare providers. Specifically, the HIPAA Privacy Rule may be summarized as follows.

- It requires that patients receive a clear written explanation of how their health information is used, kept, and disclosed.
- It requires that patients be permitted to see and obtain copies of their records and to request amendments to those records. Also, a history of disclosures of their records must be accessible to the patients.
- It specifies that patient consent is required before sharing protected health information for treatment, payment, or healthcare operations purposes. In addition,"authorization" is required when the healthcare information is to be used for nonroutine and most nonhealthcare purposes.
- It specifies that, except for uses or disclosures for purposes of treatment, payment, or healthcare operations, patient consent to use and disclosure of protected health information may not be required and must not be coerced by providers and health plans.
- It provides patients with recourse in the event of HIPAA violations.

The security standards... define administrative, physical, and technical safeguards to protect the confidentiality (safe from wrongful access), integrity (safe from alteration), and availability (safe from loss) of electronic protected health information. The standards require covered entities to implement basic safeguards to protect electronic protected health information from unauthorized access, alteration, deletion, and transmission. The Privacy Rule, by contrast, sets standards for how protected health information should be controlled by setting forth what uses and disclosures are authorized or required and what rights patients have with respect to their health information. [http://www.cms.hhs.gov/hipaa/hipaa2/regulations/security/03-3877.pdf]

The HIPAA Security Rule applies only to electronic data, which includes storage media (hard drives, magnetic disks and tapes, optical disks) and transmission media (Internet, dial-up lines) (McCartney, 2003). The Security Rule includes the administrative policy and physical and technical requirements summarized below (McCartney, 2003).

Required administrative policies include the following.

- Security management
- Security official
- Risk analysis
- Identification and response to a security incident

- Sanction policy
- Information system activity review (audit)
- Contingency plan for data backup, system failure, environmental disaster recovery, and emergency situations (includes requirement to create and store retrievable exact copies of electronic patient data)
- Procedures to authorize access to protected health information
- Security training

Required physical safeguards include these items.

- Policies that limit physical access to the facility, workstations, electronic devices, and media
- Policy that details the movement and disposal of any electronic protected health information

Required technical safeguards include the following

- Each user has a unique user name or number for identification and authentication of permission to access protected health information.
- Activity, in an electronic file, of any user must be permanently recorded, able to be examined at a later date, and be nonrepudiatable (individual cannot deny accessing the information).
- Automatic logoff is in place.
- Encryption is part of the system.
- Integrity safeguards ensure that electronic protected health information are clearly represented in the original format, complete, correctly identified, retrievable, and have not been altered, destroyed or wrongfully transmitted.
- Corroboration (evidence that protected health information has not been altered) is built into the system.

Nurses must be knowledgeable about HIPPA and how it relates to their individual practice. Organizations and institutions have developed policies and procedures specific to their situation. If you are not aware of the policies and procedures related to protected health information in your work setting, contact the nursing administration in your institution.

In Canada, the federal government and all provinces have passed freedom of information and protection of privacy legislation to protect personal information in the public sector. Common provisions in these laws include guidelines for the collection, use, and disclosure of personal information. Four provinces have passed legislation specific to health information. There is a federal initiative to develop national legislation to deal specifically with the privacy, confidentiality and security requirements of the electronic health record. Additionally, the Canadian Organization for the Advancement of Computers in Health (COACH) has published Guidelines for the Protection of Health Information (2004). These guidelines provide an overview of key issues related to the development and implementation of security and privacy programs for healthcare organization and legislators.

The European Union passed a data protection directive, Directive 95/46/EC, in 1995 (http://europa.eu.int/comm/internal_market/privacy/index_en.htm). The Directive covers the processing of personal data and free movement of the data. Several countries have moved to supplement this broad legislation with laws that provide strict privacy safeguards for medical data. In the United Kingdom, the Data Protection Act, passed in 1998 (http://www.hmso.gov.uk/acts/acts1998/19980029.htm), categorizes information relating to an individual's physical or mental health as sensitive data, requiring special efforts to protect its privacy.

Nursing Responsibilities

The components of privacy protection in a healthcare information system are not mutually exclusive but are highly interrelated and interactive. As patient advocates, nurses must be vigilant in protecting patient privacy. Nurses must initiate and participate in the evaluation of the privacy protection in new or existing computerized patient information systems. The following questions might be useful in guiding such an evaluation.

- What is the mechanism for restricting entry to main computer system areas?
- How are the terminals "locked"—that is, by card, key, or password?
- What security is provided for media storage areas? Will a librarian be available to control access? Will stored materials ever be allowed to leave the storage area?
- What provision is made to protect data in the event of fire, destruction of the area, and the like?
- What control is used to establish who can view, enter, or alter data?
- Are certain terminals designated for access to specific data sets only (e.g., dietary)?
- Is the sign-on done by department, unit, or individual? Are codes a combination of alphanumeric symbols?
- Is an audit trail available through a transaction log to process the time and identification code of each log-on?
- What mechanism(s) exists for encrypting personal data?
- Is there a mechanism whereby a terminal is identified before information goes out?
- Do statistical reports identify individuals in any way?
- Is an oath of secrecy or a signed statement on ethical position necessary for staff members who are not governed by a code of ethics (e.g., those who process and store the data)?
- Does the duty of confidentiality transfer from direct caregivers to data processors?
- How are data-processing personnel screened for jobs? How is their responsibility for confidentiality emphasized? What are the consequences for inappropriate release of data?

- When personnel leave, what happens to their password?
- What agency is used to test the security of the system?
- How are security breaches reported (by whom, to whom)? Who has authority to take disciplinary action when security breaches occur?
- Who has overall responsibility in the institution for confidentiality of information?
- Who is responsible for keeping the public informed of the purpose, use, and existence of computerized records?
- Who is responsible for establishing, updating, and enforcing written policies and procedures?

Knowledgeable nurses advocate their institution's or organization's compliance with the following criteria, which the literature identifies in relation to both new and existing computerized health information systems.

- The use of passwords and identification codes is essential. Controlled terminal access can be used in conjunction with the measures described here; by itself, however, it does not appear to be adequate. Passwords should be changed at regular intervals and as necessary. The same password should not be repeated to eliminate the employees using old passwords to gain access to wrong information.
- Limits on the collection and recording of information must be established. Individual institutions will formulate policies in this regard. As individuals, nurses need to assess the relevance of the information they record.
- When entering data, we need to ensure that the information is accurate. This has always been essential; but because of the qualities of automated records, the potential harm of inaccurate charting currently has an even greater impact on the patient.
- When developing policies regarding privacy, confidentiality, and a system's security, the patient must be the prime concern. To facilitate this objective, a patients' rights representative is a great asset.
- Informing the public when implementing a new hospital information system is important. Part of the public awareness campaign should include its impact on privacy. This method may cause unwarranted concern, but the public is now aware of the system's implementation and potential, both positive and negative aspects. Also, the more introductory information given to the public about the system, the more likely it is to accepted.
- Before the input of an individual's data into a system, the patient must be informed that computerized medical records are operational in the institution. To withhold this fact from a person is an invasion of the patient's privacy.
- When using information for research, a consent is absolutely essential. Information should not be identifiable.
- The system and its controls must be reviewed at regular intervals, and audits must be performed by an independent party.
- At present in Canada, medical records are the property of the hospital. A study on personal privacy performed in the United States recommends

that patients have a right to see their own records and, furthermore, be able to make amendments as necessary to maintain their accuracy. Legislation is necessary to change this policy. Making the medical record the property of the individual allows patients to have access to their own medical records. Access to the record should be available anytime and anywhere. The patient could then assess its accuracy. Provisions would have to be made enabling the individual to make amendments to the record. Patient ownership of records is an issue in itself but is beyond the scope of this section and is not being addressed further.

- With the implementation of computerized medical records, an entire new department of staff has access to the patient's record. These are the information systems personnel. A "code of ethics" should be formulated for them regarding privacy and confidentiality of the information. The document should be signed by each employee to obtain its full impact in maintaining confidentiality.
- Government legislation is necessary in the area of database linkages to control data transfer from one system to another and to control data uses. As previously stated, because of the potential harm to the individual and the institution, strict policies need to be enforced for governing both the access and use of information.
- Education of all personnel in the area of patient privacy and confidentiality is imperative. It is especially important for persons who are new to the healthcare system and involved with patient care records for the first time (e.g., information systems personnel). Education is an essential part of the maintenance of privacy and confidentiality. Professionals who are traditionally critical of automated medical records accept the system more readily if they are educated about how security is maintained. Regular intervals of inservice must be carried out to inform the staff of new developments in this area.

References

Barber, B. (1997). Security and confidentiality issues from a national perspective. In: *Patient Privacy, Confidentiality and Data Security: Papers from the British Computer Society Nursing Specialist Group Annual Conference.* Lincolnshire, UK: British Computer Society, pp. 61–72.

Bowen, J.W., Klimczak, C., Ruiz, M., & Barnes, M. Design of access control methods for protecting the confidentiality of patient information systems in networked systems. *Journal of the American Medical Informatics Association: Symposium Supplement*. Nashville: Haanlley & Belfus, 1997:46–50.

COACH—Canada's Health Informatics Organization. (2004). *Guidelines for the Protection of Health Information.* Toronto: COACH.

Data Protection Act. (1998). http://www.hmso.gov.uk/acts/acts1998/19980029.htm.

European Data Protection Directive. (1995). http://europa.eu.int/comm/internal_market/privacy/index_en.htm.

Follansbee, N. (2002). Implications of the Health Information Portability and Accountability Act. *Journal of Nursing Administration 32*(1):42–47.

Health Information Portability and Accountability Act. (1996). http://www.hhs.gov/ocr/hipaa/.

Hoy, D. (1997). Protecting the individual: Confidentiality, security and the growth of information systems. In: *Sharing Information: Key Issues for the Nursing Profession*. Lincolnshire, UK: British Computer Society, pp. 78–87.

McCartney, P.R. (2003). HIPAA and electronic health information security. *The American Journal of Maternal Child Nursing, 28*(5):333–334.

McKenzie, D.J.P. (1996). Healthcare trend improves security practices. *In Confidence.*, May/June, pp 1–3. http://www.ahima.org/publications/1a/May-June.inconf.html.

Miller, D.W. Internet security: What health information managers should know. *Journal of AHIMA*. 1996, September, 4 pg. Online. Available: http://www.ahimma.org/publications/2f/sept.focus.html.

Organization for Economic Cooperation and Development (OECD). (1980). *Guidelines on the Protection of Privacy and Transborder Flows of Personal Data.* Paris: OECD.

Personal Information Protection and Electronic Documents Act. (1980). http://www.privcom.gc.ca/legislation/02_06_01_e.asp.

Trossman, S. (2003). Protecting patient information: healthcare facilities gear up for privacy regulations. *American Journal of Nursing 103*(2):65–67.

Additional Resources

DiBenedetto, D. (2004). AAOHN and CMSA develop joint position paper on HIPAA and confidentiality. *Case Management 9*(2):106–108.

Mills, M.E. (1997). Data privacy and confidentiality in the public arena. *Journal of the American Medical Informatics Association: Symposium Supplement.* Nashville, TN: Hanley & Belfus, pp. 42–45.

Muller, L. (2004). HIPAA: Demonstrating compliance. *Case Management 9*(1):27–31.

Murray, P.J. (1997). "It'll never happen to me": Revisiting some computer security issues. *Computers in Nursing 15*(2):65–66, 70.

Olsen, D.P. (2003). HIPAA privacy regulations and nursing research. *Nursing Research 52*(5):344–348.

Roberts, D.W. (2003). Privacy and confidentiality: The Health Insurance Portability and Accountability Act in critical care nursing. *AACN Clinical Issues: Advanced Practice in Acute Critical Care 14*(5):302–309.

Websites of Interest

American National Standards Institute Home Page: http://www.ansi.org
Canada Health Infoway: http://www.infoway-inforoute.ca/home.php?lang=en
Canadian Institute for Health Information: http://www.cihi.ca
United States Privacy Laws by State: http://www.epic.org

16
Ergonomics

A major concern for nursing informatics is ergonomics. The word "ergonomics" comes from the Greek words *ergo*, meaning work, and *nomos*, meaning law. Ergonomics, a relatively new science, looks at the application of physiological, psychological, and engineering principles to interactions between people and machines. Ergonomics attempts to define working conditions that enhance individual health, safety, comfort, and productivity. This can be done by recognizing three things: the physiological, anatomical, and psychological capabilities and limitations of people; the tools they use; and the environments in which they function.

As the use of computerized nursing information systems increases, ergonomics is of increasing interest to nurses in their dual role as users of computers and as healthcare providers. Nurses are concerned with how computer workstations or handheld computers affect the provision of patient care (see Chapters 7 and 8) and the nurse as an individual. These concerns include the physiological aspects (i.e., physical comfort), cognitive aspects (i.e., comprehension of displayed information), and practical aspects (i.e., infection control when using computers at the bedside). Ergonomics standards play a key role in improving the usability of systems and addressing many of the concerns identified here. The standards provide guidance to decision makers in the procurement of systems and systems components that can be used effectively, efficiently, safely, and comfortably. Ergonomics standards themselves do not guarantee good, design, but they do provide a means of identifying interface quality in design, procurement, and operational use. International standards for display screen equipment are being developed by the International Organization for Standardization (ISO). The ISO recommendations are developed by working groups whose members are representatives of the national standards bodies of member countries. There are 17 parts to the standard related to work with visual display terminals (VDTs). Many of these parts are still works in progress. More information regarding ISO standards can be obtained at http://www.iso.ch (for a fee) or at www.usabilitynet.org/tools/r_international.htm.

The following is a list of the various parts of ISO 9241 Ergonomics Requirements for Office Work with Visual Display Terminals (VDTs).

- Part 1: General introduction
- Part 2: Guidance on task requirements
- Part 3: Visual display requirements
- Part 4: Keyboard requirements
- Part 5: Workstation layout and postural requirements
- Part 6: Environmental requirements
- Part 7: Display requirements with reflections
- Part 8: Requirements for displayed colors
- Part 9: Requirements for nonkeyboard input devices
- Part 10: Dialogue principles
- Part 11: Guidance on usability specification and measures
- Part 12: Presentation of information
- Part 13: User guidance
- Part 14: Menu dialogues
- Part 15: Command dialogues
- Part 16: Direct manipulation dialogues
- Part 17: Form-filling dialogues

There is work in progress to develop ISO AWI 18789 (Ergonomic requirements and measurement for electronic visual display), which will revise and replace ISO 9241 Parts 3, 7, and 8 and ISO 13406 (Ergonomic requirement for work with visual displays based on flat panels (www.usabilitynet.org/tools/r_international.htm).

Detailed discussion of ergonomics and the ISO standards is beyond the scope of this text, but the next section addresses selected areas directly related to nurses.

Nursing Computer Workstation

The nursing computer workstation has two components: hardware (the physical equipment) and software (the programs required to enter, retrieve, and process information). Both components affect the quality of patient care and the physical and psychological comfort of the nurse. The hardware normally has a way to enter data and commands and a way to display data and results. How this is accomplished primarily affects the physical comfort of the nurse. The quality of patient care is determined by how accurately data can be entered and how easily retrieved information can be interpreted and comprehended by the nurse. The effect of the presence of bedside terminals on the patient–nurse relationship has not been well documented.

Video display terminals are the usual point of contact between the nurse and most computerized nursing information systems. VDTs are the devices that show both input to, and output from, the central processing unit. Information is typed on the keyboard and presented on the display screen for verification by the operator before being transmitted to the computer. Output from the computer is presented to the operator in the same fashion, that is, as an image generated on the display screen.

Physiological Concerns

Much research has been done regarding the physiological aspects of VDT workstations. The terms VDT, video display unit (VDU), video matrix terminal (VMT), cathode ray terminal (CRT), and monitor are synonymous. Some users of VDTs complain of ergonomic shortcomings such as strained postures, poor photometric display characteristics, and inadequate lighting conditions. Others claim that the complaints are symptoms of a health hazard requiring immediate measures to protect the health of operators. The National Institute for Safety and Health (NIOSH) in the United States has sponsored extensive research concerning a variety of ergonomics-related topics. These reports are available through the NIOSH website (http://www.cdc.gov/niosh/homepage.html). Additional reference articles, current journal listings, and related conferences can be accessed at the ERGOWEB site (http://www.ergoweb.com). A VDT workstation checklist is available at the ERGOWEB site that is useful for nurses and employers to evaluate the ergonomics of fixed workstations. The following sections provide an overview of ergonomic concerns related to nursing informatics.

Eye Strain

Screen Resolution

The displayed size of the characters on the screen can contribute to eyestrain. The character's image is generated on the display screen by a cathode ray tube. The cathode ray tube used in computer terminals is identical to those found in television sets. It is essentially a glass vacuum tube encased in a lead seal with an electron gun in opposition to a phosphor-coated screen. High-voltage electricity is used by the electron gun to generate a stream of electrons that can be directed to any display screen location. This electrical excitation of the phosphors eliminates the point on the screen at which the slender beam of electrons is being focused. A scanning mechanism generates letters and characters using a dot matrix pattern. The number of horizontal and vertical dots, called pixels, in the matrix determines the resolution of the character. The ranges for high-, medium-, and low-resolution screens continue to change with each advance in technology.

Flicker

Flicker on the screen also causes eyestrain. Two characteristics of the screen play a crucial role in reducing flicker: persistence and refresh rate. *Persistence* is the length of time the phosphors remain illuminated after being electrically excited. The *refresh rate* is the frequency with which each point on the surface of the screen is reilluminated by electrical excitation. The refresh rate must be frequent enough so persistence of the phosphor is sustained; otherwise, the displayed characters seem to fade away. Flicker occurs when the refresh rate is too low. The operator then notices the decay in the phosphor's illumination before it is reexcited. In this case, the operator can identify pulsating luminescence in the display. The presence of flicker causes eye and mental fatigue for operators. Refresh rates of 70 Hz (cycles per second) are usually sufficient to prevent perceptible flicker on screens having light characters on a dark background, thereby reducing eye strain (ISO, 9241, Part 3, 1996).

Color

The color of the display does not seem to be a major physiological factor. The choice of the phosphor to be used in the screen is determined by the phosphor's grain, its luminescence, its color, and its persistence (rate of decay). There is considerable disagreement whether amber or green phosphors provide better legibility and color contrast. Generally, it is agreed that lighting conditions determine which is best in specific situations. Usually, green is preferred for highly illuminated rooms and amber for less well lit areas. Often the choice of color is more a matter of personal preference than of scientific determination considering the lighting conditions in most work environments.

Glare

Glare also contributes to eyestrain among users. Although lighting conditions do not appear to influence the choice of screen phosphor color, they are of considerable ergonomic significance in relation to glare. Glare occurs when the range of luminances in the visual field is too great (e.g., when bright sources of luminares, windows, or their refracted images fall within the field of vision). Glare causes distractions, visual discomfort, reduced legibility, and reduced visual acuity. Engineers have attempted to reduce glare on display screens using three methods: etched glass and filters, optical coatings, and position of the screen. Etched glass and filters do reduce glare but also tend to simultaneously reduce legibility by defocusing the characters and reducing character brightness. In fact, some filters have been found to increase the operator's awareness of screen reflections. Optical coating of the screen glass has been found to be an effective but expensive solution for glare. The most effective, least expensive means of reducing glare is simply to make sure that the screen can be moved and positioned so reflections are no longer visible. This can be accomplished by placing the screen at right angles to the source of light and by ensuring that the display screen is an independent, adjustable unit.

Contrast

Contrast examines how the use of color compatibility affects human performance under the effect of reflected glare. Performance may be improved by selecting proper color combinations. Most displays use light characters on a darker background (negative presentation). In general, white on black, white on blue, or amber on black is preferable to using black on white or white on yellow. Such displays appear to flicker less but suffer from reduced contrast between characters and background as a result of high ambient light levels. The contrast between the brightness of the image and the brightness of the background is a key factor in determining the legibility of images on a VDT. It is recommended that the contrast ratio of characters and background on CRT screens be large, at least 3:1 and up to 15:1 (ISO, 9241, Part 3, 1996). As individual preferences for both brightness and contrast vary, the controls for these components should be effective over the range of lighting and environmental conditions experienced at the workstation.

Posture

The presence of rotating, tilt, and swivel mechanisms to allow adjustment of the screen is also important in helping the operator maintain proper posture. As illustrated in Figure 16.1, NIOSH recommended that the keyboard be 29 to 31 inches from the floor. The center of the display screen should be 10 to 20 degrees below the user's vertical eye level. The angle between the upper and lower arm should be between 80 and 120 degrees. The user's wrist angle in using the keyboard should be less than 10 degrees, and ample leg room must be available. It has also been found that swivel chairs with adjustable seat height and independent back support are helpful. Compliance with these criteria reduces or prevents the pain or stiffness in the neck, shoulders, and lower back that results from poor posture at the workstation.

The user's workspace should be arranged so the eye to display screen viewing distance is between 17 and 25 inches (see Fig. 16.1), depending of course on the user's eyesight. To reduce eye strain induced by eye refocusing, the screen, keyboard, any any text that is being copied should be at the same distance from the operator's eyes. Another factor that has been shown to create itching, burning, and dry and irritated eyes is the warm airflow created by floppy disk drives and terminal fans which often seems to be aimed at the user's face.

The previously described postural concerns relate solely to seated workstations. Little research has been reported relating to clinical workstations.

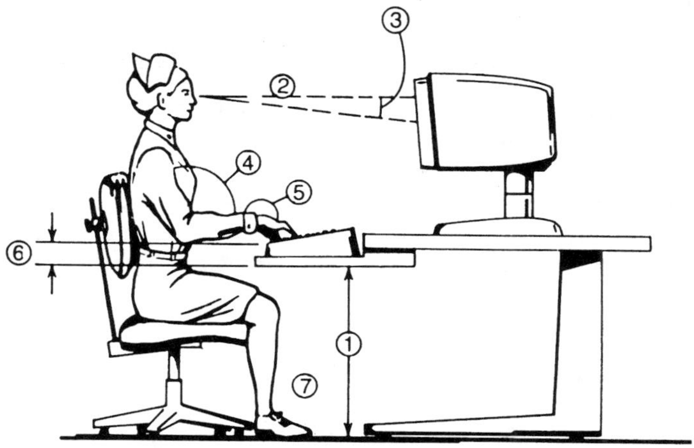

FIGURE 16.1. National Institute for Occupational Safety and Health (NIOSH) specifications for visual display terminal (VDT) use show (1) height of keys at 29–31 inches; (2) optimal viewing distance 17–25 inches; (3) screen center 10–20 degrees below the plane of the operator's eye height; (4) angle between upper and lower arm 80–120 degrees; (5) wrist angle less than 10 degrees; (6) keyboard at or below elbow height; (7) ample leg room. (From Computers Medicine 2, no. 5, September 1982, with permission.)

Although general laptop guidelines have been articulated, there is no reporting of the ergonomic considerations of their use in clinical settings. Additionally, there is no research related to the ergonomic aspects of personal digital assistant (PDA) use (Nielsen and Trinkoff, 2003). Ergonomic concerns arising from bedside or notebook technology have also not been described in the literature.

Cumulative trauma disorder (CTD), also know as repetitive stress injury (RSI) is a major concern for nurses as the amount of time spent working on computers increases (Berner and Jacobs, 2002: Nielsen and Trinkoff, 2003). Interventions can be put into place in both work flow process development and workstation engineering to limit the risk of injury to nurses from their work with computers.

Other Health Concerns

The major debate surrounding cathode ray terminals is the question of potential radiation hazards. In North America, extensive testing was undertaken by NIOSH: measurements of ionizing and nonionizing radiation, analysis of workroom air for contaminants, administration of a questionnaire on health complaints to employees, and evaluation of ergonomic aspects in the workplaces. On the basis of this study, Murray et al. (1981) stated that "the results of these tests demonstrated that the VDT operators included in this investigation were not exposed to hazardous levels of radiation or chemical agents." NIOSH further concluded that routine monitoring of VDTs was unjustified. A similar position has been adopted by the Consumer and Clinical Radiation Hazards Division, Health and Welfare Canada (Charboneau, 1982). Since these landmark studies, the literature has been largely silent on this issue.

Responsible nurses monitor the literature and exercise a judicious use of caution and informed professional decision making to recognize media-generated hysteria and rebuttal by parties with vested interest.

Psychological Concerns

The psychological aspects of computer ergonomics have been much less thoroughly researched and studied than the physiologic aspects. To some extent, this situation is to be expected because physiologic aspects are more easily measured and quantified than are the psychological aspects of computer use. However, as hardware costs decrease, as more software is developed, and as the physiologic aspects of ergonomics are addressed, greater attention is being directed toward the psychological aspects of ergonomics (Helander and Tham, 2003: Riva, 2003). Unfortunately, the psychological aspects of the human–machine interface continue to be approached in a highly subjective, emotional, and personal fashion.

Human–Machine Interface

The latest techniques in computer program development consider the user's cognitive abilities, including memory load, visual scanning, and formulation of mental models. These techniques make it easier for the user to enter data and comprehend information. These techniques address the following issues.

- Dialogue design: intelligent or adaptive interfaces
- Input methods: windows, icons, mouse, and pointer environments
- Screen design: graphical–user interfaces
- Attention-getting techniques: use of color
- Consistency in the appearance of screen information, error messages, and system usage

Also, these techniques meet the subjective criteria by which their advocates evaluate them. However, further research is required to determine if they meet the psychological ergonomic needs of other users.

Variety of Input/Output Media

There has been a move away from total reliance on the keyboard for input and the monochrome display for output. Individuals can use speech for both input and output, color graphics, physiologic probes, and computer mice to facilitate keyboard use. There are also touch screens used for data entry. Pen-based notebook systems offer yet another form of a more naturalistic input device. Moreover, natural speech recognition programs offer another naturalistic approach to input and output. Many users new to the computing environment find a greater degree of psychological comfort in using input devices not requiring keyboarding/typing skills (see Chapter 2 for a description of these input media).

Research Needs/Opportunities

A psychological aspect of computing ergonomics that remains largely unstudied is the impact of a computerized workstation on individuals' behavior within an organization. We simply do not yet know the full effects on people when they work in a highly automated environment and, subsequently, have less need and opportunity for human contact. Interpersonal relationships, group dynamics, personal stress levels, anxiety levels, and productivity among personnel in such organizations are unexplored. It is imperative that this kind of information be sought without delay.

The potential of bedside systems to affect the nurse–patient relationship must also be researched. As new technology is developed, there is an ongoing need to evaluate not only the effectiveness of the technology but also the ergonomic effects on both nurses and patients.

References

Berner, K., & Jacobs, K. (2002). The gap between exposure and implementation of computer workstation ergonomics in the workplace. *Work 19*:193–199.

Charbonneau, L. (1982). The VDT controversy. *The Canadian Nurse* October:30.

Helander, M., & Tham, M.P. (2003). Hedonomics—affective human factors design. *Ergonomics 46*(13/14): 1269–1272.

Murray, W.E., Cox, C., Moss, C., & Parr, W. A. (1981). *Radiation and Industrial Hygiene Survey of Video Display Terminal Operation.* Cincinnati: National Institute of Occupational Safety and Health.

Nielsen, K., & Trinkoff, A. (2003). Applying ergonomics to nurse computer workstations: Review and recommendations. *CIN: Computers, Informatics, Nursing 21*(3):150–157.

Riva, G. (2003). Ambient intelligence in health care. *CyberPsychology & Behavior 6*(3):295–297.

Additional Resources

Croasmun, J. (2003). Taking the oxymoron out of ergonomic laptops. *Ergonomics Today* September 19, 2003.

Piccoli, B. (2003). A critical appraisal of current knowledge and future directions of ergophthamology: Consensus document of the ICOH Committee on "Work and Vision." *Ergonomics 46*(4):384–406.

Seghers, J., Jochem, A. & Spaepen, A. (2003). Posture, muscle activity and muscle fatigue in prolonged VDT work at different screen height settings. *Ergonomics 46*(7):714–730.

17 Disaster Recovery Planning

Disaster recovery planning (DRP) is many things to many people. To some, it is planning how to recover or replace damaged computer systems in organizations that range from a single nurse practitioner's office practice to a multisite hospital group. To others, it is planning how to maintain critical hospital/nursing functions during interruptions in computer service. To still others it is planning how to avoid those interruptions, and to yet others it is planning an organization's response to any emergency or crisis situation.

Disaster recovery planning is, of course, all these things and more. In its broadest sense, DRP encompasses all measures taken to ensure organizational survival in the event of a natural or manmade calamity and to minimize the impact of such an event on the organization's staff, patients, and bottom line. Disaster recovery planners are faced with an intimidating array of terms, techniques, and technologies: hot sites, cold sites, warm sites, mobile recovery, off-site storage, electronic vaulting, uninterrupted power supply, T1 links, Megastream, satellite transmission (see Glossary). What does this have to do with nursing informatics?

In this examination of DRP, the focus is on data, both paper-based and electronic, while recognizing the many other areas required of a comprehensive contingency plan. Nursing has traditionally not been involved in DRP. However, as nurses come to depend more and more on information technology, they must become involved in developing disaster recovery plans to safeguard patient care (Simpson, 2001). The disaster recovery plan is an extensive, inclusive statement of actions to be taken before, during, and after a disaster. The plan must be regularly tested and updated to ensure the continuity of operations and the availability of critical data and processes in the event of a disaster. The goal of the planning process is to minimize the disruption of operations and ensure a measure of organizational stability and orderly recovery after a disaster (Simpson, 2001). In all organizations or facilities, a formal planning method is needed to ensure quality, consistency, and comprehensiveness of disaster recovery contingency plans. Informal, ad hoc, and (worst of all) "it will never happen to us" approaches must absolutely be avoided. It should also be noted that DRP is not a one-time, finished product but a process that must continually be used to update the contingency plans as elements in the organization change.

In the United States, the Health Insurance Portability and Accountability Act (HIPAA) of 1996 final security rule that must be implemented by April 2005 requires that every health organization implement documented policies and procedures addressing disaster recovery and contingency planning (http://www.hipaadvisory.com/action/security/disasterrecov.htm) (Lucas and Adams, 2004). Healthcare organizations are also required to test the plan to ensure that it promotes restoration of systems, networks, and data following a disaster (Simpson, 2001).

Planning Process

The disaster recovery contingency planning process includes these steps.

- Risk identification: Which problems might occur?
- Risk analysis: What would be their impact?
- Risk prioritization: Which problems are the most critical?
- Risk reduction: How can I reduce the impact of the problems?
- Risk management planning: How will I apply this to the project?
- Risk monitoring and testing: How effective is our risk control?

The interaction of these activities is shown in the flowchart in Figure 17.1.

Planning Team

A fundamental premise of all types of planning applies to DRP: Plans are best developed by those who must implement them in the event of a disaster. A planning committee, including representatives from all functional areas of the organization, the operations manager, and the data-processing manager should oversee the development and implementation of the plan. Many organizations additionally appoint a contingency planner to work with a planning committee. Developing such a plan can be done completely in-house with assistance from an external specialized disaster software or storage vendor or by hiring an external disaster planning consultant. Often a combination of these strategies provides the best value during the planning process. There are numerous software products available to guide a planning committee through the process. There are also national and regional professional organizations of disaster recovery consultants that can provide guidance to novice planners. Access to a variety of disaster planning information, terminology, conference announcements, sample plans, and links to other related organizations is available at the websites of the *Disaster Recovery Journal* (http://www.drj.com) and the Disaster Recovery Information Exchange (www.drie.org).

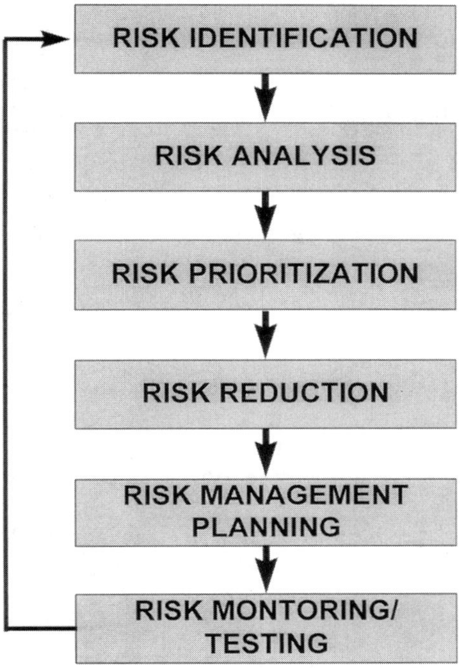

FIGURE 17.1. Disaster recovery contingency planning process.

Risk Identification

Many risk assessments start with a group of project personnel gathering together to make a list of potential risks. In general, this is not an effective starting point for risk identification. It constrains the identified risks to those that each individual thought was worth raising at the time. Many issues that are not considered as risks are not raised, but such issues can combine in complex ways and develop into critical risks. The way to avoid this trap is to "brainstorm" the issues surrounding the project.

Obvious risks may be extracted from the list of issues produced. The remaining issues are kept for analysis. Further risks may be identified from analysis of project plans. Other techniques such as decision drivers exist. This method looks at the major decision points in the project and is intended to identify when the decision may be driven by inappropriate influences. Application of these techniques should ensure that most of the risks surrounding the project are identified, including all the critical risks. The following hazard analysis checklist identifies some potential sources of risk that users of nursing information technology should consider (Simpson, 2001; Wold and Shriver, 1997).

Possible Sources of Hazards

Natural Threats

- Climate: Which materials in your collection are the most sensitive to extremes and fluctuations in temperature? Do you get heavy or prolonged snowfall, rainfall, or severe storms?
- Topography: Is your building beside a lake or river? Is your basement below water table level? Is your area prone to avalanches, landslides, or earthquakes?

Technical Threats

- Building structures: Has the roof a skylight, roof access, and drains? Are there water pipes running through the records area?
- Dangerous goods: Are there any gas cylinders, solvents, or paints stored near the records? Are staff trained in the correct handling of dangerous goods?
- Internal services: Are plumbing, electrical wiring, fire detectors, fire extinguishers, and security measures regularly inspected and maintained? Are there up-to-date plans and drawings of them? Are duplicates stored safely somewhere else?
- Utility services: For which ones are you responsible? How about sewers and telephones? Have you up-to-date plans of their locations, including master switches? Is there a backup? What about power outages? Does the facility have an uninterruptible power system (UPS)? Is water pressure adequate for fighting fire?
- Information systems: Are there alternate systems available if there is a malfunction or failure of the CPU? Failure of system software? Failure of application software?

Human Threats

- Is unauthorized access possible to either the physical site or information systems?
- What safeguards are in place related to bomb threats, extortion, burglary, work stoppage, termination or resignation, or computer crime?

Risk Analysis

Records

When performing the risk analysis, consider the value of the records, both paper and electronic, that need to be protected. Several factors affect the value of a record. Consider the following.

1. How much did it cost to create that record in the first place? What would it cost to recreate it now?
2. Does the information protect the rights of individuals, research, or the business interests of the agency?
3. Is the information complete, or would other documents be necessary if action had to be taken.
4. How available is it? If the information could be obtained from another source without too much delay, its value is reduced.

When assessing the value of your essential records for insurance purposes, there are two approaches.

- Recreating the information: Calculate the cost of gathering the information from scratch (e.g., by research, surveys, drafting) and then the cost of producing and reproducing it. This is estimated by the number of man-hours × $/hour for the project.
- Reproducing only: Calculate the cost of duplicating your essential records now for off-site storage, or the cost of reproducing your off-site records for use after a disaster. The most visible form of information is paper, closely followed by magnetic and film records.

One thing is certain: It would cost much less to duplicate now than to recreate later, after the information has been destroyed. For example, if you were to lose 100 cubic feet of records, it might cost $10,000 to recreate the information. If you have off-site backup copies, however, the only additional cost is for transportation. It is necessary to keep reproduction to a minimum and to use the most reasonable means of reproduction consistent with the purpose or use of the information on the records. Remember, it is the information you are insuring, not the media. Before any reproduction is undertaken, consider the following questions.

1. Could the original record be stored at a safer location without causing great inconvenience?
2. Is the record available elsewhere, in a field office, in another department, or with the government, for example?
3. Would an extract or synopsis of the records meet the need, rather than a copy of the entire original record?
4. Does a summary type of record fulfill the need, or is the original record necessary? For example, using personal history cards instead of the personal file.
5. Are the records available now in printed or prepared form, such as annual reports, machine-run or extra typed or printed copies?

Processing

There is also a need to analyze the risk related to delivery of service in the event of a computer-related disaster. Computers are involved in the automatic delivery of intravenous medications, delivery of supplies throughout many hospitals, and even regulating everything from lights and heating to elevators. The risk exposure of all these systems must be considered during contingency planning. From a nursing perspective, there is extensive experience of the disruption caused when even one computerized intravenous delivery system malfunctions. Project the impact of a large-scale electrical or computer technology problem in an intensive care unit if thorough contingency planning has not taken place.

Risk Prioritizing

Risk prioritization is all about determining "risk exposure" (Baxter, 1991).

$$\text{Risk exposure} = (\text{probability of unsatisfactory outcome}) \times (\text{loss, if outcome is unsatisfactory})$$

The components of "unsatisfactory outcome" may be cost, schedule, performance, and support; the problems may even relate to system evolution. Determining risk exposure provides the disaster planning project manager with a prioritized list of risks. Those near the top require immediate action, whereas the bottom part of the list consists of risks that would be costly but unlikely to occur, or risks likely to occur but would cause little loss. The type of risk reduction strategies used depend on the type of risk analysis performed. Where quantitative analysis has been used, a range of parameter values may be investigated so the project manager can select an appropriate "level" of risk for a given likely outcome.

In all cases, the cost of reducing the risks must also be considered. A ratio may be calculated that is known as the "risk reduction leverage." This ratio assesses the risk exposure before and after the risk reduction processes have been carried out and compares them with the cost of those processes. A relative cost–benefit measure can then be achieved when it is applied to the prioritized risk list. This helps with planning risk reduction activities and may lead to a decision to "live with some risks."

Risk Reduction

Physical Prevention

Physical prevention requires a thorough audit of all facilities to identify areas where paper-based or electronic data are created and stored. The audit reviews the presence or absence of factors such as those listed as natural or technical treats. For example, identifying where water lines are found in relation to the organizations' computer servers is important to prevent flooding from broken water pipes. Installing and maintaining fire detection and extinguishing systems act to reduce the spread of fire. A risk reduction audit must be comprehensive and intentional if a disaster recovery plan is to be well informed and therefore well formed.

Procedural Prevention

Procedural prevention includes activities relating to security and recovery, performed on a day-to-day, month-to-month, or annual basis. Examples include maintaining up-to-date backup copies of all computer files; annual verification of User IDs and passwords; maintaining a system for storing backup copies in a place discrete from the source computer; and scheduling inspections and testing of smoke detectors, sprinkler systems, and fire extinguishers.

Procedural prevention also includes an examination of human resources policies. Procedures to remove the user accounts of terminated employees prevents retribution. Additionally, resignations must be handled in a similar way to ensure that no one who is not a current employee has access to an organization's data. The goal of procedural prevention is to define activities necessary to prevent various disasters and ensure that these activities are performed as required.

Recovery Options

Before a plan can be formalized, the planning committee must evaluate all the available recovery options. Such options include the following.

- Off-site data storage at hot sites, warm sites, or cold sites
- Reciprocal agreements for data storage with other organizations
- Multiple data centers and multiple computers
- Consortium arrangements with many organizations sharing data storage

The key to evaluating recovery strategies is to identify the strategy that works best for your organization rather than opting for the newest and latest rage in recovery technology that does not provide a best match for your operations.

Disaster Recovery Plan

Document a written plan. DRP involves more than off-site storage and backup processing. Organizations must develop written, comprehensive disaster recovery plans that address all its critical operations and functions. It is essential that nurses are involved in this process so the data-processing needs related to patient care in whatever setting are represented.

With the growth in complexity of organizations and the threats to those organizations, DRP has become increasingly complicated. Many organizations find it necessary to devote a separate department to this task or to hire outside consultants to work with them to develop and maintain a disaster recovery plan.

A disaster recovery plan should contain all the information necessary to maintain the plan and execute its action steps. Use of a standard format for all departmental planning allows easy access to information and ongoing maintenance of the plan. The following areas should be considered when developing a disaster recovery plan.

Part 1: *Introduction and statement of purpose*: State why the plan has been written and what it intends to achieve. You should say something about who developed it and how it is to be kept current.

Part 2: *Authority*: Document the authority for the preparation of the plan and subsequent action. In this part, you also designate who is to be responsible for the records during the emergency (i.e., who will coordinate the execution of the plan and the line of succession).

Part 3: *Scope of the plan*: This part generally has three sections.

- *Events planned for*: Itemize each type of emergency event dealt with in the plan. For each, indicate the circumstances under which the event might occur and indicate what its expected impact on the department could be. List the most serious or most likely events first.
- *Locations planned for*: If the department's records are located only at one site, this section may not be required. However, if more than one site or building is involved, indicate here which sites are covered by the plan and the circumstances under which the plan might or might not apply to each site. Alternatively, if it is more practical, separate plans can be developed for each site or building. The following equipment should be considered: mainframe computer system, personal computers, bedside systems, data communications, and voice communications.
- *Relationship to other plans*: If the organization has other action plans, such as a medical emergency plan or a fire reaction plan, it is usually a good idea to describe how all plans relate to and supplement each other and to indicate the circumstances under which they may be executed individually or simultaneously.

Part 4: *Emergency procedures*: Business resumption planning theory usually suggests that vital records be backed up and stored off-site. However, in practice, there are always documents too bulky or too valuable to be copied. There are also documents where only the original will do, and then there is always work in progress. To be realistic, contingency plans should address the probability of having to retrieve vital material from an evacuated site. Other contents of this section includes these points.

- Note is to put the plan into action, under what circumstances the plan is to be fully or partially executed, and how all the actions will be carried out.
- The location of the emergency operations center (EOC) is specified. It is a predetermined meeting site for the disaster action team.

- A floor plan showing the locations of the essential records for all sites must be included.
- Detailed procedures for contingency processing at an alternate site (i.e., fixed location hot site, mobile facility) must be in place and written down.
- Detailed procedures for establishing voice and data communications with the alternate processing site must be in place.
- Sample testing schedules and procedures, including types of tests, test participants, team test responsibilities, and test forms are included.
- Include maintenance procedures for keeping the plan current.

The disaster recover plan should also address the following questions.

- *Storage*: Are vital documents stored in a fireproof room/vault/cabinet? Is the fire rating sufficient? Is it rated for magnetic media? Is it waterproof?
- *Security*: Will the room/vault/cabinet be closed in an emergency? How can you secure documents if they have been retrieved?
- *Access*: How can you arrange access to a cordoned off building? Who would be assigned to retrieve the material?
- *Identification*: If you were allowed to retrieve only one box of material, how would you identify the most urgent or critical one?
- *Restoration*: If your documents are charred or soaked, do you know how to restore them?

Appendices

Use as many appendices as may be needed to include information vital to the success of the plan. These may change so often, however, as to make its inclusion in Parts 1 to 4 impractical. Suggested subjects follow.

- A staffing chart of the department, an organization chart showing the department's relationship to other departments (e.g., city government or other outside governing authority), and a chart illustrating the disaster control organization within the department. Other organizational charts may illustrate the department's relation to local civil preparedness authorities and to disaster and welfare agencies, including the Red Cross.
- Call-up lists of key personnel who are valuable to execution of the plan; include name, title, address, telephone numbers, and the duties assigned to each.
- Instructions for contacting outside organizations, such as the fire department; the police department; local electric, gas, water, and telephone companies; hospitals and ambulance services; plumbers; electricians; locksmiths; glass companies, guard and janitorial services; exterminators; attorneys; and any other key people or agencies that might be of assistance. State why each is to be called and what service each is expected to render. It is critical to keep these lists current; review them at regular intervals (at least annually).

- An inventory of essential records and the priorities for their protection. The estimated cost of creating or reproducing valuable records for off-site storage.
- A summary of the arrangements that have been made for relocating the records. It includes the names of persons to be contacted when temporary space is needed and information about alternative space in case the primary space is suffering from the same disaster.
- Instructions for ensuring the emergency operation of the building's utilities and for service and operation of vital building support systems.
- Probably the most important appendix is a list of resources that might be needed in an emergency. There should also be a list of local suppliers. Record the supplies and materials you would need, what they are to be used for, who is to buy them, who is to use them, and where they can be found. Record your arrangements for borrowing materials, equipment, and personnel from other departments, how to transport items, and whom to call. List specialists who can be called on for assistance in preserving damaged record materials.
- The final appendix should be a glossary of special terms that are used in the plan so all its users are speaking the same language.

Plan Testing and Maintenance

After all the effort taken to develop a disaster recovery plan, many organizations make the mistake of thinking that the process is "finished." The contingency plan must be audited and tested on a regular basis to know that proposed processes serve the purpose of protecting the data and processes of the organization should a real disaster occur.

Because organizations change continually, disaster recovery plans must also be dynamic. A process must be included for regularly updating the plan. Most disaster recovery plans require a complete review of all procedures every 5 years that focuses on refining the requirements, exploiting new technology, and using a fresh approach to consider new solutions to old problems. With regular testing and an annual audit, the plan should be effective in processing critical data after a catastrophe occurs.

Summary

Disasters such as fires, earthquakes, hurricanes, power blackouts, and floods will continue to occur. Less dramatic disasters, such as power "bumps" or broken water pipes, also claim data vital to patient care. To minimize losses, hospitals, clinics and individual practitioner's offices must establish and maintain effective data recovery contingency plans. Healthcare agencies should identify the most suitable plan for their organization, obtain management's commitment to the plan, and then implement the plan. Nursing must ensure that information vital to patient care is considered during DRP.

It is truly rare when a facility must implement its disaster recovery plan. However, maintaining a current reliable and tested plan gives an organization the best possible response when calamity does strike.

References

Baxter, K. (1991). Avoiding the inevitable. *The British Journal of Health Care Computing 8*(2):33–34.

Lucas, B., & Adams, S. (2004). Roadmap to HIPAA: Keeping occupational health nurses on track. *AAOHN Journal 52*(4):169–178.

Simpson, R. (2001). What to do before disaster strikes. *Nursing Management 32*(11):13–14.

Wold, G.H., & Shriver, R.F. (1997). Risk analysis techniques. *Disaster Recovery Journal 7*(3):1–8 (http://www.drj.com/new2dr/w3_030.htm).

Additional Reading

Anonymous, (2002). Calm during crisis. *Health Management Technology 23*(11):42–44.

Barnes, J. (2004). The business continuity planning cube. *Disaster Recovery Journal 17*(2) (http://www.drj.com/articles/spr04/1702-16p.html).

Hensel, J. (1999). Hurricane and earthquake planning. *Occupational Health and Safety 68*(10):222–224.

Huser, T. (2003). Flaming car in lobby tests hospital plans, employees. *Disaster Recovery Journal 16*(1) (http://www.drj.com/articles/win03/1601-11.html).

Lewis, S. (2003). Disaster recovery planning for information technology functions. *Nursing Homes 52*(2):50.

McCartney, P.R. (2003). HIPAA and electronic health information security. *The American Journal of Maternal Child Nursing 28*(5):333.

Reinert, J. (2004). Data recovery completes disaster recovery. *Disaster Recovery Journal 17*(2) (http://www.drj.com/articles/spr04/1702-15p.html).

Roden, K. (2004). Building a business case for disaster recovery planning. *Disaster Recovery Journal 17*(3) (http://www.drj.com/articles/sum04/1703-19.html).

Vecchio, A. (2000). Plan for the worst before disaster strikes. *Health Management Technology 21*(6):28–30.

Websites of Interest

Disaster Recovery Information Exchange: www.drie.org Information Systems Security Association: www.issa.org

18 Implementation Concerns

WITH CONTRIBUTIONS BY ELEANOR CALLAHAN HUNT, SARA BRECKENRIDGE SPROAT, AND REBECCA RUTHERFORD KITZMILLER

Successful implementation of a clinical information system depends on a variety of factors, but the two most important issues are not related to the technology but to organizational and people issues (Lorenzi et al., 2004). This chapter focuses on improving and responding to organizational and people issues. Promoting user acceptance by identifying and responding to resistance against information systems, optimizing communication, and managing change effectively mitigate both of these issues.

Resistance to Information Systems and Computers in Healthcare

The adoption of technology requires users to change how they work. Organizational change places great demands on staff members. Change creates uncomfortable situations where staff faces the unknown and where their coping skills may not be effective. In 1982 Ball and Snelbecker examined the reasons why healthcare professionals—nurses, physicians, and technologists alike—have been slow in adopting computers and information technology. Their research resulted in identification of the following major factors contributing to resistance: oversell by vendors, unrealistic expectations, changing traditional practices, insufficient nursing involvement, fear of embracing new approaches, and fear of the unknown. The results of this classic study continue to be applicable in today's healthcare environment (Adderly et al., 1997; Despont-Gros et al., 2004; Doyle and Kowba, 1997; FitzHenry and Snyder, 1996; Lorenzi et al., 2004; Marasovic et al., 1997).

Oversell by Vendors

The first general reason for resistance to innovative technology is a tendency of some vendors to overstate the capabilities of or to oversell their product.

The contents of this chapter are opinions of the authors only and do not reflect those of the US Army Medical Department or the US Army.

Of course, not every vendor or salesman oversells every time. Nonetheless, this general statement describes vendor conduct in dealing with some clients in the healthcare field. All too often the computer has been presented as a panacea for all healthcare's organizational and overall management problems.

Until recently, healthcare professionals were unschooled in computer use and tended to believe naively that the vendor had the perfect solution to all problems. Often health professionals who were either too trusting or too overwhelmed by technology turned decision-making power over to information systems personnel, who knew little of the health professionals' information needs and work flow. This practice typically has led to serious communication problems between technology vendors, end-users, and those who assume responsibility for the design and implementation of these systems. This breakdown in communication impairs the potential quality of the system and hampers future progress in the basic use of computers in healthcare.

Unrealistic Expectations

A second source of resistance stems from unrealistic expectations regarding the capability potential of computer systems. This attitude is unfortunate because it leads to inappropriate goals for what computer systems can do. At other times, it tends to mask otherwise desirable and feasible contributions. For example, the computer may be viewed as a universal remedy for administrative or political problems—a method to decrease the number of errors and improve patient outcomes. When promises and expectations of the system do not magically fix processes or procedural problems, healthcare professionals are disappointed and blame the computer system. Often problems are not related to the technology but to issues that may be deeply engrained in the organization and have nothing to do with automation. In some cases, however, a 40% to 60% solution may have been achieved, which in itself should be viewed as a monumental advance. However, healthcare professionals who may have been promised an unrealistic 100% solution are then blinded to the benefits and are disappointed and disillusioned with the technology. As a consequence, the entire project may be discontinued, the 40% to 60% success abandoned, and future projects not even attempted.

Inappropriate expectations of a system include the following (Hunt et al., 2004).

- Solutions to ancient procedural problems
- Technology will make the organization profitable
- Magically improve the quality of care
- Provide the data to justify staff
- Reduce the patients' length of stay in hospital
- Reduce the staff
- Ensure regulatory compliance

Many hospital organizations struggle with processes surrounding verbal or telephone orders. In general, a verbal/telephone order is given to a nurse from a licensed, independent provider. The nurse then writes the order onto an order document. As a safety measure, the provider or its designate reviews the order within 24 hours to ensure that is was accurately recorded and co-signs the document. The Joint Commission on Accreditation of Hospital Organizations (JCAHO) evaluates this safety process. Healthcare organizations have looked to computerized provider order entry as a means to decrease or eliminate verbal/telephone orders or to provide a mechanism to remind providers to co-sign the order within 24 hours. Unfortunately, these same organizations often fail to address the healthcare processes, which promote the use of verbal/telephone orders in the first place and as a result fail to see a benefit from an installed system. For example, a way to improve this process is to provide or improve access in areas where verbal and telephone orders flourish. This includes using handheld wireless devices at patient bedsides or in the emergency department or allowing providers to access the system when outside of the organization, in their homes or offices. Promoting and facilitating use of the system at the place and point in time when care decisions are being made decrease the use of telephone orders.

Users' unrealistic expectations typically lead to mixed feelings and resistance concerning computer technology. If clinicians and hospital administrators have little experience with selecting, configuring, installing, and maximizing the use of computers and information technology, they may relinquish control to a systems specialist. Although a systems specialist may be expert in using and installing computerized information systems, they are likely to be inexperienced in understanding the care process and helping users recognize processes that must change and in working through those changes. Failing to develop a partnership between clinical experts and technology experts promotes a situation in which users do not buy into the system's use and thus implementation fails.

Changes in Traditional Procedures

It is difficult to move an organization forward with current technology and trends. Many are reluctant to move beyond the decade in which they were schooled. For example, clinicians who are used to viewing themselves as experts and are asked to learn new processes and skills may be uncomfortably pushed into a situation in which they are not the expert and they resist. However, today's healthcare environment with complex patient care demands high-tech, integrated healthcare systems to manage the data and demands that clinicians reevaluate their healthcare processes (Hunt et al., 2004). Nursing has a traditional set of rules, laws, ethics, and codes of confidentiality. Computers and information technology can pose threats to long-established, sound procedures in nursing. Computerization has an impact on all of this, just as all types of innovations appear to pose a major threat when first introduced. The key here is to leverage the positive uses of technology and limit negative influences.

For nurses, skepticism is a most desirable professional trait. Nurses are entrusted with the welfare of their patients; and in that context, being skeptical about new fads and resistance to change in one's mode of practice is well founded. The nurse may perceive that the patient is endangered by the use of a clinical system when they lack confidence in its use. To counter this perception, involving nursing users at the beginning can educate them and identify potential problems. This combination is powerful in that it "buys in" the nursing users as well as developing a mutual level of trust. Just as nursing implements best care practices based on demonstrated evidence and efficacy, clinical information systems are coming to represent "best practice," and nurses are recognizing this as an advantage and embracing it.

The use and early adoption of advanced technology has created a perceived generational gap among healthcare providers. The older generation is seen to be technophobic, leading to a lack of integrated vision and integrated systems (Tan, 2001). Despite the general acceptance of technology into all aspects of our lives, fear of technological change does persist in our workplace. As healthcare providers become increasingly overwhelmed by information and demands on their time to provide quality care to patients, they are looking for solutions. Addressing technophobic fears is vital to success. Technophobia is not the only fear the project team should anticipate. Consider these five concerns, which lead to resistant behavior among staff members (Tan, 2001).

- As the organization expects to become more efficient when using automation, staff members may fear losing their jobs.
- Information systems impact both formal and informal communication patterns.
- Peer pressure and previous experience with system implementation can also influence the organizational climate, promoting success.
- Individual reaction to system implementation depends on the individual's overall personality and cultural background.
- Management techniques used to implement systems directly affect users' perceptions.

Involving nursing users throughout the selection and implementation process mitigates potentially resistant behaviors.

Insufficient Involvement of Nurses

It is absolutely imperative to insist on clinical involvement at every step of healthcare information system installation. Each clinical user group has a role to play in the selection, implementation, and successful use of an information system. Administrators and nurses need to be adequately and consistently involved in critical decisions about the use of information technology.

Only involving hospital top management in new information technology choices has proven detrimental to the success of computer installations in health centers. Ensure appropriate representation and involvement from all users when developing short and long range plans for selection and installation of information systems.

In the past, management has treated implementation of a patient or hospital information system the same as installation of a telephone system or an air conditioning system. There was a gap in understanding of the potential impact to the whole organization. Now, decision-makers realize the major responsibility in deciding how technology tools are deployed. Without nursing and clinician involvement combined with competent consultants, accurate vendor contracts, responsible systems analysis, and an involved administration, the potential of technological systems cannot be fully realized. The ongoing nursing shortage has made it more difficult to obtain access to nursing end-users at a time when it is becoming imperative to install technology that affects those very same end-users. As a result, involvement has to become more creative instead of allowing nurses to be cut out of the loop because of time commitments. One method for overcoming this time demand is that, instead of requiring attendance at committee meetings, leverage the technology to create web portals that allow links, distribution of documentation, access to power point presentations, and interactive discussion boards to elicit information without tying up clinicians' time. Nurses must recognize that input may need to be provided outside of normal working hours and is just as important as reading healthcare literature outside of working hours to stay on top of healthcare trends. Include technology as part of your continuous learning and self-education.

Embracing New Approaches

In many cases resistance occurs when personnel insist on holding onto what they know and existing systems, rather than exploring new technologies. Although "new" is not necessarily better, such resistance can preclude advances in nursing and patient care. A common tendency is to view a particular function solely in terms of existing systems characteristics rather than to recognize alternative ways of how patient care may be improved. It is not adequate to use new technologies simply to complete old tasks faster (see Chapter 13). Instead, technology is being used to transform the entire caregiving process.

The problem of managing and accessing medical records provides a typical illustration. The medical record is designed to provide a single location where clinicians can document the care they provide and use the information from other clinicians to make decisions. Unfortunately, most of this documentation remains on paper, posing many problems: sizable storage challenges, expensive maintenance and reproduction costs, inaccessibility to all care venues in which a clinician makes decisions. Expanding the paper-based system has not solved these issues. Computerized information systems as a communications controller and file manager provides greater flexibility in the functions and use of medical record systems. However, computer technology should also aid in finding the best means for maintaining and gaining access to needed information.

The objective of any medical record is to document information about the care of patients. It is ideally accessible to all of the healthcare team who collaboratively provide high-quality care. Such collaboration and communication require data storage, access, and retrieval among a number of health professionals on the team. Unfortunately, traditional medical records systems operation is sometimes dictated by existing legacy systems, which determine how information can be stored and retrieved. Computerized methods bring invaluable patient data to the physician and nurse at the point where decisions are being made, resulting in better care. Through the paradigm shift of documenting at the point of care, it is now possible for computer technology to provide healthcare providers with information about patients when and where it is needed. Having electronically captured data has eliminated the need for eight different members of the care team each to ask patients the same questions for medical histories, allergies, and demographics. It has allowed nurses to use standards-based objectives to chart, reducing the overall time required to document the care provided.

Fear of Leaving Paper and of the Unknown

Another form of resistance is linked to the traditional, time-tested reliance and trust of printed material. We sometimes fail to recognize that the printed word has limitations. Paper-based records are available to only one person at a time, they are not up-to-the-minute accurate, data are not backed up, and what is written is only as good as the person's memory and handwriting. This affects healthcare providers by limiting their ability to review current, necessary patient care documentation when making decisions. Computer-based information systems not only provide storage and retrieval of information, they afford new opportunities for increasing knowledge and research through data mining and data collection. It is through quality training, consistent use, and positive reinforcement that clinicians will move from paper to electrons to chart a patient's course.

Duplication of effort is one of the most expensive yet least measured cost expenditures in healthcare organizations. When working with customers who are considering doing away with paper, ask the following questions (Kriegel and Brandt, 1996).

- Does the paper provide value to the client in terms of improving quality or service?
- Does the paper improve productivity or cut costs?
- Does anybody read it? More important, does anyone use it to make a decision?

The answers to these questions should unite and guide users to recognize how to streamline paper processes. Streamlining provides users with additional resources to accomplish their critical missions. This may be enough to motivate support of an automated system (Hunt et al., 2004).

Seldom has an individual given a more concise analysis of the acceptance or acknowledgment of change within a traditional system or discipline than did Machiavelli in 1513. His analysis on the establishment of new systems is as follows.

> It must be remembered that there is nothing more difficult to plan, more doubtful of success, nor more dangerous to manage, than the creation of a new system. For the initiator has the enmity of all who would profit by the preservation of the old institutions and merely lukewarm defenders in those who would gain by the new ones.

Change fails because of people, plain and simple. Change brings people face to face with their biggest fears: failure, humiliation, ridicule. Change is uncomfortable, it is unpredictable, and in a healthcare setting it is viewed as risky. Recognize that fear is an incredibly strong motivator (Hunt et al., 2004; Kriegal and Brandt 1996). Once recognized, however, it can be used to assist in the change process.

Management of Change

After all other sources of resistance have been identified and mitigated, the focus shifts toward change management. There is a tremendous amount of research, stories, and journal articles that address change management in the healthcare and business literature. This section touches on a few change management theories, describing their application in clinical system implementation.

It is important to recognize that an organization is like any other social system and change—where everything and everybody's actions are interrelated (Hunt et al., 2004). All departments in an organization are integrated and interdependent. Implementing change in one department affects the function of another. It is also likely that change, although embraced in one department, may be completely resisted by another. Additionally, there may be other changes occurring within the organization that affect or will be affected by the proposed system implementation. Managers must completely assess the effects of change on the entire organization and develop a plan to motivate each department to participate in the implementation and adapt to change (Hunt et al., 2004). Roger's theory of diffusion of innovation suggests that some never adopt the change (Hilz, 2000). Where you need to concern yourself is if the active resistor(s), or laggard(s), is in an area of influence or a management position. Otherwise, once enough areas and users are using the system, the rest naturally follow. Reaching that tipping point is key to implementing change successfully (Gladwell, 2000).

One way to reach this tipping point, where the rest of the implementation follows with less resistance, is to foster a collaborative relationship among nurses, physicians, other health professionals, and information technology (IT) professionals. This relationship can be developed while selecting, designing, and configuring the system and can be continued through maintaining the system. The common goal that all want to achieve is to be able to deliver cost-efficient, high quality patient care.

The team can motivate each group affected by the system by identifying how the system benefits them and fulfills personal and organizational goals. This is critical to creating motivated team members, users, and stakeholders; and it obtains the "buy-in" that is crucial to user system acceptance. Motivation for change is the key to overcoming resistance. Tapping into users' feelings that "there must be a better way"and educating and involving the users leads to users who are motivated to participate in the change. When people burn with enthusiasm, they take risks, go the extra mile, and fully commit themselves to change (Kreigel and Brandt, 1996). Failure to communicate is the greatest threat to the success of any project, especially IT projects (Lorenzi et al., 2004).

Another major aspect to collaboration between key team members is to communicate effectively a plan that includes the positive effects offered by the change as well as the dire circumstances should the status quo prevail. This may mean that the "sacred cow" must be addressed. A sacred cow (a term used in business) is an outmoded belief, assumption, practice, policy, system, or strategy that inhibits change and prevents responsiveness to new opportunities. A sacred cow uses valuable resources and limits productivity, innovative thinking, and creativity, thus hampering an organization's ability to respond to changing market conditions. According to Kriegel and Brandt (1996),

If it doesn't

- Add value to the customer
- Increase productivity
- Improve morale

.... It "moos"!

While anticipating the broad scale implementation of computerized information systems in healthcare institutions and agencies, it is fast becoming clear that such transformation is frequently complex and always accompanied by a shift in values and priorities that can conflict with vested interests. Can you think of a few sacred cows that are alive in your organizations, schools of nursing, and other workplaces? Implementing a clinical system without recognizing and addressing at least a few of these sacred cows puts your implementation at risk.

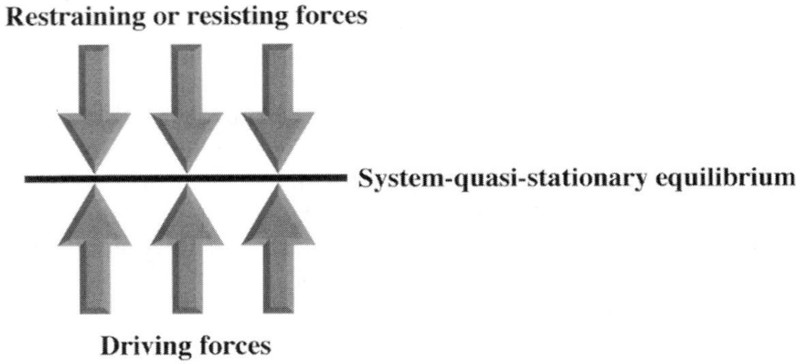

FIGURE 18.1. Lewin's dynamic balance of forces.

Most IT-related degree programs have many technical requirements but few require courses in communication, psychology, and organizational behavior. As a result, communication is not necessarily in the forefront of the IT staff's skills, but it is high among nursing skills. This is one of the reasons nurses make such great project leaders—they are trained to collaborate, communicate, multitask, and document. Combine effective technical skills with strong communication skills when working on IT projects, as individuals need all these characteristics to be successful (Hunt et al., 2004; Schwalbe, 2002).

Another theory that is applicable when implementing change is Lewin's (1969) classic work suggesting that behavior in an institutional setting is not a static habit or pattern but a dynamic balance of forces working in opposite directions within the social-psychological space of the institution (Fig. 18.1). Lewin identified three stages for accomplishing changes in behavior: unfreezing the existing equilibrium, moving toward a new equilibrium, and refreezing the new equilibrium. To initiate the unfreezing of the equilibrium, there are three strategies.

- Increase the number of driving forces
- Decrease the number of resisting forces
- A combination of the two preceding factors

The nursing profession is beginning to experience the profound impact computers and information systems ultimately will have on nursing practice and patient care. Previously, nurses were faced with the possibility of having change thrust on them from others outside of the profession. Resistance to change brought on by the introduction of healthcare information systems merely results in increasing the resisting forces that produce consequential increase in the driving forces (e.g., societal trends, government, and administration). Ultimately, because the driving forces in this case also have the power and authority, change would be instituted but probably be accompanied by increased tension, instability, and unpredictability. This is unacceptable to nurses who, as patient advocates, are committed to using every means at their disposal to ensure the highest quality care for patients. Computers and information systems are only one tool to be used to achieve this goal. No longer is the question "Should the nursing profession resist automation?" Given present societal, governmental, and technical trends, the change to and expansion of computerized information systems in healthcare agencies is inevitable. The question now becomes one of coping with the resisting forces within and among the profession so the end result is a stable, predictable, rational approach to improving the quality of nursing practice and thus the quality of patient care.

Nursing is the single largest group of care providers in any healthcare organization. The ability to influence the entire organization positively when choosing and installing computer-based systems is a major factor in implementation success. Consider the historical roots of the nursing profession. Nursing's roots in the military and hierarchical religious nursing orders meant change was by command rather than cooperation. This approach is still seen in many community practices but is slowly changing as today's nurses, who are academically prepared professionals, are establishing collaborative relationships with the rest of the care team. The impact this has on implementation is that nurses no longer accept change simply on the basis of position authority. They now expect to have input and demand to know the business and scientific bases for the change. Also expected is that change is based on knowledge, logic, and research rather than on whim and emotion. Nurses expect greater sophistication from their leaders in the use of skills and strategies for introducing change that affect nursing practice. Numerous nursing authors have reported their strategies and experiences in implementing such change. Repeatedly, the importance of the following factors is identified (Adderly et al., 1997; Despont-Gros, et al., 2004; Doyle and Kowba, 1997; FitzHenry and Snyder, 1996; Hostgaard and Nohr, 2004; Hunt et al., 2004; Lorenzi et al., 2004; Marasovic et al., 1997).

- Involve nursing early in planning change that affects all departments.
- Involve users actively in planning.
- Designate a person in the nursing department at the senior management level to coordinate the implementation process in the nursing department.
- Designate the nursing implementation coordinator as liaison between the nursing department and other departments.
- Establish a user committee in the nursing department chaired by the nursing implementation coordinator; include the enthusiastic, the uncommitted, and the mildly negative on the committee.
- Make resource people available as consultants to the nursing implementation coordinator.
- Develop a training program that includes an explanation of the rationale for computerization, nurses' responsibilities related to the new system, the

expected effect of the system on nurses and nursing care in the organization as well as actual use of the system.
- Use professional colleagues and peers to train others (i.e., a core group of trained nursing users train nursing staff to use the system).
- Time the training to occur just before the new system goes "on-line"; allow sufficient learning time; provide training time to all shifts.

Summary

Computers and information systems are as much a part of nursing practice today as the stethoscope. Resistance to change is normal for humans but can be easily overcome if health personnel and IT specialists launch a collaborative effort. Through early cooperation and free exchange of ideas, information systems technology can facilitate major advances in improving patient care, and nurses are showing that they willingly embrace it.

References

Adderly, D., Hyde, C., & Mauseth, P. (1997). The computer age impacts nurses. *Computers in Nursing 15*(1):43–46.

Ball, M.J., & Snelbecker, G.E. (1982). Overcoming resistances to telecommunications innovations in medicine and continuing medical education. *Computers in Hospitals 3*(4):40–45.

Despont-Gros, C. Fabry, P., Muller, H., Geissbuhler, A., & Lovis, C. (2004). User acceptance of clinical information systems: A methodological approach to identify the key dimensions allowing a reliable evaluation framework. *Medinfo 2004*, pp. 1038–1042.

Doyle, K., & Kowba, M. (1997). Managing the human side of change to automation. *Computers in Nursing 15*(2):67–68.

Gladwell, M. (2000). *The Tipping Point: How Little Things Can Make a Big Difference*. Boston: Little Brown.

FitzHenry, F., & Snyder, J. (1996). Improving organizational processes for gains during implementation. *Computers in Nursing 14*(3):171–180.

Hilz, L.M. (2000). The informatics nurse specialist as change agent: Application of innovation-diffusion theory. *Computers in Nursing 18*(6):272–281.

Hostgaard, A.M., & Nohr, C. (2004). Dealing with organizational change when implementing EHR systems. *Medinfo 2004*, pp. 631–634.

Hunt, E, Breckenridge-Sproat, S., & Kitzmiller R. (2004). *The Nursing Informatics Implementation Guide.* New York: Springer.

Kriegel R, & Brandt D. (1996). *Sacred Cows Make the Best Burgers: Paradigm-Busting Strategies for Developing Change-Ready People and Organizations*. New York: Warner Books.

Lewin, K. (1969). Quasi-stationary social equilibria and the problem of permanent change. In: Bennis, W.G., K.D. Benne, & R. Chin (eds.) *The Planning of Change.* New York: Holt, Reinhart, pp. 235–238.

Lorenzi, N., Smith, J., Conner, S., & Campion, T. (2004). The success factor profile for clinical computer innovation. *Medinfo 2004*, pp. 1077–1080.

Machiavelli, N. (1513). *The Prince*. Translated by George Bull (1961). New York: Penguin.

Marasovic, C., Kenney, C., Elliott, D., & Sindhusake, D. (1997). Attitudes of Australian nurses toward the implementation of a clinical information system. *Computers in Nursing 15*(2):91–98.

Schwalbe, K. (2002). *Information Technology Project Management*, 2nd ed. Boston: Course Technology.

Tan, J.K.H. (2001). *Health Management Information Systems: Methods and Practical Applications*, 2nd ed. Gaithersburg, MD: Aspen.

19
A Process Redesign Approach to Successful IT Implementation

Paul E. Pancoast
With contributions by Carole Stephens, Diana Domonkos, and Lee Lavergne

> There is nothing more difficult to take in hand, more perilous to conduct, or more uncertain in its success, than to take the lead in the introduction of a new order of things, because the innovator has for enemies all those who have done well under the old conditions and lukewarm defenders in those who may do well under the new.
>
> —Niccolò Machiavelli in *The Prince*

A large integrated healthcare system decides to embark on an aggressive "transformation" project to accomplish several major objectives.

- Improve patient safety and quality
- Become more patient-centric
- Improve continuity of care across the delivery system
- Make life easier for caregivers and patients
- Reduce care variation and unnecessary expenses

They decide that information technology (IT) is a key enabler, and they invest $25 million in new software, hardware, and vendor-supplied consulting over a 4-year period. The investment includes, among other things, a new central data repository for electronic health records, patient registration and scheduling software, enterprise-wide networking, clinical documentation for nursing, computer-based physician order entry and results reporting software, implementation of new care guidelines, and physician remote access to patient records.

After 4 years and $30 million, the project is behind schedule. The consultant estimates that it will take an additional year and a half and $5 million to complete. The applications that have been installed are working, but nothing has improved. Physician and nurse productivity has declined. Nurses complain that their workload has increased. Users are disgruntled with the Information Systems Department and are asking when the systems will be fully operational. The chief financial officer is asking what the organization has gained by the substantial investment. The cheif executive officer wants to know how it happened. The chief information officer has resigned. Senior management wants to bring in a new consulting firm to help rescue them.

As the example illustrates, many IT implementations fail because attention is not paid to how workflow and processes are affected when new technology is put in place. Sometimes people are not able to adjust to the new processes, or the new processes are not appropriately designed to improve workflow efficiency. As a result, the systems are just not used. Redesigning processes before installing a new IT system is more cost-effective than doing the reverse.

This chapter introduces the reader to the concepts of project management, process redesign, and change management in the context of healthcare organizations undergoing IT implementations. Process redesign cannot successfully occur without concurrent change management, and project management is also an integral component. Descriptions of the major stages and phases of these three activities are provided.

Background

In 1991 the U.S. Institute of Medicine (IOM) published *The Computer-Based Patient Record*, recommending that electronic health records (EHR) be widely adopted for use within the next 10 years (Dick et al., 1991). Six years later, a revised and updated edition was released, reiterating the need and updating the progress. By 2003, best industry estimates of EHR use in the United States were 20% in hospitals, 10% in physician offices, and 5% in ambulatory clinics (http://www.healthcare-informatics.com/reports/industry20.pdf).

In 1999, the IOM released *To Err is Human: Building a Safer Health System* (Kohn et al., 1999). This report summarized two major studies about patient safety in the United States, showing that between 44,000 and 98,000 patients die each year owing to medical errors. In 2001 the IOM published *Crossing the Quality Chasm: A New Health System for the 21st Century*, again reiterating the need for change. This report noted that "The American healthcare delivery system is in need of fundamental change . . . the frustration levels of both patients and clinicians have probably never been higher. Yet the problems remain." (Committee on Quality of Healthcare in America, 2001).

Our current healthcare delivery system has a number of problems.

- Lack of information for clinicians when they need it
- Healthcare processes that allow avoidable errors to occur
- Inefficiencies and system waste

The solutions are available to correct these problems, so why have we not adopted them? Implementing a new healthcare information system is a complex endeavor that requires a significant shift in thinking and policy.

Process redesign (reengineering) makes quantum changes to core business processes, allowing much greater performance improvements than can be achieved by incremental change. Process redesign means evaluating the desired outcome and changing the way that outcome is attained. This usually involves much more than merely streamlining the existing processes and removing unnecessary steps. It often means completely revising peoples' job descriptions, removing existing tasks, and adding new ones. Process redesign is necessary for organizations to take full advantage of technological solutions. Process redesign is usually perceived as threatening by the people it affects. If process redesign is so difficult and painful, why do it at all? In healthcare, we simply no longer can accept the status quo. Healthcare requires a major shift in thinking, policy, and processes. The only way to accomplish the needed changes is through process redesign.

Key Definitions

- *Process*—the method by which a task is accomplished. Processes can involve several people from several departments. For instance, the process by which a medication is ordered for an inpatient by their physician is as follows.
    1. Physician decides what order to place.
    2. Physician finds the chart (or asks a nurse or resident to find the chart).
    3. Physician finds the order sheet in the chart.
    4. Physician writes the order on the sheet and signs it (or tells the nurse, resident, or unit secretary to write the order).
    5. Physician gives the chart to the unit secretary (or to the resident or nurse to give to the unit secretary).
    6. Unit secretary puts the chart in the stack to be processed.
    7. Later....
    8. Unit secretary opens the chart to the orders section.
    9. Unit secretary reads the order (and may ask the nurse or secretary to decipher the handwriting).
    10. Unit secretary transmits the order to pharmacy using a computer order system, fax, telephone, or courier for example, depending on the specific process at the hospital).
    11. Pharmacist receives the order and processes it (which includes sending the medication to the patient's unit).
    12. Nurse receives the medication.
    13. Nurse administers the medication to the patient.
    14. Nurse records the medication administration in the medication administration record (MAR).
    15. Nurse charts the medication administration, the patient's response, and (we hope) the lack of reaction to the administration.
- *Project management*—Project management includes planning, scheduling, organizing, monitoring, budgeting, and reporting for all aspects of a project.

Approaches to Changing Healthcare Delivery

There are two major components involved in change related to the implementation of any information system in the healthcare delivery system:

- *Process redesign* (process reengineering, process transformation) means changing the processes by which tasks are accomplished to achieve greater accuracy and efficiency. Typical tasks include registering a patient, medicating a patient, documenting clinical information, replenishing stock supplies, and billing for services.
- *Change management* is helping people adjust to the changes they face as a result of process redesign and IT implementation.

Information Technology Implementation

Information technology implementation refers to installing hardware and software applications. However, many IT implementations do not provide the anticipated value to an organization. People are unable to adjust to the new processes, or the new processes are not appropriately designed to improve workflow efficiency; hence the systems are not used.

There are two approaches a healthcare system can take when implementing information technology to improve healthcare delivery. One approach is commonly known as a "plain vanilla" installation, which consists of: (1) purchasing an IT system; (2) installing the technology into the healthcare system; (3) determining how the new IT system can be used to improve healthcare delivery; and (4) trying to convince people to use the new IT system. This approach is preferred by some EHR vendors because it requires little customization of the applications and can be performed more quickly. Unfortunately, this type of installation often results in disappointment on the part of the purchasing healthcare system because the new IT system does not meet the needs of the healthcare system. Many IT systems installed "off the shelf" have some (many) of their functionalities 'turned off' shortly after the system goes "live."

Process Transformation

The second approach is commonly described as process transformation. It requires more work but usually results in more effective outcomes and a satisfied healthcare system. This approach involves the following.

1. Determining exactly what the healthcare system hopes to accomplish
2. Looking at the clinical and business processes that need to be changed to accomplish those goals
3. Deciding how the healthcare system's "future state" will look
4. Redesigning the processes to reflect the "future state"

5. Building (or modifying) the EHR applications to work with those redesigned processes
6. Training the people whose "worlds will change" when the new EHR system is installed
7. Installing the EHR system
8. Evaluating how well the new EHR system meets the organizational needs

Process transformation requires the integration of process redesign and change management with the IT implementation. A key success factor for process transformation is that it must be sponsored and managed from the highest organizational levels.

Process Redesign Methodology

Most EHR vendors have teams of consultants who specialize in assisting healthcare organizations to implement the vendor's applications and systems. These teams are primarily focused on preparing the installation site to receive the EHR application. If a healthcare organization wants the system customized to their specific requirements, it must assemble a team to manage the process redesign component. Healthcare systems rarely have specific teams in place who are skilled in process transformation activities; these activities are not a part of the regular activities of a healthcare organization. When healthcare systems do not have outside help during a "system install," they may end up frustrated, as illustrated in the opening example. Healthcare consulting companies may be called in to fill this gap.

Healthcare consulting companies perform four types of activity for their clients.

- *Strategic planning*: establish a vision of how the organization will deliver and manage care in the future; understand how technology can help to achieve this vision; and develop a roadmap of the initiatives required to reach the vision
- *Process redesign and system selection*: determine how the processes of the healthcare system will change to accomplish the organizational goals; select a suitable EHR vendor to provide an IT system that can help reach those goals
- *Implementation*: determine how the IT system "build" (the "look and feel" of the applications) should be performed; use the healthcare system vision to drive the IT system installation
- *Optimization*: after an IT system is installed, making the functions of the IT system meet the needs of the healthcare organization

Project management is the art of bringing together ideas, people, and physical resources in a productive manner to achieve specific objectives. One of the most important success factors for a healthcare system transformation project involving millions of dollars and hundreds of employees is to know exactly what the project will accomplish and all the steps needed to complete the project before starting. All credible project managers use a project management methodology to manage the projects, from the initial planning phase through to the project wrap-up. Using a standardized, consistent methodology for project management allows the project to proceed in a predictable, reliable manner. Choice of project management methodology depends on the personal preference of the user; all commercially available project management methodologies have similar components and can be used successfully.

Success can be defined by certain factors.

- Clearly defined and agreed-upon project objectives
- Tools and methods to support project management
- Project completed on time and within budget
- Delivery of consistent level of quality
- Project outcomes accepted by the organization

Common stages in project management methodologies include the following.

1. *Project initiation.* Project charters and documentation as well as methods and tools are put in place for sharing knowledge about the project prior to the project start-up to ensure that the project team has the information needed to plan for project launch. The intent of this stage is to ensure that everyone on the project shares the same expectations. Organization structure for the project is created, and members of the project team are recruited. The best methodologies include all key stakeholders in the organization on the teams and committees.
2. *Project launch.* Kick-off meetings orient the team and organization to the project, the tools, and the methodologies to be used to accomplish the objectives.
3. *Ongoing project management.* Methods, tools, and templates facilitating the management of project plans, risks and issues, meetings, and documentation are clarified.
4. *Ongoing communication.* Communication of project expectations, activities, and progress across the organization is used throughout the project.
5. *Project completion.* The objectives and expectations of the project are achieved, including final documentation and project information.
6. *Project review.* A debriefing is held, and the lessons learned are identified.

There are a number of major phases in a process redesign project. The exact sequence and the staff used to accomplish these phases may vary depending on whether the project is being managed and staffed internally, or if external consultants have been called in to assist with the project. Effective project management throughout these phases is essential to achieving project goals. Detailed discussion of each of these phases is beyond the scope of this book.

Change Management

Process redesign is about changing the way people do things. Change management is about helping people deal with these changes. Redesigning the processes by which people do their work can improve efficiency and productivity as well as reduce waste, but it may be perceived as frightening or even threatening. The most common reaction to a process redesign project is resistance. When processes change, the people who perform those processes have to change as well. It is difficult for people to accept change until they understand both the organizational and personal implications. It is important to reiterate that "change management" refers to managing peoples' reactions to change, not to managing changes in software and technology.

Senior executive leaders of an organization who embark on a major process redesign project have certain concerns.

- How long will it take to accomplish?
- How much will it cost?
- What will be the return on investment (ROI)?
- How will this affect our customers (patients and family members in the case of healthcare organizations)?

When employees think about organizational change, or process redesign projects, they have specific concerns.

- Will I still have a job, or will I be "downsized"?
- What will my new responsibilities be?
- Do I have the necessary skills and knowledge to be able to perform my new tasks?
- Will I have time to eat during my lunch break?

Although employees want their organization to be successful and to make the changes needed to maintain a competitive edge, they are also concerned about how those changes will affect them personally. Change management programs are needed to help the employees adjust to the changes that occur in conjunction with process redesign projects. Process redesign projects that do not include change management programs are difficult to complete and may result in a significant loss of skilled employees. The best and brightest of the employees are in demand and have no trouble finding another position with an organization they believe is "safer" as an employer. Often such projects are abandoned before they achieve success.

There are five major principles that must be followed for a successful change management program.

1. *Change management must come from the top.* Just like a successful process redesign project, a successful change management program must clearly originate from the senior executive levels. The decision to change the organization must come from the top decision-makers of the organization. The

senior executives not only must kick off the change management program, they must continue to be seen as fully involved in the program throughout its duration.

2. *Change management must be supported throughout the organizational hierarchy; managers must become agents of change.* Change management begins at the top and continues down through each hierarchical layer until it reaches the regular workers in an organization. Because the natural reaction to change is resistance, the managers must be educated by their supervisors about the change. They must understand the organizational implications as well as the personal implications of the impending changes. When the managers are comfortable with the new notions, they can act as change agents to the people they manage. Each level of the organizational hierarchy must understand and accept the upcoming changes; then they can act as change agents to the level below them.

3. *Change managers must communicate a vision throughout the organization; they must show an existing problem that needs to be corrected.* People need to understand the organizational reasons for change. Although the change may be difficult, it is easier to accept when the need for change is understood. People are more willing to make personal sacrifices for the organization if they believe those sacrifices will make the organization more stable and more likely to be a reliable employer. The vision communicated by the change managers should clearly explain the current problem and how the changes will rectify matters. This information should come from the senior executive level (Hiatt and Creasy, 2003). Most individuals wish to hear organization-specific information from people most familiar with the organizational workings.

4. *Change management programs must address the needs and concerns of all the employees. Change managers must listen as well as talk.* Often managers have a specific message they are tasked with communicating to a list of employees. They go to each of the individuals in turn and tell them the message. Each of these individuals may then be tasked with giving the same message to another list of employees. Unfortunately, after the first cycle of "communications" the true meaning of the message has been lost. Communication implies two-way interaction. A good change manager gives the message and then asks employees what they heard. During this process, the employee can ask questions and express their concerns. Often their questions have nothing at all to do with the proposed process changes; their questions are personal: Will I still have a job? Will I have enough hours? Am I going to have to get new training or learn new skills? For the project to go smoothly, each employee needs to understand the process and to have his or her questions answered.

5. *The change must be reinforced and must become part of the corporate culture: "That's how we do things around here."* It is crucial to the organization's long-term success that the change be reinforced. Managers and employees must understand that the process changes are permanent—that

they cannot just go along for a couple weeks and then resume "business as usual." Process redesign projects usually cost millions or tens of millions of dollars. A hospital cannot afford to invest these resources in a major project and then fall back into the previous routines.

There are five specific phases of a change management program. A successful change manager recognizes these phases and addresses the important issues in each.

1. *Awareness of impending change.* During this phase, the affected people become aware that change is imminent, and that the change is going to affect them. It is preferable for the awareness to come from respected, authoritative sources than from the rumor mill. People prefer to hear of major organizational movements from the leaders of the organization, than from their colleagues. Ideally, this event occurs during the early project phase of the business process redesign. Too often change management activities are added as an afterthought when implementation of the redesigned processes encounters problems. Initiating change management early helps ensure smooth implementation.

2. *Acceptance of need for change.* Most people resist impending change. "Why fix it if it isn't broken?" Change management includes an educational program that contains explanations of the reasons for change for everyone in the organization. There must be communication (two-way dialogue) between the employees and their immediate supervisors about the need for change. Once people understand the reasons for the change, they are able to accept the need for change. Acceptance of need for change must occur on both emotional and intellectual levels. It is crucial that there be communication between the supervisors and employees—that the supervisors do not merely "give their spiel" and move along. This phase is crucial for the employees to be able to express their anxieties and concerns and to obtain answers to their questions. This must filter from top to bottom. Initially, the senior leadership educates the top-level management about the change; then senior management educates the middle management; middle management educates the direct supervisors; and so on.

3. *Knowledge of the process of change.* After the organization has made the decision to move forward with the upcoming change, people begin to learn how their world will change and what they must do to accommodate the changes. In the best case, people from the organization help design the new processes they will use. Even if they are not involved in the design phase, there are new policies and procedures to learn. Employees must learn how they will work in the new environment and become comfortable with the new procedures.

4. *Process of change.* Managing change occurs on two levels: the organizational level and the individual level. The strategies for implementing the business process redesign occur at the organizational level. The include

evaluating the scope of change, assessing the organization's ability to adapt to new processes, and determining the timing and content of messages to be communicated. Enabling employees to accept and embrace the new processes occurs at the individual level. This is where the role of the change agent becomes heavily people focused. Creating and maintaining clear channels of communication helps the change agents hear the employees' fears and concerns and address those concerns before resistance to the new processes becomes hardened throughout the organization. In an ideal organization, each employee ultimately learns the skills needed to manage change at the individual level. The entire organization thus has recreated itself as change-embracing and is able to adapt quickly to business course changes. This is the ideal. Most organizations must settle for creating an active body of change agents who can be called into action when process changes are planned.

5. *Reinforcement of change.* After the new processes have been successfully implemented and accepted, it is essential to continue to monitor the environment to ensure that there is no slipping back into "the old ways." When difficulties are encountered while doing something new, it is human nature to revert to prior behaviors. Those behaviors had become automatic, requiring less thinking and attention; and even if they were awkward, slower, or clumsy, the employee could get the job done. At this reinforcement stage, the change agent must provide support to the individual, evaluate the failure points for the organization, and participate in ongoing process redesign planning to further improve acceptance. It is important to note that reinforcement of change is of major significance for sponsors of change at the leadership level of the organization. Too frequently these leaders assume that their job is done and they turn their attention to something else. Employees may perceive this to mean that there is no longer support for the "new ways."

To achieve consistently the business objectives of the organization for improved reaction time and time to market, for example, and to retain skilled individuals and permit them to function effectively in an organization, it is essential to be familiar with and employ change management principles whenever process redesign occurs. Process redesign and change management are the twins of effective organizations today.

Summary

Healthcare organizations today must adapt new technologies to improve their ability to provide safe and efficient care to patients. Technology is available that can make dramatic improvements in current healthcare processes, but technology cannot be implemented successfully without adequate organizational preparation. This preparation involves redesigning current processes to make optimum use of the technology and helping people deal with the changes brought by the redesigned processes. Process redesign is a method of improvement that requires organizations to redesign the processes by which their tasks are completed. When process redesign occurs, the lives of people who perform those redesigned tasks are affected. Change management is needed to help people adjust to these changes in their lives. Together, process redesign, information technology implementation, and change management can dramatically improve the delivery of healthcare.

References

Committee on Quality of Health Care in America. (2001). *Crossing the Quality Chasm: A New Health System for the 21st Century.* Washington, D.C.: Institute of Medicine, National Academy Press.

Dick, R.S., Steen, E.B., & Detmer, D.E. (eds.) (1991). The Computer-Based Patient Record. Washington, D.C.: Institute of Medicine, National Academy Press.

Hiatt, J.M., & Creasey, T.J. (2003). Change Management: The People Side of Change. Loveland, CO: ProSci Learning Center.

Kohn, L.T., Corrigan, J.M., & Donaldson, M.S. (eds.) (1999) To Err is Human: Building a Safer Health System. Washington, D.C.: Institute of Medicine, National Academy Press.

Website of Interest

http://www.healthcare-informatics.com/reports/industry20.pdf (accessed August 10, 2004).

Part V
Professional Nursing Informatics

20
Nursing Informatics Education: Past, Present, and Future

WITH CONTRIBUTIONS BY SUSAN K. NEWBOLD, JO ANN KLEIN, AND JUDITH V. DOUGLAS

Today's healthcare environment continually places increasing demands on nurses to communicate, share data, and synthesize information through the use of information systems, with or without the assistance of computers (Chapman et al., 1994; Ngin and Simms, 1996). In addition to having knowledge of information systems, nurses who are computer literate have the opportunity to use the power and efficiency of computer systems to play an important role in enhancing patient care delivery, offering safe care, and shaping nursing practice. In July 2004, Dr. Charles Safran, President of the American Medical Informatics Association, announced at the National Health Information Infrastructure Conference in Washington, DC that 6000 informatics nurses would be needed to support patient care delivery in the United States.

Computer-literate nurses are defined as licensed nurses who demonstrate competence in understanding and using computer hardware, software, terminology, and operating systems (Saba and McCormick, 2001). In today's information age, nurses are expected to keep pace with rapidly advancing technology. Appropriate utilization of computers and information systems can help nurses make well informed decisions regarding management and patient care issues. It is therefore critical that education in the use of computerized healthcare knowledge systems be included as an important component of basic, as well as advanced, nursing curricula.

Nurse educators are expected to teach how to develop, retrieve, and implement electronically stored data to optimize information-dependent clinical decisions. Also, the nurse educator is expected to provide guidelines concerning newly emerging nursing knowledge and ways that this knowledge can be accessed. This need requires the nurse educator to keep abreast of the advancing technology on a theoretical as well as practical basis.

The intent of this chapter is to explore the development of graduate-level nursing informatics education from its inception to the present, with an emphasis on the importance of computer and information literacy as an integral part of the educational program. After discussing the evolution of nursing informatics education and incorporating an existing nursing informatics model, goals and objectives for future nursing informatics education are suggested.

A review of the literature provides a historical overview of nursing informatics education, including a discussion of the recognition of nursing informatics as a formal specialty by the American Nurses Association (ANA) with certification through the American Nurses Credentialing Center. Through this recognition, the specialty of nursing informatics has assumed standards of practice that should be integrated into the graduate-level nursing informatics educational curriculum. Studies that have been conducted to determine the educational needs of nursing informatics students were also examined.

Review of the Literature

Historical Overview of Nursing Informatics Education

During the 1980s, nurses who were involved in informatics were primarily self-educated because of the small number of formal graduate programs available to prepare nurses to work in this specialty. During that time, the number of faculty involved in these graduate programs was small enough that they could independently network in an effort to exchange course content. Education focused on teaching the use of computers as a tool for word processing, spreadsheet analysis, graphics production, and statistical applications (Arnold, 1996). These early programs addressed only the nature of information systems and their selections for nursing practice (Graves et al., 1995; McGonigle, 1991).

In 1988, Dr. Barbara Heller was instrumental in establishing the first graduate program in nursing informatics at the University of Maryland School of Nursing in Baltimore. The focus of this formalized program included an understanding of nursing informatics science and systems theory in a clinical and management context, with particular emphasis on its impact on nursing practice (Romano and Heller, 1990).

The Maryland program was developed in close collaboration with the university's information services division, headed by Dr. Marion J. Ball, who worked with the School of Nursing to launch their technology-assisted learning centers, develop an outside advisory board for the program, and initiate innovations in the curriculum. Together with Dr. Kathryn Hannah, she contributed the major initial texts for the program (Ball and Hannah, 1984, Ball et al., 1988, 1995; Hannah et al., 1999).

A second graduate school program followed in 1990 when the University of Utah initiated a nursing informatics program that focused on the transformation of nursing data into information to support clinical decision making.

Students learned about nursing informatics theory, design and analysis of clinical nursing systems, clinical nursing database design, decision support, and administration of clinical nursing information systems (Arnold, 1996). This program followed on the heels of a discontinued grant-funded summer postdoctoral seminar for nursing informatics that began at Utah during the summer of 1988 and ended before the opening of that university's graduate program in nursing informatics.

Since the inception of Utah's graduate-level nursing informatics program, a lack of federal funding has limited the development of other, similar programs. Funding resources are critical for providing adequate computer hardware, software, support services, faculty, and individual implementation strategies for these programs.

In September 1998, the New York University School of Nursing, under the direction of Dr. Barbara Carty, began a program with a nursing informatics graduate track. This program includes theory and clinical applications with multiple preceptorship experiences encompassing all aspects of nursing informatics.

The University of Colorado Health Sciences Center School of Nursing offers a Master of Science program in nursing designed to prepare nurses for advanced practice roles. In addition, they offer a post-master's certificate with specialization in healthcare informatics, and a post-bachelor's healthcare informatics certificate program.

Despite a lack of funding for new programs, the need for nursing informatics courses has been recognized by other nursing schools. These educational institutions have integrated nursing informatics courses in their undergraduate and graduate curricula in the form of required courses, electives, conferences and continuing education workshops. Furthermore, the traditional classroom has expanded beyond its walls to include distance education, telemedicine, and continuing education offerings. Excelsior College is the first program to offer a nursing masters program focused on nursing informatics that is totally online. The program, which began in 1999, offers a Master of Science degree in nursing administration with an emphasis on clinical informatics that is accredited by the National League for Nursing. A 17-credit post-bachelor's certificate can also be obtained in clinical informatics.

In 2003 The University of Arizona College of Nursing began to offer a doctorate in nursing with one option for study being healthcare informatics. Students can study online except for an intensive 2-week presession each year.

Continuing Education in Nursing Informatics

The University of Maryland School of Nursing hosts an annual Summer Institute in Nursing Informatics. In addition to invited speakers, attendees can make presentations and posters. Exhibitors and networking events are included in this 3-day event. Preconference and postconference workshops are offered, including the Weekend Immersion in Nursing Informatics. Other organizations that offer yearly continuing education for nursing and healthcare informatics include the American Medical Informatics Association (www.amia.org) and the Healthcare Information and Management Systems Society (www.himss.org). The Canadian Nursing Informatics Association (www.cnia.ca) also offers nursing informatics education and links to other educational offerings.

Recognition as a Nursing Specialty

In 1992, nursing informatics was formally recognized as a nursing specialty by the American Nurses Association. This recognition of nursing informatics as its own specialty was followed by the development of nursing informatics standards of practice, which were published by the American Nurses Association in 1995 and revised in 2001. These standards require that informatics nurses acquire and maintain current knowledge in nursing informatics practice (American Nurses Association, 2001). To achieve this, the informatics nurse is required to seek additional knowledge and skills appropriate to the practice setting by participating in educational programs and activities, conferences, workshops, interdisciplinary professional meetings, and self-directed learning. Thus, nursing informatics educators are needed to provide appropriate learning opportunities. The standards also suggest that each informatics nurse keep a record of his or her own learning activities and seek certification and recertification when eligible.

Nursing informatics certification became available in 1995 through the American Nurses Credentialing Center (ANCC). Major topics on the certification examination include (1) system analysis and design; (2) system implementation and support; (3) system testing and evaluation; (4) human factors; (5) computer technology; (6) information/database management; (7) professional practice/trends and issues; and (8) theories (ANCC, 2004).

To be eligible to take the nursing informatics certification examination, applicants are required to have a baccalaureate or higher degree in nursing or related areas, maintain licensure, and have 2 years of active experience as a registered nurse. In addition, each candidate must have a minimum of 2000 hours of experience in the field of nursing informatics during the 5 years before taking the examination. In lieu of this experience, 12 semester hours of academic credit in informatics in a nursing graduate program and a minimum of 1000 hours in informatics nursing may be substituted (ANCC, 2004). Since 1997, the certification examination has been available by computer at 55 testing facilities throughout the United States. It was the first computerized ANCC certification examination, and to date more than 1000 nurses have been certified.

Nursing Informatics Graduate-Level Education Today

Many educational and practice institutions have initiated programs to prepare nurse clinicians simply as users of automated systems, and others are preparing healthcare information systems specialists. Despite the increased use of computer systems in nursing informatics, the management component of informatics presented by Graves and Corcoran (1989) remains essential. The nursing informatics student is still taught to have the "functional ability to collect, aggregate, organize, move, and represent information in an economical, efficient way that is useful to users of the system" (Graves and Corcoran, 1989).

Today, nurses can take advantage of the virtual classroom where the educational process occurs outside the formal classroom setting. In this environment, use of telecommunication technologies through computer-based intranets, extranets, and the Internet make innovative multimedia teaching possible. This teaching methodology is ideal for students who require flexible class schedules secondary to work and family obligations. The virtual classroom, as an interactive process, enables nursing students and their teachers to utilize telecommunication software applications such as interactive video instruction, electronic mail, bulletin boards or newsgroups, and chat conferencing as a learning milieu. To supplement virtual classroom activities, students are guided to utilize the Internet, where databases of nursing and healthcare information and other applicable learning resources can be accessed from school and home computers. It is therefore the responsibility of nurse educators to train students to access, retrieve, and implement this growing base of virtual learning tools and to provide feedback to students regarding their success in implementing these tools. O'Neil et al. (2004) have offered a practical step-by-step process to take nurse educators through the necessary steps to transform a traditional course into an on-line or partially online course.

Studies Examining Nursing Informatics Educational Needs

As early as 1990, when no formal nursing informatics program existed at their school, the Computing Advisory Council (CAC) at The University of Texas Health Science Center School of Nursing at San Antonio made recommendations for integration of nursing informatics into graduate research coursework (Noll and Murphy, 1993). At that time, it was recommended that students achieve the following areas of competence upon completion of the graduate program, regardless of their major: (1) analyze and select relevant information sources; (2) access existing Internet resources for nursing and related disciplines; (3) extract, manage, and organize data; (4) analyze the nurse's role in data security and integrity; (5) analyze the impact of nursing information systems; (6) evaluate and use appropriate software for advanced practice; and (7) demonstrate information transfer between computer systems (Noll and Murphy, 1993).

These programs, which incorporate nursing informatics coursework in their graduate level curricula, confirm that achieving computer competence is not easy for all the participants. Magnus et al. (1994) participated in a graduate course titled "Nursing Informatics" at the Hunter–Bellevue School of Nursing that emphasized the integration and use of computer and information technology as it related to the management and processing of data, information, and knowledge to support nursing practice and the delivery of care. At that time, there was noted resistance to using computers because of fear of the unknown. Magnus and her classmates suggested that participating in the course helped diffuse the "mystery" surrounding the material (Magnus et al., 1994). Noll and Murphy (1993) reported that integration of nursing informatics material with hands-on application facilitated learning. In addition, students noted that information about software packages, particularly bibliographic databases, was extremely helpful and would be useful in the development of their graduating theses.

A study conducted by Saranto and Leino-Kilpi (1997) identified and described computer skills required in nursing and what should be taught about information technology in nursing education. A three-round Delphi survey was conducted with a panel of experts representing nursing practice, nursing education, nursing students, and consumers. The experts agreed that nurses must know how to use the computer for word-processing purposes as well as for accessing and using hospital information systems and electronic mail (e-mail). Nurses must also be aware of system security and show a positive attitude toward computers. Conclusively, the study determined that hospital information systems and nursing informatics should be integrated into laboratory and hospital training (Saranto and Leino-Kilpi, 1997).

In 1996, Dr. Jean Arnold, then associated with the College of Nursing, Rutgers, the State University of New Jersey, conducted a survey among 497 respondents in a northeastern metropolitan area to determine the informatics needs of professional nurses. The subjects primarily represented informatics specialists, nurse educators, and nurse managers, many with masters or doctoral degrees. Respondents were asked to indicate their current knowledge and desired knowledge of nursing informatics in 23 content areas that are included in the ANCC nursing informatics certification examination.

The survey revealed that 73% of the respondents were interested in returning to school to earn certification in nursing informatics, and 59% were interested in a graduate degree (Arnold, 1996). Decision support, integration of nursing informatics, advanced nursing informatics, decision analysis, and graphics presentations were the content areas most highly ranked by informatics nurses. In addition, informatics trends and issues information were the foremost educational needs identified by informatics nurses in the survey. The results reported by informatics nurses in both areas differed from the responses by nurse educators and nurse managers, suggesting that position titles and responsibilities have an impact on a subject's interest in advanced education in addition to the subject's use of computer applications (Arnold, 1996).

As a result of her survey, Arnold recommended that informatics nursing curricula content include "graphic presentation of data, decision support, electronic communications, integration of nursing informatics within basic and other specialty programs, critique of computer-assisted clinical data analysis, and expert knowledge acquisition" (Arnold, 1996). She also recommended including review courses for the informatics certification examination and emphasized the need for more graduate and continuing education programs to meet the increased demand for informatics knowledge.

Staggers et al. (2002) also conducted a Delphi study to determine the areas of competence needed for nurses in the field of information technology. Their research revealed 305 such competencies proposed for nurses at four levels of practice: the beginning nurse, the experienced nurse, the informatics nurse, and the nurse innovator.

Future of Nursing Informatics Education

Clearly, there is a need to standardize graduate nursing informatics curricula based on the standards of nursing informatics practice defined by the ANA, nursing informatics certification requirements defined by the ANCC, and utilization of a nursing informatics model such as that developed by Saba and McCormick (2001) incorporating the suggested adaptations.

For the nurse educator to teach and reinforce this newly acquired nursing informatics knowledge effectively, computer systems should be readily available at all sites where nursing education occurs or clinical decisions are made, and in any place where nursing is practiced. Students must be allowed to experience situations where computer applications related to nursing informatics can be used, which includes utilization of the virtual classroom.

One of the primary barriers to utilization of the virtual classroom in nursing informatics education has been the speed with which telecommunication and computer technology has been developing, resulting in frequently changing software and hardware requirements and a financial investment that many schools are not able to sustain. It is hoped that as the cost of computer hardware and accompanying software systems continues to decline, computerized educational modalities and clinical information banks will become more readily accessible.

The development of nursing informatics curricula for graduate-level nursing students demands that the minimum standards be based on an understanding of the ANA's nursing informatics standards of practice. Optimally, the curricula is based on the understanding and application of the ANA's nursing informatics standards of practice in addition to the requirements for achieving certification in nursing informatics through the ANCC.

To achieve these goals, there must be practical application of the presented information systems theory. This should include not only additional educational experiences but also substantial hands-on experience through preceptorship arrangements. First-hand experience ensures that all master's level nursing informatics graduates have a high level of competence in both theory and practice. Because this is such a crucial goal, coursework should continue to focus on computer applications and related issues in nursing practice, nursing administration, nursing education, and nursing research.

Defining an Educational Model for Graduate-Level Nursing Informatics

Not only is there a need for more nursing informatics programs, a need also exists for an educational framework to promote standardization and structure in the nursing informatics curricula. Because the specialty is so new, there has been limited research regarding the development of models specifically designed for nursing informatics education. Utilization of educational models would provide the needed framework not only for theoretical education but also for practical applications.

Riley and Saba's nursing informatics education model (NIEM) is an educational application aimed at undergraduate students that can be adapted for graduate students. The model can fulfill the need for a theoretical and practical framework in addition to meeting the desired requirements of informatics nurses cited in Arnold's survey (Saba and McCormick, 2001).

The NIEM emerged and evolved with the development of computer technology in the healthcare industry. As illustrated in Figure 20.1 NIEM identifies three dimensions of content that comprise nursing informatics computer science, information science, and nursing science. NIEM further identifies the educational outcomes that must be addressed in the three domains of learning: cognitive, affective, and psychomotor. Once the objectives are achieved in each domain of learning, students can integrate nursing informatics into their nursing roles. This integration of knowledge and competence in nursing education requires that a program include content, hands-on application, and attitude. The model supports the integration of computer and information technology into nursing education to enhance critical thinking skills and provide an active learning experience. Confidence, psychomotor skill level, and knowledge attainment are enhanced in the process. An advantage of using this model is the ability for the student nurse to make decisions in simulated case studies without risk to the patient (Saba and McCormick, 2001).

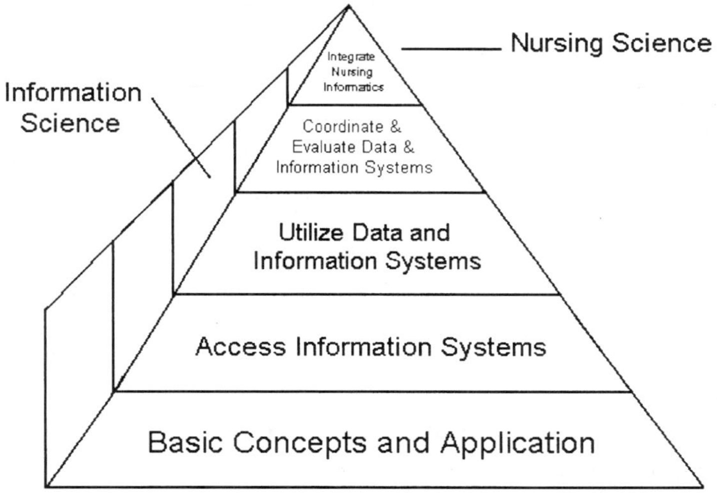

FIGURE 20.1. Riley and Saba's nursing informatics education model (NIEM). (From Saba V, McCormick K. *Essentials of Computers for Nurses.* New York: McGraw-Hill, 2001, p. 558, with permission.)

As summarized here, NIEM's objectives occur in four steps. Because basic computer skills are germane to fundamental nursing education, the first step gives students the knowledge and technical skills to function effectively (Lawless, 1993; Saba and McCormick, 2001). Computer application content at this level includes concepts of computer hardware and software as well as computer system components. Students are required to use a word processing program for assignments and to format documents in American Psychological Association (APA) format. System content includes the use of computerized databases and search engines for reference material (Saba and McCormick, 2001). Although it is hoped that all students entering a graduate-level program are proficient in basic computer skills and applications, this step provides the needed content and practical experience for those students entering graduate-level programs with little or no computer knowledge.

Saba and McCormick (2001) recommended that the nursing informatics student have knowledge of word processing, database, presentation, and spreadsheet software programs in addition to bibliographic retrieval using CD-ROM software as well as Internet searches. This hands-on computer experience is augmented by the assignment of e-mail addresses and required subscription to a class e-mail discussion group, which can be utilized for discussion and assignments. Nursing literature supports the use of e-mail as an informal exchange of communication to help new computer users cope with the stress of using new technology and to enhance critical thinking skills (Magnus et al., 1994; Todd, 1998).

The second step of Riley and Saba's model involves application of computer technology to document and access health information for the purposes of patient assessment. On an undergraduate level, Riley and Saba introduce the Saba Home Healthcare Classification of Nursing Diagnosis and Intervention in the classroom to develop patient care plans and in the hospital patient information system for recording care (Saba and McCormick, 2001).

At the graduate level, step 2 can be adapted to include organizational theory and associated computer applications, such as utilization of Microsoft Project software for project management simulation. In addition, students can apply computer applications to healthcare financial management coursework to determine staffing needs, cost–benefit ratios, and budgets. It is during step 2 that this author suggests the electronic health record (EHR) be introduced, particularly in regard to classification systems and taxonomies, managed care, and the social, legal, and ethical issues associated with the EHR.

The third step of the Riley and Saba model introduces undergraduate students to advanced concepts utilizing existing information systems in clinical agencies to plan and implement patient care (Saba and McCormick, 2001). On a graduate level, this step can be adapted to include telecommunications in healthcare with an emphasis on understanding the policy development that led to the current trend toward telemedicine and telenursing applications in addition to its utilization. Also, knowledge about system requirements and design and development applications should be imparted through actual student experience working in venues such as outpatient agencies, vendors, hospital information system departments, and consulting firms.

Riley and Saba's fourth and final step requires students to integrate computer technology into nursing care. It includes evaluation, quality improvement, multidisciplinary collaboration, and utilization of available resources with the technology. In addition, students are required to examine the social, legal, and ethical issues they encounter through the use of computer technology (Saba and McCormick, 2001).

This final step has been integrated into earlier steps of the graduate-level adapted model. Therefore it is suggested that the fourth step be revised to include implementation of a full systems analysis. To achieve this, the student must work on a systems development life cycle in a preceptor-based practicum real-life experience during the course of a 1-year internship. This plan would allow the student to benefit from long-term hands-on experience under the guidance of an experienced practitioner. In turn, this experience, coupled with earlier short-term practical experience, would enable students to claim credible nursing informatics experience when searching for employment after graduation.

Clearly, Riley and Saba's model is adaptable and can be applied to all levels of nursing informatics education. Because the practice of nursing informatics can occur in any area where nurses practice, this model is applicable in all practice settings (Lange, 1997). It is therefore a realistic model for standardizing nursing informatics education methodology.

Summary

Informatics knowledge, in this age of information, is necessary for growth of the nursing profession. The number of available nursing informatics graduate-level programs is increasing, but the informatics expertise of faculty members to teach in those programs is critical if the nursing profession is to meet the challenges presented by integration of this rapidly advancing technology into healthcare. Therefore the graduate-level nursing informatics educational environment must continue to strive to become a forum where educator and student meet in an expanded capacity made possible by an increase in the integration of computer competence in the nursing informatics curricula.

This practice does not undermine the importance of noncomputerized systems in the field of nursing informatics but responds to the challenge of keeping pace with the changing regimen. By creating a pilot nursing informatics program utilizing the suggested adaptations of Riley and Saba's NIEM, increased computer and information literacy and competence can be achieved in a graduate-level nursing informatics program. Therefore it is suggested that research be conducted to determine the effectiveness of such a program to (1) measure the effectiveness of the proposed program in relation to improving computer literacy and therefore increasing competence; (2) determine the feasibility of developing an actual program; and (3) add to the current knowledge base about nursing education curriculum requirements for nursing informatics graduate-level programs.

Once validated through research, this proposed model can serve as a guideline for schools of nursing that are in the process of considering, planning, developing, or implementing graduate-level nursing informatics curricula.

References

American Nurses Association. (2001). *Scope and Standards of Nursing Informatics Practice.* Washington, D.C.: American Nurses Publishing.

American Nurses Credentialing Center (ANCC). (2004). *Informatics Nurse Certification Examination.* http://www.nursingworld.org/ancc/certification/cert/certs/informatics.html.

Arnold, J. (1996). Nursing informatics educational needs. *Computers in Nursing* *14*(6):333–339.

Ball, M.J., & Hannah, K.J. (1984). *Using Computers in Nursing.* Reston, VA: Reston Publishing.

Ball, M.J., Hannah, K.J., Gerdin Jelger, U., & Peterson, H. (1988). *Nursing Informatics: Where Caring and Technology Meet.* New York: Springer-Verlag.

Ball, M.J., Hannah, K.J., Newbold, S.K., & Douglas, J.V. (1995). *Nursing Informatics: Where Caring and Technology Meet,* 2nd ed. New York: Springer-Verlag.

Chapman, R., Reiley, P., & McKinney, J., et al. (2000). Implementing a local area network for nursing in a large teaching hospital. *Computers in Nursing 12*(2):82–87.

Graves, J., & Corcoran, S. (1989). The study of nursing informatics. *Image: Journal of Nursing Scholarship 21*(4):227–231.

Graves, J., Amos, L., Hueber, S., Lange, L., & Thompson, C. (1995). Description of a graduate program in clinical nursing informatics. *Computers in Nursing 13*(2):60–69.

Hannah, K.J., Ball, M.J., & Edwards, M.J.A. (1999). *Introduction to Nursing Informatics.* New York: Springer-Verlag.

Lange, L. (1997). Informatics nurse specialist: Roles in health care organizations. *Nursing Administration Quarterly 21*(3):1–10.

Lawless, K. (1993). Nursing informatics as a needed emphasis in graduate nursing administration education: The student perspective. *Computers in Nursing 11*(6):263–268.

Magnus, M., Co, M., Jr., & Cerkach, C. (1994). A first-level graduate studies experience in nursing informatics. *Computers in Nursing 12*(4):189–192.

McGonigle, D. (1991). Establishing a nursing informatics program. *Computers in Nursing 9*(5):184–189.

Ngin, P., & Simms, L. (1996). Computer use for work accomplishment. *Journal of Nursing Administration 26*(3):47–53.

Noll, M., & Murphy, M. (1993). Integrating nursing informatics into a graduate research course. *Journal of Nursing Education 32*(7):332–334.

O'Neil, C.A., Fisher, C.A., & Newbold, S.K. (2004). *Developing an Online Course: Best Practices for Nurse Educators*. New York: Springer.

Romano, C., & Heller, B. (1990). Nursing informatics: A model curriculum for an emerging role. *Journal of Nursing Education 15*(2):16–19.

Saba, V., & McCormick, K. (2001). *Essentials of Computers for Nurses, 3rd ed.* New York: McGraw-Hill.

Saranto, K., & Leino-Kilpi, H. (1997). Computer literacy in nursing: Developing the information technology syllabus in nursing education. *Journal of Advanced Nursing 25*(2):377–385.

Staggers, N., Gassert, C. & Curran, C. (2002). A Delphi study to determine informatics competencies at four levels of practice. *Nursing Research 51*(6):383–390.

Todd, N. (1998). Using e-mail in an undergraduate nursing course to increase critical thinking skills. *Computers in Nursing 16*(2):115–118.

21
The Future for Nurses in Health Informatics

With contributions by Joyce Sensmeier, Susan K. Newbold, and James Cato

Since we have entered the new millennium, the emphasis on health informatics has been increasingly growing. The focus of development, which was initially on hardware, has moved to an emphasis on application software. As the understanding of health informatics continues to evolve, however, hardware and software are increasingly recognized as merely a means to capture, transport, and transform data into information that enables caregivers to provide people with the best possible health services. This new information-rich environment also contains new and powerful tools that enable caregivers and care recipients alike to seek and use information to make health-affecting decisions and to generate new health knowledge. To gain maximum benefits from this new environment, expanded understanding of how people seek and use information by drawing on cognitive science and organizational development is essential (Ball and Nelson, 2004; Ball et al., 2004).

Visions of the Future

Haux (1998) defined a vision for medical informatics that rests on 10 aims. Ball et al. (1997) explored the implications of these aims for the nursing profession.

- *Aim 1: diagnostics—the visible human body.* Remote access to high-quality digital images supports new modes of care delivery (Dayhoff and Siegel, 1998; Zimmerman, 1995). These images can be minimized, ensure access to specialists, and create new requirements for coordinating and managing care. Other influential developments include the incorporation of images of various types into electronic patient records. Many of these advances have already taken place and continue to enhance the information available to caregivers, including nurses; and they affect the ways in which caregivers deliver care. The National Library of Medicine's Visible Man and Visible Woman are now accessible via the Internet or

CD-ROM; the availability of such images can increase knowledge of the human body and ultimately contribute to nursing assessment and intervention.

- *Aim 2: therapy: medical intervention with as little strain on the patient as possible.* Noninvasive diagnostics and minimally invasive surgery are growing significantly, thanks to laparoscopic procedures and computer-aided visualization as well as laser surgery. Clearly, these advances affect nurses involved in the procedure. When combined with other forces, they also affect nurse's involvement throughout the care process, influencing factors such as limiting the number of hospital days and changing the role of the hospital-based nurses.
- *Aim 3: therapy simulation.* Nurse educators have been leaders in using simulation-based training for their students, offering simulation laboratories to teach basic skills. Further development of simulation technologies will allow nurses to refine advanced skills. Multimedia computer–based training will supplement hands-on laboratory experiences even more in the years to come.
- *Aim 4: early recognition and prevention.* Today, increasing numbers of nurse practitioners are providing primary care, and nurse-managed clinics are becoming the mechanism for delivering affordable primary care. Both trends suggest that nursing will become responsible for patient education, working with patients to develop health behaviors that prevent illness and promote wellness. Use of the Internet and new functions, such as information prescriptions, are putting more and more tools into the hands of healthcare providers.
- *Aim 5: compensating for physical handicaps.* Devices used on an ongoing basis by patients tend ultimately to involve nursing in their support as a daily living skill. Teaching these skills has long been the concern of nursing. New informatics applications in this area will require a new level of knowledge and sophistication among nursing staff. To accomplish these goals, a revolution needs to occur in the nursing curriculum. Each nurse must have a comfort level with enabling technologies, which is not present today.
- *Aim 6: health consulting: the informed patient.* Patient education is receiving new attention. Multimedia programs guide patients when they are deciding on interventions for their condition. Moreover, videotapes, CDs, and DVDs are available for purchase in pharmacies with titles addressing conditions ranging from alcoholism to gastrointestinal ulcers. As more health-related information becomes available to consumers via the Internet, patients definitely need guidance for evaluating and using this information. Nursing has often provided this guidance in the past and will increasingly continue to do so as counselors and teachers of patients and clients. Tools provided by responsible organizations such as Health on the Net (HON) are there to help the consumers and patients make informed decisions.

- *Aim 7: health reporting.* To date, public health has relied on retrospective reports to control disease. Today the information infrastructure offers the capability to intervene in a timelier manner through ongoing surveillance of certain conditions and through programs such as clinical alerts of national the Library of Medicine (NLM) clinical alerts. The National Institutes of Health is extending the boundaries through its Human Genome Project and Gene Bank. We have yet to realize the benefits that can result from large-scale data repositories providing population-based health statistics. Nursing will play a role in using and understanding outcomes information to improve the management and quality of care. The next initiative, called the National Health Information Infrastructure (NHII), will be a transformational initiative (discussed later).
- *Aim 8: enterprise information systems.* Nurses have long been the frontline users of information systems in healthcare. Indeed the nurse is the foot soldier of our healthcare system. Clinical informatics must focus on making information tools an integral component of the care process, noticeable only by their absence. Technology should free up the caregiver, eliminating cumbersome and repetitive data entry. Increasingly, technology will need to support health professionals including nurses in a wide variety of settings in large-scale integrated health service networks. As members of the healthcare team, nurses will continue to be at the hub of patient care—even when are functioning in a telehealth/telemedicine setting.
- *Aim 9: medical documentation.* Movement toward the electronic health record (EHR) continues in the United States (NHII), Canada (Canada Health Infoway), and the United Kingdom and Australia (GEHR). In the United States, President Bush has challenged the profession to develop an EHR for every citizen within the next 10 years. The major obstacles are nontechnical: Questions remain regarding medical knowledge representation and the structure of the record. The Unified Nursing Language System (UNLS) has been integrated into the NLM's Unified Medical Language System (UMLS); SNOMED is free for use in the United States and the United Kingdom. The Telenurse project in the European Community, the International Classification of Nursing Practice initiative of the International Council of Nurses, the International Standard Known as Reference Terminology Model for Nursing (ISO 18104), and other initiatives, both national and international, are all having a major impact on electronic nursing documentation. All these activities are improving nursing documentation and thereby enhancing the visibility of the nursing contribution to patient care. Of course, data protection and patient confidentiality remain key critical issues. The Health Insurance Portability and Accountability Act of 1996 (HIPAA) has also had a major impact.
- *Aim 10: comprehensive documentation of medical knowledge and knowledge-based decisions for case management.* These efforts are closely linked to outcomes and quality assurance. Patient safety has moved to

the top of the list as an initiative that is key to the future of nursing. New ethical considerations will arise as we move to the future. How will knowledge-based systems affect issues of clinical judgment and responsibility? Clearly the nursing profession must address these issues, in both concept and practice.

Since the release of the above aims, other initiatives have taken place moving forward the agenda of healthcare information technology. In July 2004, at the National Health Information Infrastructure (NHII) Summit, Dr. David Brailer, the National Coordinator of Health Information Technology, unveiled the four goals of his office to mobilize U.S. Health Information Technology (HIT) initiatives during the current decade. Although nursing is not emphasized in these efforts, nursing must play a major role in taking these concepts from theory to practice.

- *Goal 1: inform clinical practice.* This goal focuses largely on efforts to bring electronic health records directly into clinical practice.
- *Goal 2: interconnect clinicians.* This allows information to be portable and to move with consumers from one point of care to another.
- *Goal 3: personalize care.* Consumer-centric information helps individuals manage their own wellness and assists with their personal healthcare decisions.
- *Goal 4: improve population health.* Population health improvement envisions improved capacity for public health monitoring, quality of care measurement, and bringing research advances more quickly into medical practice.

Making these efforts meaningful to the nursing profession will require extensive lobbying by nurses to increase the awareness of policy makers of the importance of nursing content in the HIT initiatives to achieve the goals of the NHII. Moreover, a major change will be required in nursing education. This means diffusing nursing informatics training throughout the nursing curriculum rather than in isolated fashion, as we have done to date. We are still training nurses the way we did 50 years ago, and we need to change our approach if these efforts are to transform the delivery of healthcare.

New Roles for Nurses in Nursing and Healthcare Informatics

As the discipline known as nursing informatics (see Chapter 1) continues to evolve within the context of health informatics, nurses can and should contribute in the areas of research, education, administration, and practice. In the area of research, nurses with appropriate preparation are already participating in developmental projects. All the major developers and vendors of computerized health information systems employ nurses as consultants, advisors, systems engineers, systems analysts, or programmers. Major research initiatives, led by nurse researchers, are underway to study the use of the Internet and the World Wide Web for delivery of patient care or education. Nurses have also participated in government-funded investigations studying the effects of the implementation of such systems on healthcare delivery and nursing practice. In addition, nurses have been extensively involved in research related to the development of international data and information standards for health data and information as well as nursing data and information. Major research effort is well underway in the uniquely nursing area related to the development of reference terminology models for nursing as a basis for information standards related to nursing clinical language and vocabulary.

Most recently, nurses are developing information management methods and tools for use in transforming health and nursing data into information. Similarly, nurses have been in the forefront of projects exploring the educational and instructional uses of large mainframe computers, personal computers, laptops, blackberries, tablets, multimedia, and the Internet. These nurses are actively involved in developing and evaluating computer hardware, software, peopleware, and multimedia materials in educational institutions and at organizations that provide patient care. In the future, nurse researchers should be initiating studies of the ergonomic and change management issues associated with the use of information technologies in nursing practice and nursing education.

Nurse administrators require computer skills, informatics skills, and informatics knowledge to fulfill their roles. In addition, these nurses should be able to select systems that help in the management of patients and staff, such as nursing documentation systems and staffing and scheduling products. Nurse administrators should also be prepared to promote and support their organizations' implementation of systems that foster patient safety and quality nursing practice.

In the area of practice, nurses have traditionally been the interface between the consumer and the healthcare system. In the application of nursing informatics, nurses with baccalaureate or master's degree preparation can and should participate in the selection and implementation of systems. Parker and Gassert (1996) long ago concluded that informatics nurse specialists (INSs) are eminently qualified to assist the healthcare industry in implementing Joint Commission on the Accreditation of Healthcare Organizations (JCAHO) standards in the clinical environment (JCAHO, 1994). In fact, Parker and Gassert (1996) asserted that INSs can function more effectively and appropriately as systems analysts in patient care settings than the nonclinical systems analyst, who may have a background in computer science, engineering, or another discipline. Nurses must articulate for the computer program designers and systems engineers the automated systems needs of healthcare professionals and consumers. A related role is that of change agent, someone who facilitates the business process design (or redesign) related to the delivery of patient care. This role enables organizations and the people in them (including nurses) to use information and information systems with the maximum degree of effectiveness and efficiency. The development and wide dissemination of Telehealth applications ultimately may provide an expanded scope of practice for nurses as the delivery of health services is transformed.

In the area of education, INSs should be teaching and interpreting the jargon and basic tenets of modern nursing for the information specialists. They should also be preparing their professional colleagues for the inevitable widespread implementation of automated information systems. This preparation can be accomplished through basic and ongoing education programs. In facilities where information systems are being installed or upgraded, nurses are and should continue to be the trainers for nurses using new or upgraded applications software. The American Nurses Association (ANA) officially recognized and defined the INS as far back as 1992 and has put in place a process for certifying INSs (Newbold, 1996).

The goal of these new roles for nurses is to create patient-centered, enterprise health information systems that meet the needs of the consumer for use in healthcare agencies and institutions. Healthcare professionals should not be required to change their patterns of practice to conform to a computer system. Thus, for information systems to best assist in the process of patient care decision making by nurses, nursing informatics must receive and respond to input from nursing. Nurses and information specialists must cooperate in the development of information systems that produce the types of information needed by nurses in their practice. Information specialists and nurses must establish a dialogue that results in each group understanding the needs and constraints under which the other functions.

As early as 1971, Singer warned that the more complex the system, the higher the cost of change and therefore the more rigid and inflexible the system becomes (Singer, 1971). Thus, caution when designing and implementing any information system is essential. Future nursing needs must be anticipated and provision made for flexibility in the design of programs in the information system selected for use. Again, a general understanding is needed between nurses and information specialists regarding the functions and limitations of computers and the dynamic nature of nursing to select flexible hardware and design-satisfactory computer programs. Only nurses can provide the input necessary to ensure that nursing needs are met by healthcare information systems.

Because of the widespread integration of nursing informatics into healthcare agencies and institutions, the role of the nurse will become more intensified and diversified. Redefinition, refinement, and modification of the practice of nursing will intensify the nurse's role in the delivery of patient care. At the same time, the nurse's role will acquire greater diversity by virtue of employment opportunities in the nursing informatics field. Nursing's contributions can and will influence the evolution of healthcare computing. The contributions of nurses are essential to the expansion and development of healthcare computing. By providing leadership and direction, nurses can ensure that healthcare computing and nursing informatics evolve to benefit the patient. That expected benefit is to expand and improve the quality of healthcare received by patients.

Role of Professional Associations

Nurses interested in having a positive impact on the development of the information management aspects of their profession are faced with the formidable task of keeping up with a body of knowledge that becomes quickly outdated. "State-of-the-art" technology changes with meteoric haste. The slightest lapse in one's monitoring of new technological developments can result in one's knowledge becoming historical.

How does an individual stay current in this field? Obviously, the professional journals and trade magazines provide an important service. Unfortunately, people on the frontiers of developing new technology and its applications are often too busy developing, with no time left for writing about their activities. Thus, a curious dichotomy is occurring. People are reverting to more informal means of communication to disseminate information about the newest developments in high-technology information processing.

Professional associations fulfill the vital function of facilitating the exchange of current information on informatics developments. Individuals involved in the health informatics field are more than willing to welcome "new blood" with fresh ideas. They are also more than eager to expound on their ideas to new listeners. Often, contact initiated on a face-to-face basis at professional association annual meetings results in establishment of an informal network of colleagues. These informal networks serve to maintain contact between conferences for the purpose of sharing information and ideas. In addition, professional associations provide a forum for the communication and exchange of ideas. Formal addresses by leaders in the field and informal discussions in the corridors and at social events during conferences facilitate this exchange of ideas. Professional associations also publish newsletters, journals, and conference proceedings. These media are aimed at accelerating wide dissemination of information about new information management methods, technology, and software and their use and applications.

Nurses with interest and expertise in health informatics should seek membership in three types of organization.

- The first is affiliation with multidisciplinary associations whose focus is health informatics. The purpose of membership in this type of organization is to maintain and expand expertise in health informatics.

- The second type of organizational membership is maintenance of affiliations with nursing professional organizations. This membership should be maintained for the dual purpose of providing leadership and sharing ideas and information about health informatics in the nursing community.
- The third type of affiliation is membership in vendor-sponsored user groups.

Multidisciplinary Professional Associations

When addressing the multidisciplinary professional affiliation, it is readily apparent that although few nurses have achieved a high level of preparation in nursing informatics and health informatics there is a growing cadre of nursing colleagues with a shared interest in this field. The value of affiliating with a multidisciplinary association lies in the scope and depth of expertise, information, and perspective available from contact with experts in health informatics. In the United States, the American Medical Informatics Association (AMIA) offers a variety of activities.

- Conducting scientific, technical, and educational meetings, one of which is the annual AMIA fall symposium
- Publishing and disseminating digests, reports, proceedings, and other pertinent documents independently and in the professional literature
- Advising and coordinating functions and matters of interest to the membership
- Stimulating, sponsoring, and conducting research into the application and evaluation of technologic systems as they apply to healthcare and medical science
- Representing the United States in the international arena of medical systems and informatics

In 1982, the nurse members of this association formed a Nursing Professional Specialty Group (PSG) within SCAMC, the organization that later became AMIA. This subgroup meets at the same time as the AMIA annual meeting and the spring congress. It is also active in promoting and facilitating communication among its members between meetings. The PSG is now known as the Nursing Informatics Working Group (NI-WG). The Mission of NI-WG is to promote the advancement of nursing informatics within the larger multidisciplinary context of health informatics. The organization and its members pursue this goal in many arenas: professional practice, education, research, governmental and other service, professional organizations, and industry. The Working Group represents the interests of nursing informatics for members in the Working Group and in AMIA and provides member services and outreach functions.

Another valuable multidisciplinary organization is the Healthcare Information and Management Systems Society (HIMSS). HIMSS is one of the healthcare industry's leading membership organizations and is exclusively focused on promoting the optimal use of healthcare information technology and management systems for the betterment of healthcare. HIMSS was founded in 1961 and currently has offices in Chicago, Washington, DC, and other locations across the United States. HIMSS represents more than 15,000 individual members and 220 member corporations that employ more than 1 million people. HIMSS frames and leads healthcare national public policy and industry practices through its advocacy and educational and professional development initiatives, which are designed to promote the contribution that information and management systems make to ensure quality patient care. After separating from the American Hospital Association in 1994, HIMSS convened its first conference and exhibition as an independent organization in Phoenix, Arizona, with 248 exhibitors and 6300 attendees. During the past decade, this annual event has grown into a prime venue that focuses on healthcare information and management systems. In 2004, this event attracted more than 700 exhibitors and 20,000 attendees.

As the role of nursing in the design and implementation of information systems continues to expand, HIMSS has increased its number of educational offerings and related activities to support the needs of clinicians. During the 1990s, seminars focusing on nursing informatics topics, such as clinical documentation and medication management, and networking activities with local chapters increasingly drew nurses to HIMSS membership. In 2004, HIMSS convened its first nursing informatics symposium immediately prior to the HIMSS annual conference and exhibition, with more than 300 nurses attending. The 2004 HIMSS nursing informatics survey confirmed that nurses play a critical role in clinical documentation systems, indicating that nearly 75% of the 537 respondents were currently involved in implementing these systems. Half of the respondents were implementing computerized provider order entry (CPOE) systems or EMR systems.

Canada's Health Informatics Association (COACH) is a multidisciplinary group of healthcare and information processing professionals who are active in the area of medical informatics and healthcare computing. The purpose of COACH is to create a forum for the exchange of ideas, concepts, and developments in the information processing field within the Canadian healthcare environment. Within this framework, COACH's objectives are the following.

1. To continuing dialogue among healthcare institutions, associations, and governments relative to all health information processing applications
2. To disseminate information on applications or approaches through media such as seminars, workshops, conferences, or newsletters, thereby providing various sectors of the healthcare system with a source of information and expertise

There is a growing cadre of nurses active in COACH.

The preceding national organizations provide membership opportunities for individuals. These organizations also have counterparts in 38 other countries. On an international level, these various national health (medical) informatics societies constitute the membership of the International Medical Informatics Association (IMIA). IMIA is a nonpolitical, international, scientific organization whose mandate is the open exchange of scientific information and assistance in health informatics between member countries. IMIA defines itself as an international and world representative federation of national societies of health informatics and affiliated organizations. IMIA does not have individual members, although there may be several delegates from each country as observers; each country has only one designated representative with one vote.

The IMIA has long held the position that "the term 'medical informatics' is a compromise between several relevant adjectives and is considered synonymous with 'health informatics.'" IMIA's prime function is educational relative to the dissemination of knowledge of health information processing. IMIA accomplishes its educational objectives through the following groups.

1. Triennial Medinfo conferences, which have been held in Stockholm (1974); Toronto (1977); Tokyo (1980); Amsterdam (1983); Washington, DC (1986); China and Singapore (1989); Geneva (1992); Canada (1995); Seoul (1998); London (2001); and San Francisco (2004). These large conferences provide an excellent review of the state of the art of medical informatics. Information on forthcoming Medinfo conferences can be found at their Web site, http://www.hon.ch/medinfo.
2. Working groups on special topics such as nursing, education, electrocardiographic processing, and confidentiality, security, and privacy.
3. Working conferences, of which more than 30 have been held in the past 15 years.
4. By far, the largest special interest group is the nursing informatics group, which also meets every 3 years and will meet next in Seoul in 2006; in Helsinki in 2009; and in North America in 2012.

The IMIA also represents the International Federation of Information Processing (IFIP) in the health informatics field to such organizations as the World Health Organization (WHO), the World Medical Association, and at world conferences such as the Alma Ata WHO/UNICEF conferences on primary healthcare. Finally, IMIA disseminates knowledge by means of publications, particularly the IMIA Year Book, now on a CD, and distribution of Medinfo and working conference proceedings. Additional information is available from the IMIA web site (http://www.imia.org).

In the fall of 1982, following an IMIA-sponsored working conference on the impact of computers on nursing, the IMIA general assembly accepted the proposal that an international working group on nursing be formed (see Chapter 3). Working Group 8 provides an international focus for activity in nursing informatics and an international core of interested and committed people who work toward implementing IMIA objectives regarding nursing. In 1985, the first meeting of this group was held in Calgary, Canada. The working group organizes an international symposium at 3-year intervals. Each symposium produces a volume of proceedings to provide the widest possible distribution of the information presented at the meeting. Information on the special interest group and its nursing informatics symposia can be found on their Web site at http://www.gl.umbc.edu/~abbott/nurseinfo.html.

Nursing Professional Organizations

The second type of membership that nurses interested in healthcare computing should maintain is their affiliation with the nursing professional associations. The importance of this type of membership is in the obligation of professionals to share their expertise and knowledge with colleagues. The banding together of nurses with expertise in nursing informatics in national nursing organizations raises other members' awareness of this aspect of nursing. It also provides a contact point for nurses desiring to expand their knowledge in this area.

The Canadian Nursing Informatics Association (CNIA, 2005) (http://www.cnia.ca) is the culmination of efforts to catalyze the emergence of a new national association of nurse informaticians. Its mission is to be the voice for nursing informatics in Canada. The goals of CNIA are as follows.

- To provide nursing leadership for the development of nursing/health informatics in Canada
- To establish national networking opportunities for nurse informaticians
- To facilitate informatics educational opportunities for all nurses in Canada
- To engage in international nursing informatics initiatives
- To act as a nursing advisory group in matters of nursing and health informatics
- To expand awareness of nursing informatics to all nurses and the healthcare community

CNIA is associated with COACH through a strategic alliance that enables CNIA to represent Canadian nurses in the IMIA Nursing Informatics Working Group (see below). CNIA also holds affiliate group status with the Canadian Nurses Association.

Another example of this second type of organization is CARING—also known as the Capital Area Roundtable on Informatics in Nursing. CARING has been based in the Washington, DC area for more than 22 years. It is the most geographically dispersed national nursing informatics group, with nearly 1000 members in 50 states and 16 countries, and is active in promoting education, networking, and job opportunities (Newbold, 2004).

Recently CARING and 17 other organizations formed the Alliance in Nursing Informatics. This group is now developing its mission and objectives and will unite the various nursing informatics groups in the United States. It is planned that the focus is to be on political and research activities, which are underserved by the other individual groups.

The Nursing Informatics Collaboration Task Force (NICTF) was recently convened to provide a forum for regional and national nursing informatics groups that are working together to guide the design and lead the implementation of clinical systems. The task force was formed through the efforts of the Nursing Informatics Working Group of the AMIA, the professional nurses represented by the HIMSS, and the ANA. The NICTF, in one of its first joint efforts, provided testimony to the President's Information Technology Advisory Committee (PITAC) during an open meeting on April 13, 2004. Nurses represent the largest group of organized professionals in healthcare in the United States. Nurse informaticists are fulfilling a critical role in creating an effective healthcare information infrastructure, developing clinical nursing documentation and information systems, developing research agendas, and educating others in nursing informatics. The NICTF continues to expand its scope of activities following successful initiatives such as the nursing informatics symposium at Medinfo 2004 and participation in the 2005 annual HIMSS conference and exhibition.

Vendor-Sponsored User Groups

Practically all major vendors of software applications for healthcare encourage and support the establishment of formal organizations for users of their products. This type of affiliation facilitates the exchange of ideas and approaches among users of similar software applications. This practice also prevents duplication of effort related to experience with use of a particular software application. It also provides a forum for users to communicate with the vendor about changes or upgrades to the software. All of the major vendors vendor have such a group, such as Eclipsys Users Group with emphasis on Nursing (EUN), Cerner, and Siemens.

Summary

Nurses find professional organizations valuable for the positive impact they provide on the information processing aspects of their profession. Participation in three types of organizations—multidisciplinary, nursing, vendor-sponsored—is highly recommended.

This chapter considered the trend toward new roles for nurses as a result of the widespread use of computer-based enterprise health information systems. Without question, new roles for nurses will continue to develop. At the same time, the current role of the nurse is changing. The survival and advancement of the profession, however, depend on nurses abandoning their previous professional stance of passive reaction and adopting a new anticipatory, proactive position. Nursing must be prepared to exploit information technology fully and to participate actively in information management to advance the practice of nursing.

References

Ball, M.J., & Nelson, R. (eds.) (2004). *Consumer Informatics in a Cyber Healthy World*. New York: Springer-Verlag.

Ball, M.J., Douglas, J.V., & Hoehn, B.J. (1997). New challenges for nursing informatics. In: Gerdin, U., Tallberg, M., & Wainwright, P. (eds.) *Nursing Informatics: The Impact of Nursing Knowledge on Health Care Informatics.* Amsterdam: IOS Press, pp. 39–43.

Ball, M. J., Weaver, C., & Kiel, J. (Eds.). (2004). *Health Information Management Systems*. New York: Springer-Verlag.

Canadian Nursing Informatics Association (CNIA). (2005). http://www.cnia.ca (accessed February 7, 2005).

Dayhoff, R.E., & Siegel, E.L. (1998). Digital imaging within and among medical facilities. In: Kolodner, R.M. (ed.) *Computerizing Large Integrated Health Networks: The V.A. Experience.* New York: Springer-Verlag.

Haux, R. (1997). Aims and tasks of medical informatics. *International Journal of Biomedical Computing*, Joint Commission on the Accreditation of Healthcare Organizations available http://www.jcaho.org/.

Newbold, S.K. (1996). The informatics nurse and the certification process. *Computers in Nursing 14*(2):84–88.

Newbold, S.K. (2004). *CARING: An International Group for Informatics Nurses*. MedInfo 2004. San Francisco.

Parker, C.D., & Gassert, C. (1996). JCAHO's Management of information standards: the role of the informatics nurse specialist. *Journal of Nursing Administration 26*(6):13–15.

Singer, J.P. (1971). Hospital computer systems: Myths and realities. *Hospital Topics 4*(9), (January).

Zimmerman, K.L. (1995). Clinical imaging: Applications and implications for nursing. In: Ball, M.J., K.J. Hannah, S.K. Newbold, & J.V. Douglas, (eds.) *Nursing Informatics: Where Caring and Technology Meet, 2nd ed*. New York: Springer-Verlag, pp. 320–330.

Appendices

Appendix A
Generic Request for Proposal

We are pleased to offer the Request for Proposal in electronic format on the publisher's Web site, which can be found at **http: //springeronline.com/0-387-26096-X**.

XYZ Health Services

REQUEST FOR PROPOSAL

For an

Advanced Clinical Information System

Date

NOTE: Proposal Submittal Deadline: XYZ P.M., mm/dd/yyyy

Table of Contents

Appendix B
Nursing Informatics Special Interest Groups

Susan K. Newbold

Alliance for Nursing Informatics
Area: United States
Contact: Connie J Delaney (connie-delaney@uiowa.edu) or Joyce Sensmeier (JSensmeier@himss.org)

American Medical Informatics Association (AMIA)
4915 St Elmo Avenue, Suite 401
Bethesda, MD 20814 USA
1-301-657-1291
mail@amia2.amia.org

American Medical Informatics Association (AMIA) Nursing Informatics Working Group
(www.amia.org/working/ni/main.html)

American Nursing Informatics Association (ANIA)
(www.ania.org)

Australian Nursing Informatics Special Interest Group
Health Informatics Society Australia, Inc.
413 Lygon Street
East Brunswick, VIC Australia 3057
61-3-9388-0555, 61-3-9388-2086 (fax)
hisa@hisa.org.au

Brasilian Nursing Association Nursing Informatics Group at Brazilian Nursing Association (GEINE)
Contact: Heimar F. Marin (heimar@denf.epm.br) or Christine Cunha (icris@denf.epm.br)

British Computer Society Nursing Specialist Group
(See also NPIG)
(www.bcsnsg.org.uk)
Editor ITIN (editinnur@bcs.org.uk). Also treasurer.nsg@bcs.org.uk

Canadian Nursing Informatics Association (CNIA)
www.cnia.ca

Capital Area Roundtable on Informatics in Nursing (CARING)
www.caringonline.org

European Federation for Medical Informatics–WG 5 Nursing Informatics in Europe
www.nicecomputing.ch/nieurope/index.htm

Patrick Weber, Chair, IMIA representative (patrick.weber@nicecomputing.ch)
Paula M Procter, Vice Chair (p.procter@sheffield.ac.uk)
Denise Barnett, Secretary (101630.2751@compuserve.com)

Health Informatics New Zealand (HINZ)
www.hinz.org.nz
PO Box 32 515
Devonport, Auckland, NZ
admin@hinz.org.nz
Chairperson (chairperson@HINZ.org.nz)
Administration manager (secretary@hinz.org.nz)

Healthcare Informatics Society of Ireland Nursing Special Interest Group
www.hisi.ie/html/nursing.htm

Health Information and Management Systems Society (HIMSS)
HIMSS
230 East Ohio, Suite 600
Chicago, IL 60611, USA
1-312-664-4467 (tel); 1-312-664-6143 (fax)
himss@himss.org
See www.himss.org for the 41 chapters (www.himss.org/asp/chapters.asp)

International Medical Informatics Association (IMIA) Special Interest Group on Nursing Informatics (SIGNI)
(www.imia.org/ni/index.html)

IMIA NI Education Working Group (http://welcome.to/imia-ni-education)

IMIA-SIG-NI WG on Open Source Nursing Informatics
(www.osni.info/html/index.php)

National League for Nursing
61 Broadway, New York, NY 10006, USA
1-800-669-1656, 1-212-363-5555
nlninform@nln.org

National League for Nursing (NLN) Nursing Educational Technology Information Management Advisory Council (ETIMAC)
http://www.nln.org/aboutnln/AdvisoryCouncils_TaskGroups/etimac.htm

NURSINFO Hong Kong
Helen Sit Wing-Fun (sithwf@ha.org.hk)

Nursing Informatics Special Interest Group of the GMDS
The German Association of Medical Informatics, Biometry, and Epidemiology [Deutsche Gesellschaft fuer Medizinische Informatik, Biometrie und Epidemiologie (GMDS)]
Matthias Hinz, Vice Chairman of the NI SIG
Institute for Medical Informatics
Fetscherstrasse 74
D-01307 Dresden,
Germany hinz@imib.med.tu-dresden.de

Nursing Professions Informatics Group (NPIG)
United Kingdom
www.nhsia.nhs.uk/npig/

Perinatal Information Systems User Group (PISUG)
International
Debbie Aiton, PISUG President (DEBAITON@aol.com)

Spanish Society of Nursing Informatics and Internet (SEEI)

http://www.seei.es
seei@seei.es

Swiss Special Interest Group Nursing Informatics (SIG-NI)
Patrick Van Gele (pvangele@chuv.hospvd.ch)

Appendix C
Sources of Additional Healthcare Informatics Information

Books and Internet

American Nurses Association. (2001). Scope and Standards of Nursing Informatics Practice. Washington, DC: ANA.

Androwich, I.M., Bickford, C.J., & Button, P.S. et al. (2003). Clinical Information Systems: A Framework for Reaching the Vision. Washington, DC: American Nurses Association.

American Nurses Association. (2005) Informatics Certification Examination Information (www.nursingworld.org/ancc/certification/cert/exams/TCOs/BSN27_Infor_TCO.html).

Ball, M.J., Hannah, K.J., Newbold, S.K., & Douglas, J.V. (eds) (2000). Nursing Informatics: Where caring and technology meet, 3rd ed. New York: Springer. See the entire series of Healthcare Informatics books by Springer. (www.springeronline.com).

Womack, D., Newbold, S.K., Staugaitis, H., & Cunningham, B. (2004). Technology's role in addressing the nursing shortage: innovations and examples. (http://maryland.nursetech.com/F/NT/MD/NursingInnovations2004.pdf).

Journals and Magazines

Advance for Health Informatics Executives
ADVANCE Newsmagazines/
Merion Publications, Inc.
2900 Horizon Drive
King of Prussia,
PA 19406
Tel. 800-355-5627
subscribe@merion.com

Advance for Health Information Professionals
ADVANCE Newsmagazines/
Merion Publications, Inc.

2900 Horizon Drive
King of Prussia, PA 19406
Tel. 800-355-5627
subscribe@merion.com

The British Journal of Healthcare Computing & Information Management
Tel. +44 1932 821723; Fax +44 1932 820305
subscriptions@bjhcinfo.demon.co.uk

CIN: Computers Informatics in Nursing
Lippincott Williams & Wilkins
PO Box 1620
Hagerstown MD 21741
Tel. 1-800-638-3030 or 1-301-223-2300

Health Informatics Journal
Sage Publications
2455 Teller Road
Thousand Oaks, CA 91320
Tel. 805-499-9774 or 800-818-7243; Fax 805-499-0871 or 800-583-2665

Journal of AHIMA
233 N. Michigan Avenue, Suite 2150
Chicago, IL 60601-5800
Tel. (312) 233-1100
journal@ahima.org

Journal of the American Medical Informatics Association (JAMIA)
Hanley & Belfus, Inc.
Customer Services Department
6277 Sea Harbor Drive
Orlando, FL 32887-4800
Tel. 800 654-2452 Toll-free (U.S. and Canada); 407-345-4000 (outside the U.S. and Canada); 407-363-9661
elspcs@elsevier.com

JHIM: Journal of Healthcare Information Management
230 East Ohio Street, Suite 500
Chicago, IL 60611-3269
Tel. 312-664-4467; Fax 312-664-6143
www.himss.org

Healthcare Informatics
4530 West 77th Street, Suite 300
Minneapolis, MN 55435
Tel. 612-835-3222

Health Data Management
118 South Clinton Street, Suite 700
Chicago, IL 60661-3628
Tel. 312-648-0261

Health Management Technology
Nelson Publishing/Health Management Technology
2500 Tamiami Trail North
Nokomis, FL 34275
Tel. 941-966-9521

Hospitals & Health Networks
737 North Michigan Avenue
Chicago, IL 60611-2615
Tel. 312-440-6800
http://www.hhnmag.com/hhnmag/index.jsp

Modern Healthcare
360 N. Michigan Avenue, 5th Floor
Chicago, IL 60601-3806
Tel. 312-649-5350 or
312-649-5297

Nursing Education Perspectives
61 Broadway
New York, NY 10006
Tel. 800-669-1656 or 212-363-5555

Nursing Economic$
Anthony J. Jannetti, Inc.
East Holly Avenue, Box 56
Pitman, NJ 08071-0056
Tel. 856-256-2300;
Fax 856-589-7463

Nursing Management
Lippincott Williams & Wilkins
PO Box 1620
Hagerstown, MD 21741
Tel. 1-800-638-3030 or
1-301-223-2300

Appendix D
Professional Societies

American Academy of Nursing
555 East Wells Street, 11th Floor
Milwaukee, WI 53202-3823
Tel. 414-287-0289; Fax 414-276-3349
info@AANnet.org

American Association of Colleges of Nursing
One Dupont Circle NW, Suite 530
Washington, DC 20036
Tel. 202-463-6930
http://www.aacn.nche.edu

American Medical Informatics Association (AMIA)
Nursing Informatics Working Group
4915 St. Elmo Avenue, Suite 401
Bethesda, MD 20814
Tel. 301-657-1291
http://www.amia.org

American Nurses Association Council on Nursing Services and Informatics
America Nurses Association
600 Maryland Avenue, Suite 100 West, SW
Washington, DC 20024-2571
Tel. 202-651-7000
http://www.ana.org

Canadian Organization for the Advancement of Computers in Health (COACH)
2 Carlton Street, Suite 1304
Toronto, Ontario M5B 1J3, Canada
Tel. 416-979-5551
http://www.coachorg.com

Healthcare Information and Management Systems Society (HIMSS)
230 East Ohio Street, Suite 600
Chicago, IL 60611-3201
Tel. 312-664-44677
http://www.himss.org

IEEE Computer Society
1730 Massachusetts Avenue NW
Washington, DC 20036
Tel. 202-371-0101
http://www.iccad.com/ieee.html or http://www.computer.org/

International Medical Informatics Association (IMIA)
Nursing Informatics Special Interest Group
Ulla Gerdin, RN, Chair
Swedish Institute for Health Services Development (SPRI)

Box 70487
Stockholm, Sweden
Tel. 011-46-8-702-4600
ulla.gerdin@spri.se
http://www.imia.org

Medical Group Management Association
104 Inverness Terrace East
Englewood, CO 80112
Tel. 303-799-1111
http://www.mgma.com

Midwest Nursing Research Society (MNRS)
10200 W. 44th Avenue, Suite 304
Wheat Ridge, CO 80033
Tel. 720-898-4831
http://www.mnrs.org/

National Institute of Nursing Research
31 Center Drive, Room 5B09, MSC 2178
Bethesda, MD 20892-2178
http://www.nih.gov/ninr/

National League for Nursing Council on Nursing Informatics
National League for Nursing
61 Broadway
New York, NY 10006
Tel. 800-669-1656 or 212-363-5555
http://www.nln.org
nlninform@n/n.org

Sigma Theta Tau International
Honor Society of Nursing
550 West North Street
Indianapolis, IN 46202
Tel. 317-634-8171
http://www.nursingsociety.org/

Society for Medical Decision Making
1211 Locust Street
Philadelphia, PA 19107
Tel. 215-545-7697; Fax 215-545-8107
http://www.smdm.org

Appendix E
Academic Informatics Programs Worldwide

Programs in the United States

Arizona School of Health Sciences (Mesa, Arizona)

Centers for Disease Control (Atlanta, GA)
Public Health Informatics Fellowship Program (Epidemiology Program Office)

Cleveland Clinic (Cleveland, OH)
Medical Informatics Fellowship (Division of Medicine/ Department of General Internal Medicine)

College of St. Scholastica (Duluth, MN)
Health Informatics

Columbia University (New York, NY)
Dental Informatics, School of Dental and Oral Surgery

Columbia University (New York, NY)
Medical Informatics (Graduate School of Arts and Sciences)

Dalhousie University (Halifax, Nova Scotia, Canada)

Drexel University (Philadelphia, PA)
Institute for Healthcare Informatics (College of Information Science and Technology)

Duke University (Durham, NC)
Clinical Informatics (Department of Community and Family Medicine, Division of Medical Informatics)

Duke University (Durham, NC)
Nursing Informatics (School of Nursing)

East Carolina University (Greenville, NC)
The Brody School of Medicine, Telemedicine Center, Advanced Telemedicine Training

Eastern University (St. Davids, PA)
School of Professional Studies, Nursing Informatics Certificate Program

Emory University (Atlanta, GA)
Department of Biostatistics, MSPH Program in Public Health Informatics

Excelsior College (Albany, NY)
Clinical Systems Management/Healthcare Informatics (Graduate and Certificate Programs in Nursing and Allied Health)

George Mason University (Fairfax, VA)
School of Computational Sciences (Bioinformatics Programs)

George Washington University Medical Center (Washington, DC)
School of Public Health and Health Services

**Harvard Medical School* (Boston, MA)
Center for Clinical Computing, Beth Israel Deaconess Medical Center; *Brigham & Women's Hospital/Harvard Medical School*, Decision Systems Group, Brigham and Women's Hospital; *Massachusetts General Hospital/ Harvard Medical School*, Laboratory of Computer Science, Massachusetts General Hospital

Indiana University
Indianapolis, IN
School of Informatics-Bioinformatics/Chemical Informatics/Human-Computer Interaction

---

* Harvard-MIT-NEMC Research Training Program,
Joint Division of Health Sciences & Technology:

Decision Systems Group, Brigham and Women's Hospital
Children's Hospital Informatics Program, Childrens Hospital Medical Center
Center for Clinical Computing, Beth Israel Deaconess Medical Center
Laboratory of Computer Science, Massachusetts General Hospital
Division of Clinical Decision Making, Informatics and Telemedicine, New England Medical Center
Medical Computer Science, Massachusetts Institute of Technology

Massachusetts Institute of Technology (Cambridge, MA)
Clinical Decision Making Group
Laboratory for Computer Science/Harvard-MIT Division of Health Sciences and Technology

Medical College of Wisconsin and the Milwaukee School of Engineering (Milwaukee, WI)
Medical Informatics

Montana Tech/University of Montana (Butte, Montana)
Medical Informatics
College of Math and Sciences

Mount Sinai-NYU Health System (New York, NY)
Medical Informatics
Division of Clinical Informatics Mount Sinai-NYU Health System IT and Center for Medical Informatics, Department of Medicine, Mount Sinai

National Library of Medicine (Bethesda, MD)
Medical Informatics Training Program
Lister Hill National Center for Biomedical Communications

New England Medical Center/Tufts University (Boston, MA)
Division of Clinical Decision Making, Informatics, and Telemedicine, Department of Medicine

New York University (New York, NY)
Nursing Informatics
Division of Nursing

Oregon Health and Science University (Portland, OR)
Department of Medical Informatics & Clinical Epidemiology, School of Medicine and Biomedical Information Communications Center

Philadelphia VA Center for Health Equity Research and Promotion (CHERP) (Philadelphia, PA)
Medical Informatics Fellowship

Regenstrief Institute for Healthcare (Indianapolis, IN)
Medical Informatics Fellowship
Indiana University School of Medicine

Saint Louis University (St. Louis, MO)
Nursing Informatics
School of Nursing

Stanford University (Stanford, CA)
Stanford Medical Informatics
School of Medicine

State University of New York (Brooklyn, NY)
Medical Informatics

University of Alabama at Birmingham (Birmingham, AL)
Health Informatics Program
Department of Health Services Administration

University of Arizona (Tucson, AZ)
Systems Management/Informatics
College of Nursing

University of California–Davis (Davis, CA)
Medical Informatics
School of Medicine

University of California–Irvine (Irvine, CA)
Informatics in Biology and Medicine
Department of Information & Computer Science

University of California–San Francisco (San Francisco, CA)
Biological and Medical Informatics

University of Colorado Health Sciences Center (Denver, CO)
Healthcare Informatics
School of Nursing

University of Illinois at Chicago (Chicago, IL)
Biomedical and Health Information Sciences
College of Applied Health Sciences

University of Illinois at Chicago (Chicago, IL)
School of Public Health

University of Iowa (Iowa City, IA)
Nursing Informatics
College of Nursing

University of Maryland (Baltimore, MD)
Nursing Informatics
School of Nursing

University of Medicine and Dentistry in New Jersey (Newark, NJ)
Biomedical Informatics
School of Health Related Professions

University of Miami (Miami, FL)
Medical Informatics

University of Michigan (Ann Arbor, MI)
School of Dentistry

University of Michigan Health Center (Ann Arbor, MI)
Department of Pharmacy Services

University of Minnesota (Minneapolis, MN)
Health Informatics
Division of Health Computer Sciences

University of Missouri (Columbia, MO)
Health Management and Informatics
School of Medicine

University of Nebraska Medical Center (Omaha, NE)
College of Nursing

University of New Mexico (Albuquerque, NM)
Health Sciences Library and Informatics Center

University of North Carolina (Chapel Hill, NC)
Division of Medical Computing and Informatics
School of Medicine, Biomedical Engineering

University of Pittsburgh (Pittsburgh, PA)
Pittsburgh Biomedical Informatics Training Program
Nursing Informatics
Dental Informatics

University of South Florida (Tampa, FL)
College of Nursing

University of Texas Houston Health Science Center (Houston, TX)
Health Informatics
School of Health Information Sciences

University of Utah (Salt Lake City, UT)
Department of Medical Informatics, School of Medicine

University of Utah (Salt Lake City, UT)
Clinical Informatics
College of Nursing

University of Victoria (Victoria, BC, Canada)
Health Information Science
School of Health Information Science

University of Virginia (Charlottesville, VA)
Health Evaluation Sciences

University of Washington (Seattle, WA)
Department of Medical Education and Biomedical Informatics, Division of Biomedical & Health Informatics

University of Wisconsin (Madison, WI)
Department of Biostatistics & Medical Informatics
Medical School

Vanderbilt University (Nashville, TN)
Bioinformatics Programming
Vanderbilt University Medical Center

Yale University (New Haven, CT)
Center for Medical Informatics, School of Medicine

Programs Outside the United States

Australia

University of New South Wales
Sydney, Australia
Master of Health Informatics
Degrees available: Masters (available from 2004), PhD in Health Informatics

University of Tasmania
Launceston, Australia
Department of Rural Health
Graduate program in E-Health (Health Informatics)
Degrees available: graduate certificate, graduate diploma

University of Wollongong
Wollongong NSW, Australia
Master of Health Informatics

Austria

University for Health Informatics and Technology Tyrol (UMIT)
Innsbruck, Austria
Medical Informatics
Degrees available: BSc in Medical Informatics, MSc in Medical Informatics, PhD in Medical Informatics

Brazil

Marilia Medical School
Marilla, Estate of Sao Paulo, Brazil Medical course: undergraduate

Universidade Federal de Pernambuco (UFPE)
Grupo de Tecnologias da Informação em Saúde (TIS)
Health Information Technology Group
Recife-PE, Brazil
Undergraduate course: lessons for the medical course and others health courses
Postgraduate courses: internal medicine master's program, informatics master's program

Canada

Dalhousie University
Halifax, Nova Scotia, Canada
Degree available: Master of Science (MSc)

University of Victoria
Victoria, British Columbia, Canada
Health Information Science
Degrees available: Bachelor of Science (BSc), Master of Science (MSc), PhD (by special arrangement)

University of Waterloo
Waterloo, Ontario, Canada
Education Program for Health Informatics Professionals (EPHIP)
Certificate program: online/distance education programs

Cuba

Instituto Superior de Ciencias Médicas de La Habana (ISCM-H)
La Habana, Cuba
Degree available: Master's in Health Informatics

Germany

Georg-August-University Goettingen
Applied Informatics/Health Information Officer
Goettingen, Germany
Degrees available: BSc, MSc in Medical Informatics

University of Essen
Essen, Germany
Medizin-Management with Informatics specialization
Degrees Available: Bachelor of Arts (BA), Master's (soon)

University at Leipzig/Germany
Leipzig, Germany
Institute for Formal Ontology and Medical Informationscience (IFOMIS)

Greece

National and Kapodistrian University of Athens
Athens, Greece
Health Informatics
Degrees available: Master of Science (MSc), Doctorate (PhD)

Ireland

Trinity College Dublin
Dublin, Ireland
Degree available: MSc in Health Informatics

The Netherlands

University of Amsterdam
Amsterdam, The Netherlands
Medical Information Sciences
Degrees available: Bachelor's and Master's

Peru

Instituto de Medicine Tropical Alexander Von Humbold
Universidad Peruana Cayetano Heredai
Lima, Peru
Specialized programs: Health Informatics, Telemedicine, Artificial Intelligence

United Kingdom

Centre for Health Informatics and Multiprofessional Education (CHIME)
London, UK
Degrees available: MPhil, PhD available by research in this area

Imperial College
London, United Kingdom
Degrees available: MSc in Health Informatics and Management

King Alfred's Winchester
Winchester, UK
Degrees available: Master of Science (MSc)

University College London
London, UK
Degrees available: Master of Science (MSc); diploma and certificate programs in health informatics; Graduate program (3 exit points); PG certificate; PG diploma; MSc

University of Edinburgh
Edinburgh, UK
School of Informatics, Specialism in Bioinformatics
Degrees available: Master of Science (MSc), Master's (Mres), Doctorate (PhD)

University of Sheffield
Sheffield, UK
Degrees available: certificate diploma, Master of Science (MSc), MPhil and PhD available by research in this area

University of Wales Swansea
Swansea, Wales, UK
School of Health Science, Centre for eHealth and Learning

Appendix F
Transforming Clinical Documentation: Preparing Nursing for Change

Linda Dietrich

Preplanning for Nurse Executives

- Changing an existing documentation system requires careful and deliberate planning.
- The following points must be considered when an organization changes its system. It is important to ask: What are the *reasons* we are changing the documentation system?
  1. The need to improve the quality of nursing documentation requires not only new or revised tools but also new ways of thinking. What is written contains the judgment of the writer, including analysis and evaluation.
  2. The need to reduce the amount of time in charting is critical. A charting approach that reduces the amount of time spent on charting is essential.
  3. The need to contain costs requires nurses to reexamine their documentation practices and be more efficient as well as improve any reimbursement issues related to documentation.
  4. The need to reduce duplication is essential.
  5. The emphasis on multidisciplinary care is vital, as is and the need to ensure that patients are not asked the same questions by different providers.
  6. Increasing emphasis on patient outcomes has necessitated a change in the content of nursing documentation. Care planning has taken on many forms, focusing on critical paths, care maps, and clinical pathways.
- Before making any changes in a documentation system you must first determine the desired outcome. Deciding on the desired outcome of the change directs the planning and implementation process. In addition to the above reasons to consider, the following are outcomes to

consider in conjunction with the reasons to change a documentation system.

Outcomes

1. The chart is legally sound.
2. The chart reflects the nursing process.
3. The chart describes the patient's ongoing status from shift to shift.
4. The plan of care and chart complement each other.
5. The documentation system is designed to facilitate retrieval of information for qualitively improving activities and research.
6. The documentation system supports the staffing mix and acuity levels in the current healthcare setting.

- The purpose of nursing documentation is to provide evidence that all established standards have been met. It is incumbent upon those preparing and establishing documentation systems to see that it meets statutory, regulatory, and common law as well as voluntary standards.
- Certain sources that should be consulted when designing any nursing documentation system.

1. Legal requirements
   Code of Federal Regulations
   State nurse practice acts
   State administrative codes
   Municipal codes
   Case law
   Agency legal counsel
2. Accreditation standards
   Joint Commission on Accreditation of Healthcare Organizations
   Federal health insurance program (Medicare)
   State health insurance program (Medicaid)
   Third party payers (HMOs, private insurance)
   Peer review organizations
   Federal grant agencies
3. Professional standards
   Nursing—A Social Policy Statement
   American Nurses Association—Standards of Clinical Nursing Practice (latest edition)
   National Specialty nursing associations standards of practice
   ANA Code for Nurses
   Professional literature
   National practice guidelines (AHCPR)
4. Institutional requirements
   Policies and procedures

Issues Surrounding Standardized Languages: Definition of Terms

Classification: a systematic arrangement of classes; a structural framework arranged according to similar groups
Database: A collection of interrelated files with records organized and stored together in a computer system
Data set: A collection of related data items; a directory
Data element: the smallest unit of data that has meaning without interpretation; a raw fact, material, or observation.
Language: in computing and communications, a set of characters (symbols, alphabets, codes, syntax), conventions, and rules used to convey ideas and information
Nomenclature and vocabulary: a consistent method for assigning names to elements of a system
Nursing minimum data set: an essential set of information items that have uniform definitions and categories concerned with nursing. Its purpose is to meet the informational needs of nurses in any care delivery setting through the healthcare system as well as other professionals and researchers.
Taxonomy: a method for classifying a vocabulary of terms for a specific topic according to specific laws or principles

Regarding standardized languages of NIC (interventions), NOC (outcomes), NANDA (diagnoses), and SNOMED. Remember that all of these are nomenclatures. They are not evidence-based standards that drive care. They are not documentation systems. They are not plans of care. They contribute to how you decide to orchestrate these elements in your plan of care for patients. They are not acuity systems or staff assignment systems.

There are other nomenclature initiatives (both nursing-related and non-nursing-related) that are not listed here. One example is the electronic health records (EHR) functional standards initiative, currently being led by the EHR Technical Committee (EHRTC). The goal of this initiative is to further the HL7 mission of designing standards that support the exchange of information for clinical decisions and treatments and to help lay the groundwork for nationwide interoperability by providing common language parameters that can be used to develop systems that support electronic records (http://www.hl7.org/EHR/).

General Questions for a "Preparing for Planning" Session

1. Scope—How many people and what areas/organizations do they represent?
2. What are your objectives in convening this group?

3. What are the outcomes you want to achieve at the end of this meeting?
4. Can a meeting be set up with the participants ahead of time to discuss briefly their expectations about the outcomes of the planning meeting and where they are currently with their thinking?
5. How many types of information systems (estimate) are in place already?
6. How many are undergoing a selection process?
7. Is your organization's clinical documentation system a necessary evil or a strategic asset?
8. Philosophy of management—Do any of these organizations have shared decision-making models in place?
9. What types of documentation systems are currently in place in these organizations? Narrative, charting by exception, critical paths, standardized care plans, collaborative protocols?
10. Reasons and outcomes—Are any of these more compelling than others? For example, many states want reports on nurse–patient ratios. Is this something you would expect from a nursing documentation system?
11. What are the learning needs of the group? Do you want them to do some prereading ahead of time? Can we do a quick learning needs assessment regarding their understanding of information technology and how it relates to patient care processes? Do you want them to develop a shared understanding of, for example:
    Information technology in healthcare—past and present high level
    Electronic health record—what is it, future considerations
    Clinical information systems

Thoughts on Clinical Documentation Automation for Leaders and Executives

Many executives talk about the potential benefits of automating clinical documentation. Frequently, the discussion is focused on calculating savings from reducing paper usage or reducing overtime. This approach does not take into account the breadth of benefits that automation can bring to healthcare organizations. Examples include the following.

- Prevention of complications
- Interdisciplinary integration at point of care
- Evidence-based practice patterns
- No duplications and repetitions
- Better patient outcomes
- Increased clinician job satisfaction
- Improved clinician recruitment and retention rates
- Decreased nursing overtime
- Fewer coding errors and omissions

Guidelines for Success

Lead the Charge and Stay Involved

If you believe in the quality, satisfaction, and financial benefits of automating clinical documentation, you must lead the implementation effort and stay involved in the process to the end. Staying involved is important because it takes a lot of time and effort to automate an clinical documentation system in the right way. Do not let the process slow down or stray from the stated goals.

State Your Goals Clearly

Your goals for automation should be aligned with your organization's strategic goals to ensure that everyone in your organization is pulling in the same direction. State your organization's goals for automation clearly, so you can recognize success when the goals are achieved.

- Would you like to prevent complications and reduce variability?
- Stop duplication and redundancy?
- Increase clinician retention?
- Improve patient outcomes?
- Reduce nursing overtime?
- All of the above?

Make Sure Your Clinicians Own the System

The clinicians must drive automation of clinical documentation because they are the ones who will use it. The new system must improve their lives and reflect their needs and priorities, not those of the IT department. The clinicians are the customers. Challenge them to develop a system that improves documentation and thereby improves patient care outcomes, professional growth, and the caregivers' work lives. Do not let them automate the way they have "always done it" simply to stay within their comfort zone.

Choose the Right Vendor

Select a vendor whose systems support your organization's goals for automation. If your focus is acute care, choose a vendor that has developed systems for acute care units. Make sure the vendor's software functionality aligns with your goals. Your clinicians should be the focus—and have a major say—in selecting a vendor. Find a vendor who will be your partner.

An Enterprise-Wide or Departmental Solution

- Have you considered an enterprise-wide clinical information system that can be customized to meet departmental needs?
- Will departments be allowed to purchase department-specific systems?
- Most enterprise clinical information systems have an integrated "core" component consisting of physician order entry, clinical documentation, and a medication administration record. These elements may cover most of the clinical information system requirements, but some departments (e.g., obstetrics) have distinctive needs related to their particular devices and to the integration of data from these devices into a patient's record.

References

American Nurses Association. (2004). Nursing: Scope and Standards of Practice. Washington, D.C.: Nursebooks.org.

Burke, L.J., & Murphy, J. (1995). Charting by Exception Applications: Making It Work in Clinical Settings. Albany, N.Y.: Delmar, pp. 12203–5015.

Belmont, C., Wesorick, B., Jesse, H., Troseth, M., & Brown, D. (2003). Clinical Documentation. www.HCTProject.com.

Appendix G
Research Databases of Interest to Nurses

With the assistance of Helen Lee Robertson
and Lorraine Toews

ACP Journal Club (1991–present)

- More than 1100 structured abstracts of individual published articles from core clinical journals with expert commentary on clinical relevance of study
- Covers internal medicine, psychiatry, obstetrics/gynecology, pediatrics, surgery, family medicine, public health
- Electronic equivalent to print journals *ACP Journal Club* and *Evidence-Based Medicine*

AgeLINE (1978–present)

- Bibliographic references and abstracts related to aging and middle age from interdisciplinary perspectives of psychology, economics, sociology, gerontology, public policy, business, health and healthcare services, consumer issues
- Journal articles, books, book chapters, reports, government documents
- Journal coverage includes research, professional and general interest titles
- Available at no charge from http://research.aarp.org/ageline/home.html

Alt-Health Watch (1990–present)

- Focuses on the many perspectives of complementary, holistic, and integrated approaches to healthcare and wellness
- Provides full text for articles from more than 140 international and often peer-reviewed journals, reports, and proceedings, as well as association and consumer newsletters
- Also includes pamphlets, booklets, special reports, original research, and book excerpts

AMED (Allied and Complementary Medicine Database) (1985–present)

- Bibliographic citations and abstracts covering journals in complementary medicine, physiotherapy, occupational therapy, rehabilitation, podiatry, palliative care
- Produced by the Healthcare Information Service of the British Library

- Each record includes controlled indexing terms using the *AMED Thesaurus* based on *MeSH* (MEDLINE indexing terms)

BioMed Central (2001–present)

- An independent publishing house committed to providing immediate free access to peer-reviewed biomedical research with all research articles in journals published by BioMed Central immediately and permanently available on-line without charge
- More than 100 searchable peer reviewed research journals covering general to specialist biomedical sciences, including nursing
- Available at no charge from http://www.biomedcentral.com/

CINAHL (Cumulative Index to Nursing & Allied Health) (1982–present)

- Covers the literature related to nursing and allied health
- Indexes most English-language nursing publications, primary journals in allied health fields and selected consumer health, and biomedicine journals
- Journal articles, book chapters, dissertations, proceedings, standards of practice
- Most of CINAHL's 11,000 subject headings adapted from MEDLINE's MeSH but are supplemented with more than 2000 nursing/allied health-specific headings
- More than 800,000 citations

Cochrane Database of Systematic Reviews (1991–present)

- More than 1500 regularly updated systematic reviews of primary clinical research studies prepared by the Cochrane Collaboration
- Two types: completed reviews and protocols for reviews currently being prepared
- Abstracts available at no charge from http://www.update-software.com/publications/Cochrane/

Database of Abstracts of Reviews of Effectiveness (DARE)

- Prepared by the National Health Services' Centre for Reviews and Dissemination (NHS CRD) at the University of York (UK)
- Full text structured abstracts (summaries) of systematic reviews from a variety of medical journals about the effects of interventions, each summary providing a critical commentary on the quality of the review
- Covers diagnosis, prevention, rehabilitation, screening, and treatment
- Available at no charge from http://www.york.ac.uk/inst/crd/darehp.htm

Dissertation Abstracts (1861–present)

- Searchable database listing doctoral dissertations and selected Masters theses from accredited North American degree-granting institutions
- Abstracts included for Doctoral records since 1980 and Master's since 1988
- Contains more than 1.8 million records

EMBASE (Excerpta Medica) (1980–present)

- Major biomedical and pharmaceutical database indexing more than 3500 international journals—European emphasis
- Covers drug research, pharmacology, toxicology, clinical and experimental human medicine, health policy and management, public health, occupational health, environmental health, drug dependence and abuse, psychiatry, forensic medicine
- Selective coverage for nursing, dentistry, veterinary medicine, psychology, and alternative medicine
- Uses the *EMTREE* controlled thesaurus
- More than 8 million citations and abstracts

ERIC (Education Resources Information Center) (1966–2003)

- The world's premier database of journal and nonjournal education literature
- Sponsored by the Institute of Education Sciences (IES) of the U.S. Department of Education
- Contains more than 1.1 million citations, including more than 107,000 full text nonjournal documents
- Available at no charge from http://www.eric.ed.gov/

Health and Psychosocial Instruments (HaPI) (1985–present)

- Indexes information on measurement instruments (i.e., questionnaires, interview schedules, checklists, index measures, coding schemes, manuals, rating scales, tests) in the fields of healthcare, psychosocial sciences, and organizational behavior
- More than two-thirds of tools cover medical and nursing areas such as pain measurement, quality of life assessment, and drug efficacy evaluation
- Records from the Behavioral Measurement Database Services (BMDS)
- Contains more than 105,000 records

IngentaConnect

- Comprehensive, interdisciplinary keyword-searchable collection of academic and professional research articles
- More than 17 million citations from 28,000 publications, including 6100 on-line
- Online and offline access to the full text of electronic articles available through online purchase or through subscriptions via Ingenta
- Free searching available from http://www.ingentaconnect.com/

International Bibliographic Information on Dietary Supplements (IBIDS) (1986–present)

- Collaboration between the U.S. National Institutes of Health (NIH) and the U.S. Department of Agriculture (USDA) providing citations and

abstracts from the published international and scientific literature on dietary supplements
- More than 730,000 citations from four major database sources: biomedical-related articles from MEDLINE; botanical and agricultural science from AGRICOLA; worldwide agricultural literature through AGRIS; and selected nutrition journals from CAB Abstracts and CAB Health
- Covers the use of supplements in human nutrition, fortification of foods, nutrient composition of herbal and botanical products, population surveys on dietary supplement use, the growth and production of herbal and botanical products
- Available at no charge from http://dietary-supplements.info.nih.gov/Health_Information/IBIDS.aspx

International Pharmaceutical Abstracts (IPA) (1970–present)

- International coverage to the world pharmacy literature; related health, medical, cosmetic journals, and state pharmacy journals; abstracts of presentations at major pharmacy meetings
- Topics covered: drug therapy, toxicity, and pharmacy practice as well as legislation, regulation, technology, utilization, biopharmaceutics, information processing, education, economics, and ethics
- Contains more than 350,000 records, including 10,000 references to alternative and herbal medicine
- Produced in cooperation with the American Society of Health-System Pharmacists International

MEDLINE (1966–present)

- Major English-language biomedical database produced by the U.S. National Library of Medicine (NLM) covering medicine, nursing, dentistry, veterinary medicine, allied health and preclinical sciences
- More than 12 million bibliographic citations and author abstracts from more than 4800 biomedical journals
- Uses *MeSH* (Medical Subject Headings), a hierarchical, controlled vocabulary thesaurus of biomedical terms for indexing
- Electronic counterpart to *Index Medicus*, *Index to Dental Literature*, and the *International Nursing Index*

NIOSHTIC-2

- Bibliographic database of occupational safety and health publications, documents, grant reports, and other communication products
- Supported by the National Institute for Occupational Safety and Health (NIOSH)
- Available at no charge from http://www.cdc.gov/niosh/srchpage.html

NLM Gateway

- Allows users to search in multiple retrieval systems at the NLM

- Searches MEDLINE/PubMed, TOXLINE Special (toxicology references), NLM Catalog, MedlinePlus (consumer health), ClinicalTrials.gov (clinical research studies), DIRLINE (Directory of Health Orgs), Genetics Home Reference (genetic conditions and genes), Meeting Abstracts, HSRProj (Health Services Research Projects in Progress), OMIM (Online Mendelian Inheritance in Man), and HSDB (Hazardous Substances Data Bank)
- Available at no charge from http://gateway.nlm.nih.gov/gw/Cmd

POPLINE (POPulation information onLINE) (1970–present)

- World's largest database on reproductive health, population, family planning, and related health issues
- More than 300,000 citations with abstracts to scientific articles, reports, books, and unpublished reports
- Includes links to free, full-text documents; the ability to limit searches to peer-reviewed journal articles, and many abstracts in French and Spanish
- Maintained by the Johns Hopkins Bloomberg School of Public Health/Center for Communication Programs
- Available at no charge from http://db.jhuccp.org/popinform/basic.html

PsycINFO (1967–present)

- Bibliographic database that provides abstracts and citations to the scholarly, predominantly English-language literature in the behavioral sciences and mental health
- Indexes nearly 2000 peer-reviewed journals; also books, dissertations, and other secondary publications
- More than 2 million records, including historical records back to the 1800s
- Controlled vocabulary indexing using the *Thesaurus of Psychological Index Terms*

PubMed (1950s–present)

- Developed by the U.S. National Center for Biotechnology Information (NCBI) at the NLM
- More than 15 million citations, including MEDLINE, OLDMEDLINE, "in process," and "as supplied by publisher" citations
- Includes links to sites providing full-text content, some of which is available at no charge
- Available at no charge from http://pubmed.gov

REHABDATA (1956–present)

- Produced by the U.S. National Rehabilitation Information Center
- Contains approximately 69,000 abstracts of books, reports, articles, and audiovisual materials relating to disability and rehabilitation research

- Each abstract includes bibliographic information, a 250-word abstract, and (when appropriate) information regarding the project that produced the document
- Available at no charge from http://www.naric.com/search/rhab/

Social Services Abstracts (1980–present)

- Provides bibliographic coverage of current research focused on social work, human services, and related areas, including social welfare, social policy, and community development
- Abstracts and indexes more than 1400 serial publications and includes abstracts of journal articles and dissertations and citations to book reviews
- Major areas of coverage include community and mental health services, crisis intervention, family and social welfare, gerontology, poverty and homelessness, social and health policy, support groups/networks, violence, abuse, neglect, and welfare services
- Contains almost 100,000 records

Sociological Abstracts (1963–present)

- Abstracts and indexes the international literature in sociology and related disciplines in the social and behavioral sciences
- It provides abstracts of journal articles and citations to book reviews drawn from more than 1800 serial publications and provides abstracts of books, book chapters, dissertations, and conference papers.
- Major areas of coverage include culture and social structure, evaluation research, family and social welfare, rural and urban sociology, social psychology and group interaction, studies in violence and power, substance abuse and addiction, and women's studies.
- It contains approximately 620,000 records.

Web of Science

- Web interface to the ISI citation databases, *Science Citation Index* (1945–present), *Social Sciences Citation Index* (1956–present), *Arts & Humanities Citation Index* (1975–present)
- Covers 8700 of the most prestigious, high-impact research journals in the world
- Includes searchable references to citations in the articles
- Can navigate backward using "cited references" to follow an author's prior influences and forward using "times cited" to track the work's impact on current research

Websites of Interest for Nursing Research

- Canadian Health Services Research Foundation (CHSRF) http://www.chsrf.ca/home_e.php
  - The CHSRF is an independent, not-for-profit corporation, established with endowed funds from the Canadian federal government. It promotes

and funds management and policy research in health services and nursing.
  - The site has information on research funding, research in progress, research reports, and knowledge transfer.

- Canadian Institutes of Health Research (CIHR)
  http://www.cihr-irsc.gc.ca/e/193.html
  - Canada's premier health research funding agency website, it has information on health research funding, knowledge translation, institute publications, and partnerships.

- National Institute of Nursing Research (USA)
  http://ninr.nih.gov/ninr/
  - The U.S. National Institute of Nursing Research, one of the 25 institutes and centers within the National Institutes of Health, has information on research funding and programs and news and links to related nursing organizations.

- National Institutes of Health: Scientific Resources (USA)
  http://www.nih.gov/science/
  - This subsection of the NIH website provides information on intramural research, special interest groups, library catalogs, journals, training, laboratories, scientific computing, and more.

Glossary

Acoustic coupler: A specific type of modem which uses the standard telephone set.

A/D: Analog-to-digital converter.

Analog: A computer that compares and measures one quantity with another.

ANSI: American National Standards Institute

Application program: A computer program written to solve a specific problem or perform a specific task.

Architecture: The art and science of designing and erecting buildings. Buildings and other large structures: the low brick and adobe architecture of the Southwest. A style and method of design and construction: Byzantine architecture. Orderly arrangement of parts; structure: the architecture of the federal bureaucracy; the broad architecture of a massive novel; computer architecture.

Arithmetic logic unit (ALU): Internal part of computer (found in CPU) that performs the arithmetic computations.

ASCII: American Standard Code of Information Interchange.

Assembly language: A hardware dependent symbolic language, usually characterized by a one-to-one correspondence of its statements with machine language instructions.

Auxiliary storage: Data storage other than main memory, such as that on a disk storage unit.

Backup: A duplicate copy of a file or program. Backups of material are made on disk or cassette in case something happens to the original.

Backup position listing: A list of personnel who can fill a given position, as well as alternate personnel who can fill the same position.

BASIC: Beginner's All-Purpose Symbolic Instruction Code. A popular computer language invented at Dartmouth for educational purposes. An easy-to-learn, easy-to-use language.

Batch processing: A mode of processing in which any program submitted to the computer is either run to completion or aborted. No interactive communication between program and user is possible.

Baud: Unit of measurement of transmission speed, equivalent to bits per second in serial transmission. Used by microcomputer.

Binary number system: Number system made up of the digits 0 and 1—"the language of the computer."

Bit: Binary digit (0 or 1).

Browser: A computer program which allows the user to search for data across the networks of computers which make up the Internet.

Bubble memory (data): Thin film of synthetic garnet. The bubbles are microns in size and move in a plane of the film when a magnetic gradient is present. Viewed under a microscope with a linear polarized light, the bubbles appear to be fluid circular areas that step from space to space following fixed loops and tracks.

Bug: An error in a program or an equipment fault.

Business Continuity Planning (BCP): An all encompassing, "umbrella" term covering both disaster recovery planning and business resumption planning.

Business interruption: Any event, whether anticipated (e.g., public service strike) or unanticipated (e.g., blackout) which disrupts the normal course of business operation at a corporate location.

Byte: Eight bits make up a byte (a letter, symbol, or number).

CAD: Computer-aided design.

CAD/CAM: Acronym for Computer-Assisted Design/Computer-Assisted Manufacturing, terms used by designers, engineers, and managers.

CAI: Computer-aided instruction. CAL Computer-aided learning. CAM Computer-aided manufacture.

Care map: A sequential or branching plan of the anticipated key treatments and diagnostic tests for a specific condition or medical diagnosis. IT may be used as a template for comparing the actual experience of a patient with that anticipated for the majority of patients with the same condition.

CASE: Computer Assisted Systems Engineering.

CD-ROM: Compact Disk Read Only Memory. A compact disk is round, flat and silver in colour and can contain massive amounts of information (600 megabytes or more of data, text, graphics, video, or sound).

Central processing unit (CPU): Internal part of the computer that contains the circuits which control and perform the execution of instructions. It is made up of Memory, Arithmetic/logic unit, and Control unit.

Certified Disaster Recovery Planner (CDRP): CDRPs are certified by the Disaster Recovery Institute, a not-for-profit corporation, which promotes the credibility and professionalism in the DR industry.

Chip: An integrated circuit made by etching myriads of transistors and other electronic components onto a wafer of silicon a fraction of an inch on a side.

CIPS: Canadian Information Processing Society.

Client/server: An architecture that has computers in a network assume different roles and tasks based on their particular strengths. Thus, a computer might be identified as a file server or a database server.

CNA: Canadian Nurses Association.

COACH: Canadian Organization for Advancement of Computers in Health.

COBOL: Common Business-Oriented Language.

Cold-site: An alternate facility that is void of any resources or equipment except air conditioning and raised flooring. Equipment and resources must be installed in such a facility to duplicate the critical business functions of an organization. Cold-sites have many variations depending on their communication facilities, UPS systems, or mobility (Relocatable-Shell).

COM: Computer Output to Microfilm.

Compiler: A translation program which coverts high-level instructions into a set of binary instructions (object code) for direct processor execution. Any high-level program requires a compiler or an interpreter.

Computer: An electronic device capable of taking in, putting out, storing internally, and processing data under the control of changeable processing instructions within the device.

Computer literacy: A term used to indicate knowledge of what a computer can do, how it works, how it is used to solve problems, and the limitations of a computer.

Contingency plan: *See* Disaster Recovery Plan.

Control key: Key that executes commands, in conjunction with other keys pressed simultaneously.

Control unit: Internal part of computer (found in CPU) that monitors the sequence of operations for all parts of the computer.

CP/M: Control Program/Microprocessors.

CPU: Central processing unit.

CR: Change Request.

Critical needs: The minimal procedures and equipment required to continue operations should a department, main facility, computer center, or a combination of these be destroyed or become inaccessible.

CRT: The Cathode-Ray Tube in a television set or video display monitor.

CRUD: Created, Read, Updated, or Deleted.

CSF: Critical Success Factor.

Cursor: A patch of light or other visual indicator on a screen that shows you where you are in the text.

DA: Data Administrator.

Data: Recorded facts performing arithmetic and logical process on data.

Database: An organized collection of data or information.

DB: Database.

DBA: Database Administrator.

DBMS: Database Management System.

DCE: Distributed Computing Environment.

Decision support system: A computer program devised to help a healthcare professional select the most likely clinical diagnosis or treatment.

DFD: Data Flow Diagrams.

DI: Diagnostic Imaging.

Digital: A computer that uses numbers to solve problems by performing arithmetic and logical processes on data.

Disaster: Any event creates an inability on an organization's part to provide critical business functions for some predetermined period of time.

Disaster prevention: Measures employed to prevent, detect, or contain incidents which, if unchecked, could result in disaster.

Disaster prevention checklist: A questionnaire used to assess preventative measures in areas of operations such as overall security, software, data files, data entry reports, microcomputers, and personnel.

Disaster recovery: The ability to respond to an interruption in services by implementing a disaster recovery plan to restore an organization's critical business functions.

Disaster Recovery Coordinator: The Disaster Recovery Coordinator may be responsible for overall recovery of an organization or unit(s).

Disaster Recovery Plan: The document that defines the resources, actions, tasks, and data required to manage the business recovery process in the event of a business interruption. The plan is designed to assist in restoring the business process within the stated disaster recovery goals.

Disaster Recovery Planning: The technological aspect of business continuity planning. The advance planning and preparations which are necessary to minimize loss and ensure continuity of the critical business functions of an organization in the event of a disaster.

Disaster Recovery Software: An application program developed to assist an organization in writing a comprehensive disaster recovery plan.

Disk: An external storage medium that is a flat, circular magnetic surface used to store data. The data is represented by the presence or absence of magnetized spots.

Disk drive: The device used to access or store information via a disk.

Distributed processing: Use of computers at various locations, typically interconnected via communication links for the purpose of data access and/or transfer.

Documentation: Refers to the orderly presentation, organization, and communication of recorded specialized knowledge in order to maintain a complete record of reasons for changes in variables. Documentation is necessary, not so much to give maximum utility, as to give an unquestionable historical reference record.

DOS: Disk-operating system.

DRGs: Diagnosis Related Groups. A method of costing care and treatment by grouping together cases by diagnosis or treatment method.

DSS: Decision Support System.

EDI: Electronic Data Interchange.

EDP: Electronic Data Processing.

EIS: Executive Information System.

E-mail: Electronic mail. The messages created, sent, and read between networks of computer users without having to be printed on paper.

EPROM: Erasable Programmable Read-Only Memory. A type of ROM that can be changed by means of electrical erasing.

Expert system: A computer program that stores knowledge in a special database by expressing it in the form of logical rules. The program can then logically reason, given that set of rules.

FDDI: Fibre Distributed Data Interface.

File backup: The practice of dumping (copying) a file stored on disk or tape to another disk or tape. This is done for protection case the active file gets damaged.

FIPS: Federal Information Processing Standard.

Firmware: Computer instructions that are located in Read-Only Memory (ROM). These instructions can be accessed but not altered.

Floppy disk: A flexible plastic disk enclosed in a protective envelope used to store information.

Formal Decision Table: A logical presentation of all decision paths available in the development of a computer system.

FORTRAN: Formula Translator.

Friendly: How easy a program or computer is to work with. A "user friendly" program is one that takes little time to learn, or that offers on screen prompts, or that protects the user from making disastrous mistakes.

FTAM: File Transfer, Access, and Management.

FTP: File Transfer Protocol.

FTS: File Transfer Systems.

GUI: Graphical User Interface.

Hard copy: Computer output printed on paper.

HDLC: High-level Data Link Control.

Head: Part of magnetic storage unit (Disk drive) which reads and writes information on the magnetic media.

High-level languages: Programming languages that are as close to writing English statements as possible.

HIS: Hospital Information Systems—a term used to describe overall hospital use of computers. Examples would be nurse staffing, medical records, patient admittance and discharge, patient bed control, and so on.

HMRI: Hospital Medical Records Institute.

Hot-site: An alternate facility that has the equipment and resources to recover the business functions affected by the occurrence of a disaster. Hot-sites may vary in type of facilities offered (such as data processing, communication, or any other critical business function needing duplication). Location and size of the hot-site will be proportional to the equipment and resources needed.

IC: Integrated circuit.

ICD-9-CM: International Classification of Diseases—9th rev—Clinical Modification.

IEW: Information Engineering Workbench—Proprietary product.

I/O (input/output): An Input device such as a keyboard feeds information into the computer. An Output device such as a printer or monitor takes information from the computer and turns it into usable form. Modems, cassettes, and disks work in both directions, so they are I/O devices. Input and output are also used as verbs: You input data from the keyboard.

Input: The data to be processed by the computer.

Input device: Device used to enter data to be processed by a computer (e.g., keyboard, light pen, touch screen).

Interactive video disk: A computer program uses a compact disk storing large amounts of data to provide video sequences on screen for the user to select the next sequence, or based on the answer given to a question.

Interface: A device or program that permits one part of a computer system to work with another, as when making a connection between a cassette tape recorder and the computer.

Internal memory: The internal storage of the computer. Made up of ROM and RAM.

Internal hot-sites: A fully equipped alternate processing site owned and operated by the organization.

Internet: A world-wide computer network, available via a modem and the telephone line that connects universities, government departments, and individuals. Users can send and receive e-mail, join in electronic conferences, and copy files.

IMIA: International Medical Informatics Association. It organizes a congress every three years and has a number of special interest groups composed of representatives drawn from member countries. The British Computer Society (BCS) is the member organization for the UK. The BCS Nursing Specialist Group nominates one member to the IMIA Nursing Specialist Group (SIGN).

Interpreter language: Language that converts the higher-level languages and assembler language to a language the computer machine can understand.

IPSE: Integrated Product Support Environment.

IRM: Information Resource Management.

ISDN: Integrated Services Digital Network.

ISO: International Standards Organization.

ISP: Information Systems Professional.

IT: Information Technology.

ITCH: Information Technology for Community Health (Annual Conference).

JADD: Joint Application Design and Development.

JCL: Job control language.

JIT: Just-in-Time.

K: Symbol used to express 1000. Ir a computer context it is 1024. Example 16K = 16,000 bytes; in reality it is 16,384 bytes.

LAN: abbreviation for **L**ocal **A**rea **N**etwork. Computing equipment, in close proximity to each other, connected to a server which houses software that can be accessed by the users. This method does not utilize a public carrier.

Load: To enter a program into the computer from cartridge, cassette, or disk.

Loop: A group of instructions that may be executed more than once.

Low-level languages: Programming languages that are less sophisticated than our normal English language.

LPM: Lines per minute.

Machine language: Language the computer actually understands. Nothing more than everything converted into the binary system. i.e., 0's and 1's, the presence or absence of electricity.

Magnetic tape: Flexible plastic tape, on one side of which is a uniform coating of dispersed magnetic material, in which signals are registered for subsequent reproduction. Used for registering television images, sound, or computer data.

Mailbox: An e-mail account or address, to which messages can be sent and stored, on a computer network such as Internet.

Mainframe Computer: A high-end processor, with related peripheral devices, capable of supporting large volumes of batch processing, high performance on-line transaction processing systems, and extensive data storage and retrieval.

Mark sense card: An input device that allows the operator to use a special pencil and computer readable card to input data.

Medical informatics: The discipline of applying computer science to medical processes.

Megabyte: 1 million bytes or 8 million bits.

Memory: Internal part of computer (found in the CPU) where programs and data are stored.

Metathesaurus: The combinations of several systematically arranged lists of words, their synonyms, and antonyms. A word finder to help in the identification of a language such as that used by nurses.

Microcomputer: A small inexpensive desk-top computer which uses floppy disks or small hard disk drives.

Microprocessor: Another name for the CPU chip.

Minicomputer: A larger and more powerful computer than a microcomputer, which uses large capacity hard disks, works at a greater speed, and has several hundred K of memory.

MIPS: Millions of instructions per second.

MIS: Medical (or Management) Information System (Chapter 5). A term used interchangeably with HIS; however, it specifically applies to a computerized system related to patient care as opposed to a system used by the finance department for billing financial statements, and so on.

Modem: Modulator/Demodulator. A device used to change computer codes into pulses or signals that can travel over telephone lines.

Monitor: Video device; quality of display is better than that of a television set.

MOS: Metal-oxide semiconductor.

Mouse: An input device that can be moved around over a flat surface causing the cursor to move on the screen.

MVS: Multiple virtual storage.

NANDA: North American Nursing Diagnosis Association. Its conference proceedings are published and list the currently approved diagnoses and their definitions. NANDA encourages research to identify and clarify diagnoses.

Network architecture: The basic layout of a computer and its attached systems, such as terminals and the paths between them.

Neural network model: A model on a computer system to mimic the way the human brain processes information using large numbers of neurons all working on one problem at the same time (parallel processing). Based on repeated patterns, connections are made across the computer's network of "neurons" to produce the same result each time.

NFS: Network File System.

NIC: Nursing Interventions Classification.

NIS (Nursing Information System): A term used to describe overall nursing use of computers. Examples would include source data capture, patient care plans, and use of expert systems.

NIST: National Institute of Standards and Technology.

Node: The name used to designate a part of a network. This may be used to describe one of the links in the network, or a type of link in the network (e.g., host node or intercept node)

Nursing diagnosis: A clinical judgment about individual, family, or community responses to actual or potential health problems or life processes. A nursing diagnosis provides the basis for the selection of nursing interventions.

Nursing informatics: The discipline of applying computer science to nursing processes.

Nursing Minimum Data Set (NMDS): The agreed minimum number of items of data, such as patient and nursing care elements, to be collected for managerial and government purposes. In the United States, the term may be used for the data elements identified by Werley et al. in 1985.

OA: Office Automation.

OCR: Optical Character Recognition.

OEM: Original equipment manufacturer.

Off-site storage: The process of storing records at a location removed from the normal place of use.

Omaha System: Developed by the Visiting Nurses Association of Omaha for use in community health nursing, there are three components a problem classification scheme, a problem-rating scale for outcomes, and an intervention scheme.

On-line: Being electronically connected, for example, a computer linked to a printer so that it is ready to print, or one computer linked to another computer such as over the Internet.

On-line terminal: The operation of terminals, disks, and other equipment under direct and absolute control of the central processor to eliminate the need for human intervention at any stage between initial input and computer output.

Operating Software: A type of system software supervising and directing all of the other software components plus the computer hardware.

OS: Operating system.

OSI: Open Systems Interchange. A particular technical standard that allows computers of different origins to be linked together.

OSE: Open Systems Environment.

OSF: Open Standards Foundation.

OSI: Open Systems Interconnection.

Output: Information transferred from internal storage to output device.

Output device: Devices or machines that deliver information from the computer to the operator (e.g., CRT, tape, disk, keypunched card).

Paper tape: Refers to strips of paper capable of storing or recording information. Storage may be in the form of punched holes, partially punched holes, carbonization or chemical change of impregnated material, or by imprinting.

Parallel interface: A port that sends or receives the eight bits in each byte all at one time. Many printers likely to be used in homes use a parallel interface to connect to the computer.

Parsing: The computer science term for checking the correctness of each line and the action of putting the line into proper form for next phase of program execution.

Patient classification system: There are a variety of systems, some manual, that assign either a patient's nursing problems or the nursing activities required, to a defined level of dependency on nurses for care. Some systems use nursing care plans to calculate the number of minutes of nurse time needed in 24 hours.

PC: Personal Computer.

PC-DOS: IBM's name for the Disk Operating System used in the IBM Personal Computer.

(PDQ) Cancer system: Protocol Data Query. A data retrieval system for cancer material.

Peripherals: Accessory parts of a computer system not considered essential to its operation. Printers and modems are peripherals.

Personal Health Number (PHN): A unique identifier given to individuals eligible for health services.

Physical Prevention: Special requirements for building construction as well as fire prevention for equipment components.

PIR: Post Implementation Review.

POSIX: Portable Operating System Interface for Computer Environments.

Printer: Transforms computer output into hard copy.

Program: Shortened form of "computer program." A set of stored instructions in a computer which directs the actions within the computer. See Application program.

Programmable key: Another term for user-defined key.

Programming languages: Much like French, English, and German—the grammar and punctuation accepted by the computer's input device that enables a user to communicate with the computer.

PROM: Programmable Read-Only Memory. A type of ROM that can be changed, but only with a high degree of expertise.

Proprietary software: A computer program belongs to its developer. Programs (generally) cannot be copied and freely given away, just as you cannot copy a book and give copies away.

RAM: Random-Access Memory or Read-Write Memory. This part of internal memory is known as temporary memory.

RDBMS: Relational Database Management System.

Read: To extract data from a computer's memory or from a tape or disk.

Real-time: An action or system capable of action at a speed commensurate with the time of occurrence of an actual process.

Reset: To reset the computer and its peripherals to a starting state before beginning a task. Done automatically by the disk operating system.

RFD: Request for Development.

RFI: Request for Information.

RFP: Request for Proposal.

RISE: Relationally Integrated Systems Engineering.

Risk Analysis: The process of identifying the risks to an organization, assess the critical functions necessary for an organization to continue operations, define controls to reduce exposure, and evaluate the cost of such controls.

The risk analysis often involves an evaluation of the probabilities of a particular event. Associated terms risk assessment, impact assessment, corporate loss analysis, risk identification, exposure analysis, exposure assessment.

Risk management: The discipline that ensures that an organization does not assume an unacceptable level of risk.

Robotics: General term for industrial robots used to increase production. An example is the use of computer-controlled robots in automobile assembly lines.

ROM: Read-only memory.

RPG: Report Program Generator.

SAA: Strategic Application Architecture.

SCAMC: Symposium on Computer Applications in Medical Care.

Scroll: To move a video display up or down, line by line, or side to side, character by character.

SDE: Systems Development Environment.

SDLC: Systems Development Life Cycle.

Server: A master computer into which other computers hook, so it controls a network of computers.

Soft-function key: See User-defined key.

Software: The general term for sets of computer instructions (programs) which manage the general facilities of the computer and control the operation of application programs.

SNOMED: Systematized Nomenclature of Medicine.

Source code instructions: In many microprogrammed processors, source code instructions are interpreted in the instruction register as pointers to the microprocessor programs that emulate the particular instruction set being executed. In the conventional approach, on the other hand, each instruction is decoded and executed with specific control logic wired into the machine.

SSA: Strategic Systems Architecture.

Stakeholder: Any individual or organization with vested interest in the health system.

Standards: Documented agreements containing technical specifications or the precise criteria to be used consistently as rules, guidelines, or definitions of characteristics to ensure that materials, products, processes, and services are fit for their purposes.

Storage: Usually refers to long term storage, such as storage on tape or disk.

Support: Help available from computer and software merchants. Also used as a verb to describe what products are compatible with each other.

System: A group of actions or procedures which together are logically connected by their operation and products and which accomplish a connected set of organizational objectives.

TCP/IP: Transmission Control Protocol/Internet Protocol.

Telematics: The combination of telecommunications and computing. Data communications between systems and devices.

Technical Threats: A disaster causing event that may occur regardless of any human elements.

Terminal: Device used to transmit and receive data over communications lines to and from the computer.

Top-down structure: A logical method of presenting the structure of a computer application. The initial system is the head of the structure and is subdivided into each of its component parts ultimately ending in a detailed level that allows you to go directly to programming.

TQM: Total Quality Management.

Turnkey: A term used to describe a hardware-software combination that comes in a "package." There are no changes or options; the package must be run as it is. An example is a microcomputer with a generalized software package for nurse scheduling. A "turnkey" is the opposite of a "tailored" system developed specifically for a nursing department.

Unique Lifetime Identifier (ULI): A unique identifier given to persons who receive or provide health services in Alberta.

User-defined key: A key whose function can be changed by which a command or sequence of commands can be executed with a single keystroke. Same as Programmable key and Soft-function key. Unlike a special-function key, a user-defined key may have a predefined purpose.

VDU: Visual display unit.

VDT: Video display terminal.

Video terminal: Computer terminal which shows data on a cathode ray tube (CRT), like a television tube, in letters, numbers, and so on.

Warm-site: An alternate processing site which is only partially equipped (as compared to a hot-site, which is fully equipped).

Winchester disk: A powerful form of backup storage for a computer. It is a rigid magnetic disk in a sealed container scanned by a head which does not quite touch the disk, therefore not wearing it out.

Winchester drive: A form of hard disk permanently sealed into a case.

WLMS: Work Load Measurement System.

WMS: Workload Measurement System.

Write: To enter information into memory or onto a tape or disk.

WWW: World Wide Web. A database made of linked hypertext documents originated by CERN, it exploded onto the computing scene during 1994. You call it up from a starter screen. An early browser was a program called Mosaic. WWW can provide graphics and sound but downloading these take time.

Index

Health Informatics Series

(formerly Computers in Health Care)

(continued from page ii)

Patient Care Information Systems
Successful Design and Implementation
E.L. Drazen, J.B. Metzger, J.L. Ritter, and M.K. Schneider

Introduction to Nursing Informatics, Second Edition
K.J. Hannah, M.J. Ball, and M.J.A. Edwards

Introduction to Nursing Informatics, Third Edition
K.J. Hannah, M.J. Ball, and M.J.A. Edwards

Information Retrieval
A Health and Biomedical Perspective, Second Edition
W.R. Hersh

Information Technology for the Practicing Physician
J.M. Kiel

Computerizing Large Integrated Health Networks
The VA Success
R.M. Kolodner

Medical Data Management
A Practical Guide
F. Leiner, W. Gaus, R. Haux, and P. Knaup-Gregori

Consumer Health Informatics
Informing Consumers and Improving Health Care
D. Lewis, G. Eysenbach, R. Kukafka, P.Z. Stavri, and H. Jimison

Organizational Aspects of Health Informatics
Managing Technological Change
N.M. Lorenzi and R.T. Riley

Transforming Health Care Through Information
Case Studies
N.M. Lorenzi, R.T. Riley, M.J. Ball, and J.V. Douglas

Trauma Informatics
K.I. Maull and J.S. Augenstein

Consumer Informatics
Applications and Strategies in Cyber Health Care
R. Nelson and M.J. Ball

Public Health Informatics and Information Systems
P.W O'Carroll, W.A. Yasnoff, M.E. Ward, L.H. Ripp, and E.L. Martin

Advancing Federal Sector Health Care
A Model for Technology Transfer
P. Ramsaroop, M.J. Ball, D. Beaulieu, and J.V. Douglas

Medical Informatics
Computer Applications in Health Care and Biomedicine, Second Edition
E.H. Shortliffe and L.E. Perreault

Filmless Radiology
E.L. Siegel and R.M. Kolodner

Cancer Informatics
Essential Technologies for Clinical Trials
J.S. Silva, M.J. Ball, C.G. Chute, J.V. Douglas, C.P. Langlotz, J.C. Niland, and W.L. Scherlis

Clinical Information Systems
A Component-Based Approach
R. Van de Velde and P. Degoulet

Knowledge Coupling
New Premises and New Tools for Medical Care and Education
L.L. Weed